Vincenzo Denaro

Stenosis of the Cervical Spine

Causes, Diagnosis and Treatment

With 220 Figures

Springer-Verlag
Berlin Heidelberg New York London Paris
Tokyo Hong Kong Barcelona Budapest

Professor Vincenzo Denaro
Associate Professor of Orthopedics and Traumatology
Catania University, Italy
Via A. de Gasperi 173 C
95127 Catania, Italy

Foreword by Professor Quintino Mollica
Director of Institute of Orthopedics and Traumatology
Catania University, Italy

Translated by Professor Victor Fornasier (Toronto, Canada)

Illustrated by Anna Sapuppo (Catania, Italy)

ISBN-13: 978-3-642-76205-5 e-ISBN-13: 978-3-642-76203-1
DOI: 10.1007/ 978-3-642-76203-1

Softcover reprint of the hardcover 1st edition 1991

Typesetting : Triltsch, Würzburg
31/3145-543210 Printed on acid-free paper

For Professor
Mario Boni

Foreword

Professor Vincenzo Denaro has been an active member of the Institute of Clinical Orthopedics and Traumatology of the University of Catania since 1986. It has been my pleasure, as Director, to be associated with Professor Denaro, first as a Sessional Consultant in diseases of the spine and finally, after his promotion to the permanent staff, as Associate Professor.

Professor Denaro began his postgraduate program of specialization, and hence his career, in the Orthopedic Clinic of the University of Pavia under the tutorship of Professor Mario Boni. It was the latter who directed and guided his development in studying the disease processes of the vertebral column.

In his pursuit of knowledge, he undertook additional studies in foreign clinics, including the Wellesley Hospital at the University of Toronto with Professor I. MacNab and Professor V. Fornasier. He spent a full year at the Orthopedic Clinic of the University of Paris under the guidance of Professor Roy-Camille. He derived great benefit from the clinical experience gained there and became acquainted with advanced and specialized surgical techniques specific to his field of interest.

More recently, since accepting his current appointment, he has been able to put into practice the expertise developed over 20 years of study and research. Not only does he have extensive personal clinical experience, but he very wisely undertook to maintain a thorough, complete, and accurate record of the experience gathered from his case load.

This volume is the culmination of all this effort and expertise. It unquestionably justifies the interest of those who are involved in or intend to dedicate themselves to this special area of surgery, which may sometimes be thankless, but is always challenging, requiring the fine honing of very specific and special skills.

This book brings together the various approaches and surgical techniques with a discussion of their advantages and limitations. As such it will be invaluable in the selection of appropriate management for each patient the surgeon encounters.

Prof. Quintino Mollica

Preface

The aim in preparing this work was to gather together and discuss the pathogenic factors (both organic and functional) known to participate in creating a discrepancy between the "contents" of the cervical spine (the cord and nerve roots) and its "container" (the vertebral canal), leading to what is now clinically referred to as spinal stenosis.

The discussion first considers the anatomy, biomechanical and clinical features, and instrumentation, as well as the value and significance of using current radiological imaging, all of which are essential in identifying the disease process that may be present in the patient. The approaches to the cervical spine and the specific surgical techniques available to the surgeon are then described in more detail. Great emphasis is placed on the illustrations which, the author hopes, will not only provide an understanding of the disease processes, but also describe the surgical procedures, their indications, their limitations, and the possible risks involved with each of them in a very practical way.

In presenting this book, I have adopted a relatively didactic approach that I hope will be useful to those who are new students of this discipline. I make no pretence of having been encyclopedic, nor of having dealt with every possible aspect of surgery in this area. Gaps obviously remain. The literature already contains exhaustive discussions of the pathology of the cervical spine. This work is intended to provide the reader with an understanding of the practical aspects of surgical management and a detailed description of the surgical techniques needed to deal with the various pathologies that produce cervical stenosis.

A number of contributors who helped in preparing this manuscript for the publisher must be acknowledged. Professor M. Boni was my first teacher. He taught me the first, the basic, and the essential steps in surgery of the cervical spine. I was fortunate to be able to work with him in developing many of the surgical principles and techniques discussed in this book. Professor Q. Mollica's encouragement, advice, and constant support gave me the strength to pursue and complete this undertaking. Through the friendship of Professor R. Roy-Camille I was able to learn much about internal fixation of the vertebral column. Professor A. Wackenheim provided guidance in the development of this work with practical suggestions and encouragement. My thanks are also due to Professor P. Kehr, C. Dosdat, H. Hirabayashi, A. White, M. Panjabi, A. Grasso, and F. D'Alpa for their very important contributions to specific, specialized sections of this book. I am indebted to Professor V. Fornasier, who undertook the long and arduous task of translating the entire volume, and to Anna Sapuppo, whose artistic skills are reflected in the valuable and clear illustrations that she created from my crude drawings.

Catania, July 1991 Vincenzo Denaro

Contents

Contributors

J. C. Dosdat	Polyclinique du Maine. Service de Chirurgie Orthopédique et Traumatologique. Laval. France
A. Grasso and F. D'Alpa	Neurologic Clinic. Catania University, viale A. Doria, 95100 Catania, Italy
H. Hirabayashi and K. Satomi	Keio University School of Medicine, 1-14-4 Jingumane, Shibuya-ku. Tokio, Japan 150
P. H. Kehr	25 Rue Schweighaeser, 67000 Strasbourg, France
M. M. Panjabi and A. White *	Department of Orthopaedics and Rehabilitation, Yale Medical School, 333 Cedar Street, New Haven, CT 06510
	* Department of Orthopaedic Surgery, Beth Israel Hospital, Harvard Medical School, 330 Brookline Avenue, Boston, MA 02215

CHAPTER 1

Introduction

Modern diagnostic imaging technology such as computed tomography (CT) and magnetic resonance imaging (MRI) has enabled us to achieve a better understanding of the complex aspects of diseases of the cervical spine. Stenosis of the cervical canal has become one of the more interesting and better understood areas within the wide spectrum of pathology found in the cervical segment of the spinal column. It is now possible to describe a more meaningful classification of the many clinical situations and achieve a better understanding of their pathogenesis. In the establishment of indications for surgical intervention, these new diagnostic methods have permitted the identification and definition of significant differences between disease entities and, as a consequence, have provided more specific criteria for selecting surgical approaches and developing the modern surgical techniques.

The discussion of the investigation and treatment of cervical stenosis begins with an overview of our current understanding and a definition of the entities that result from cervical stenosis. Following the chapters on anatomical and biomechanical principles, the various effects and clinical situations related to stenosis are described and classified. Clinically, emphasis is on the importance of imaging as a basis for diagnosis and for clinical and pathological correlation. Once the scope of our undertaking has been defined, including a discussion of etiological factors, we progress to a discussion of surgical techniques. Emphasis is placed on the indications for the various surgical techniques; the techniques themselves are discussed as are the practical aspects of surgical management based on personal experience. The discussion closes with a review of the complications and consequences of inappropriate surgical approaches or techniques. Being familiar with the established complications is an excellent starting point from which to develop effective measures for their prevention.

Definition

The modern definition of stenosis of the cervical spine refers to clinical situations that involve the cervical spinal cord or secondarily affect the cervical nerve roots and that are due to a disparity between the size of the spinal cord and that of the canal encompassing the cord. The causal relationships that characterize the degenerative changes in the cervical cord due to injury and extrinsic compression were described in the nineteenth century (Parkinson), 1817; Gowers WR 1892). Further discussion in this area can be found in the writings of Bailey and Casamajor (1911), Stookey (1928), and W. Brain et al. (1952). It was, however, Payne and Spillane (1957) who introduced the concept that the "initial size of the canal" was the major factor in the development of cervical myelopathy. More recently, many anatomical and radiological studies have developed our understanding of the morphology and morphometry of the vertebral canal. The use of modern imaging techniques including CT, computed tomographic myelography, and MRI has provided a more definitive understanding of the various problems; these techniques have made it possible to study the morphology of the canal in all three dimensional planes, its morphometric features such as diameter, volume, and perimeningeal space, and the state of the parenchyma of the cord, which can now be assessed without sampling or biopsy. Furthermore, the use of modern imaging techniques has demonstrated that the dimensions of the canal itself are quite independent of the height, body habitus, sex, or other general characteristics of the patient or features of the vertebral bodies themselves. This was originally described by Aboulker et al. (1965), and it is now generally accepted that the canal is very variable in its dimensions and structure.

Morphologically in normal canals there is ample perimeningeal space for the physiological housing of the cord and roots, while canals which are smaller than normal are now generally regarded as congenitally restricted and have such decreased perimeningeal space that there is no room for peridural fat. In turn these congenitally restricted canals may be restricted in a uniform and global fashion or the anomalies may consist of alterations of individual constituents of the canal such as pedicles, laminae, articular apophyses, and ligamentum flavum. Clearly one must emphasize that the narrowing of the vertebral canal is not necessarily associated with pathology of the cord or roots; it must be considered as a factor that predisposes to the development of a discrepancy in size between the cord and canal, particularly when pathological influences are introduced. These effects may be on a kinetic basis (e.g., instability) or on an organic basis (e.g., arthrosis, malunited fractures, tumors or infections). Specific and accurate measurements of the canal are important, but the relationship of the meningoneural structures within the canal to the size of the canal is much more important in the pathogenesis and pathology of the syndromes that are identified as consequences of cervical stenosis. The severity of the clinical consequences tends to reflect the extent of the discrepancy between the size of the spinal cord and the size of the canal (i.e., ratio of content to container). In other words, a pathological process of either kinetic (i.e. instability) or organic origin may remain clinically silent in a normal canal where there is space for tissue adaptation, but will produce clinical and pathological changes in a congenitally restricted canal. What in fact is reduced by spinal stenosis is the perimeningeal space that Aboulker et al. (1965) detected both intraoperatively and using gas myelography. This can be much better visualized today with CT and MRI. Clinical findings and pathological changes of the cord do not occur as long as the balance between content and container is maintained.

References

Aboulker J, Metzger J, David M, Engel P, Ballivet J (1965) Les myèlopathies cervicales d'origine rachidienne. Neurochirurgie 11:89–198

Bailey P, Casamajor L (1911) Osteoarthritis of the spine as a cause of compression of the spinal card and its roots. J Nerv Ment Dis 39:588.

Boni M, Denaro V (1982) The cervical stenosis syndrome. Int Orthop 7:185–195

Brain WR, Northfield DWC, Wilkinson M (1952) The neurological manifestation of cervical spondylosis. Brain 75:187

Gowers WR (1892) Diseases of the nervous system, 2nd edn, Vol 1. Churchill, London

Parkinson J (1817) An essay on the shaking palsy. London

Payne E, Spillane J (1957) The cervical spine. An anatomico-pathological study of 70 specimens (using a special technique) with particular reference to the problem of cervical spondylosis. Brain 80:571

Stookey B (1928) Compression of the spinal cord due to ventral extradural cervical chondromas. Arch Neurol Psychiatry 20:275

Chapter 2

Classification of Stenoses

The clinical consequences of cervical stenosis have been defined as those in which myeloradicular disease results from an imbalance between the myelomeningeal structure constituting the contents of the canal and their container, i.e., the cervical canal and all its constituents. This imbalance can result from either kinetic (functional) or organic disease. This difference in pathogenesis may be used to distinguish between organic and nonorganic or functional stenosis.

Functional Stenoses

By functional (kinetic) stenoses those cases are meant in which there is a change in the function and hence in the static physiological and biomechanical characteristics of the cervical spine that can initiate a discrepancy between the contents and the canal. This assumes by definition that correction of the kinetic effects will be sufficient not only to improve but also to correct the clinical situation. If one reviews the fundamental biomechanical characteristics of the cervical spine, then the concept of kinetic stenosis can be better understood (see Chap. 4). The ligamentous structures that regulate the movements of the first two cervical vertebrae and the ligamentous complex that forms the "motor unit" of the remaining cervical vertebrae from C3 to C7 are well known and include the anterior longitudinal ligament, the intervertebral disk, the posterior longitudinal ligament, the ligamentum flavum, the interspinous ligaments, and the interapophyseal articulations. Under physiological conditions, the excursive movements of the vertebral articulations occur within a unit where there is absolute consistency in the interrelationship of the movement to the space within the canal, i.e., a good relationship is maintained between the canal and its contents (including the spinal cord, the nerve roots, and the meningeal envelopes).

In the biomechanical function of the spinal column during flexion and extension, there is joint movement that results in a change in the diameter and the length of the spinal canal. Variations in the position of and relationships between the cord and the meninges resulting from this movement are well recognized. In flexion, the canal is lengthened in the craniocaudal plane and the posterior wall undergoes a greater lengthening than the anterior wall. At the same time, there is an increase in the anteroposterior diameter. The cord stretches and is displaced anteriorly; as a result the nerve roots assume a more vertical position and have a tendency to stretch. In extension, the canal shortens in the craniocaudal plane and there is a reduction in the anteroposterior diameter. The cord is stretched less, increasing its freedom of movement, and the nerve roots are more horizontal and more relaxed.

During extension the perimeningeal space may be reduced not only through the global reduction in the anteroposterior diameter of the canal, but also through the stenosing effect of the ligamentum flavum. The latter becomes harder, thicker, and less elastic with age. When the laminae are approximated to each other during hyperextension, the ligamentum flavum protrudes into the canal and may press on the soft tissues of the canal including both the meninges and the neural tissues. Intraoperatively it has been observed that the thickened ligamentum flavum compresses the dural sac, as can be recognized in the shape of the indentation (Aboulker 1965). It must be emphasized that the insertion of the ligamentum flavum in the laminae can be quite lateral and may reach the apophyseal joints; it is therefore an important constituent of the posterior wall of the canal and can obviously play a very important part in the pathogenesis of stenosis. In rotation and lateral flexion, the movements are combined. Maximum excursion occurs at the level of C2–C3 (Vanneuville et al. 1980). Between C3 and C7 the variability of the osteoligamentous structure of the canal is less significant since at this level the degree of tension and/or torsion of the dura mater is far more important. One must emphasize that maximum excursion of flexion and extension occurs at the metameres C4, C5, and C6, which are regarded as the "flexibility center" of the cervical spine.

It goes without saying that the greater the distance of the movement in flexion and extension, the greater will be the variation in the diameter of the canal. It has now been realized that congenitally restricted canals are characterized by lesser degrees of excursion during this movement (Babin 1970). An appropriate relationship between the movement of the neuromeningeal structures and the variation in the osseous and ligamentous constituents of the canal will be retained as long as the relationship of the neuromeningeal structures to the canal favors the former. When as a result of degenerative changes, trauma, inflammation, or arthritic diseases, there is a change in the ligamentous congruity between adjacent vertebral bodies such as to establish a degree of instability, then there may be an imposition on the requirements of the neural structures and clinical and neurological signs will occur. Such instability is defined as the loss of ability on the part of the vertebral column to maintain appropriate relationships between the vertebrae resulting in damage to the neural structures as well as establishing structural deformities (White et al. 1976).

A mild degree of such instability can result from multiple factors. One possible cause may be *degenerative pseudospondylolisthesis with arthrosis*. It is well recognized that the degenerative arthrotic process in its early stages can produce a loss of congruity between vertebral bodies leading to abnormal movement during flexion and extension. This can be seen in the frequent occurrence of retrolisthesis that may extend for several millimeters at the level of the column with the greatest physiological lordosis (C3-C4) and which is most apparent during hyperextension of the neck. The combination of the reduction in the anteroposterior diameter of the canal that occurs physiologically during extension and the protrusion of the ligamentum flavum posteriorly results in early degenerative retrolisthesis that can interfere with the normal housing of the neural structures.

Another factor may be *mild post-traumatic laxity* which permits movement between vertebral bodies of a few millimeters during flexion and extension. Joint movement exceeding 3 mm is regarded as indicating significant instability! Post-traumatic laxity (whiplash) is the frequent cause of mild cervical distortion, while ligamentous disruption would produce far greater mechanical instability.

Ligamentous laxity, as might occur in collagen diseases or rheumatoid arthritis, particularly in its early stages, results in increased joint excursion that affects the neural structures. Often the degree of serverity of this type of laxity is such that corrective conservative treatment such as muscular re-education leads to full relief of the symptoms.

Kinetic overload of a segment because of increased rigidity in adjacent vertebrae as a result of arthrodeses, trauma, or congenital stenosis also leads to instability. When two or more vertebral bodies are consolidated as a result of trauma or disease, movement in the adjacent intervertebral spaces will be exaggerated and this may result in a degree of joint laxity that produces clinical signs indicative of neuroradicular irritation. This is most common when the rigidified vertebrae are the most mobile in the neck (C4, C5, C6). This type of complicating laxity can occur in Down's syndrome and Larsen's disease (see section "Congenital Stenoses" below).

Loss of appropriate lordosis, particularly to the point of inversion, and loss of appropriate physiological posture can produce significant changes in the cervical spinal canal. Segmental kyphosis may occur affecting only two or even only a single segment of movement and possibly resulting from prematurely generalized degenerative disk disease.

Occasionally, compensatory adaptation in posture may affect the adequacy of the cervical canal. Postural changes elsewhere in the spine, either at the thoracic or lumbar levels, may influence the cervical level. However, all these anatomopathological situations produce a mild degree of change, irritation and injury to the cord that should be completely reversible with appropriate management. Part of the explanation of the mechanism of relapse in the symptoms of an early discrepancy between contents and container in the cervical column is found in the ease with which microtrauma of the neural structures may lead to localized edema. This in turn leads to increased volume of the neural structures that can worsen the original situation. This neurological deficit can be successfully treated with immobilization and rest, but may require analgesia, muscle relaxants, and anti-inflammatory agents including corticosteroids. Once the acute phase is over, one must retrain the patient to maintain the vertebral column in such a way as to avoid these mild instabilities, e.g. by strengthening the neck muscles, by improving the postural status not only of the cervical levels, but also of the entire vertebral column, and by teaching the patients to practise good overall posture and movement of the spine. Such retraining will decrease the incidence of recurrence of the symptoms in the early stages and prevent the development of more permanent and irreversible neurological deficits. In conclusion, early myeloradicular deficits resulting from spinal movement may:

- Disappear completely, if appropriately treated in the early stages. The risk of recurrence however remains indefinitely and often for the lifetime of the patient.
- Worsen, if neglected, resulting in progression towards an organic stenosis such as to produce increasing risk of permanent damage requiring surgical management.

Organic Stenoses

In a strictly morphological and anatomical sense, stenoses may be naturally classified into the congenital and acquired groups.

Congenital Stenoses

The congenital changes that decrease the size of the cervical vertebral canal can be divided into those termed idiopathic congenital stenoses, which are present from birth, and those resulting secondarily from a congenital disease, which may produce symptoms and signs during growth and development. It must be stated clearly that a purely congenital stenosis is rarely the sole cause of myeloradicular deficit symptoms. For this reason, the following discussion is somewhat theoretical and speculative. Embryologically, the size of the canal is determined by the neural structures that develop within the canal following closure of the neural arch. The somites differentiate from the mesoderm and are already located lateral to the neural canal in the craniocaudal direction very early in embryologic development (as early as the 12th day). They differentiate towards the myotomes, which are the precursors of the muscular elements, and sclerotomes, which are the precursors of the skeletal elements. The cranial portion of each sclerotome fuses with the caudal portion of the adjacent sclerotome to form a vertebra. It is at this time that ventral movement of portions of the sclerotomes results in the development of the vertebral body. A second portion of the sclerotome moves dorsally to form the vertebral arch that is in close proximity to and encases the newly formed neural canal. This latter is the mold around which these dorsal elements grow in the evolution of the posterior elements and hence of the eventual spinal canal. That the neural canal determines the development and the dimensions of the vertebral canal has been confirmed experimentally (Holtzer 1952). In order for a true congenital and idiopathic stenosis to occur, there must be interference in the normal process of development due to external factors that hinder the development from the original sclerotome of both the vertebral body and the vertebral arches while the cord and the meninges continue to develop normally. This imbalance between the development of the contents and that of the container produces a discrepancy in their relationship to each other. Only under these circumstances does injury to the neuromeningeal structures result. With this in mind, we can now identify different types of stenoses involving congenital morphological changes.

Malformations involving severe morphological deformity of the canal in the occipitocervical plane include the Arnold-Chiari malformation, congenital anomalies of the atlantoaxial joint, congenital ligamentous laxity, particulary at the odontoid process of the axis, aplasia of the articular surfaces of the atlas (Dubousset 1986), complex congenital malformation of the central to lower part of the cervical canal with listhesis of the vertebral bodies and severe structural deformity (see Fig. 9.98), and the well-known Klippel-Feil syndrome. Generally speaking, one includes in this group all the congenital fusions of the cervical column which are separated into three types:

Type 1. Massive thoracocervical vertebral fusion often associated with other skeletal abnormalities
Type 2. Fusion of one or two vertebral levels
Type 3. Cervical vertebral blocks which may additionally involve lumbar or thoracic levels

Most common are type 2 fusions, with a reported incidence on the order of 5% of all cervical lesions (Graaf 1982). This allomorphism of the cervical vertebrae will be compounded by biomechanical consequences affecting the involved elements as well as the immediately adjacent levels. In fact, in eight personal cases of Klippel-Feil type 2 stenosis as well as in similar cases from the literature (Prusic et al. 1985), the damage to the cord was ascribed to the combination of arthrotic degeneration and instability in the levels adjacent to the congenital fusion. Cord damage in such cases can also result from simple trauma without fracture but which produces distortion in hyperextension (Epstein 1983; Torg 1989).

The group of malformations without serious structural distortion of the cervical canal includes the cases of true congenital narrowing of the canal which can be narrowed in an extensive and global manner or narrowed with anomalies characterized by dysplasia or hypoplasia of one of the components of the canal. The affected constituents include:

1. The laminae; these may be dysplastic (enlarged or flattened), hypoplastic and small (with a shortening of the anteroposterior diameter), or asymmetrical (resulting in narrowing of the diameter in a single plane and fusion, i.e., mono- or bilateral synostosis; Aboulker 1965).
2. The pedicles; these are often the site of anomalies resulting in asymmetry, shortening, or unilateral thickening. The resulting asymmetrical stenosis of the canal on the side of the shortened pedicle produces a monolateral stenosis with overall narrowing of the cross-sectional area of the canal. Cases have been described in the literature where complete aplasia of the pedicles has produced instability and spondylolisthesis (Fardon and Fieldin 1981; Sakou 1982; Cox and Bennett 1984).
3. *The vertebral bodies*; there may be allomorphism of the vertebral bodies with developmental defects including hemivertebrae (transverse or longitudinal) or synostotic fusion without allomorphism, as in Klippel-Feil type 2 stenosis.

A third group consists of stenoses which result from systemic congenital disease which become manifest during growth and development. A good example of this is osteopetrosis (marble bones or Albers-Schönberg disease). Lack of normal osteoclastic function results in a wide variety of structural disorders. The allosomal dominant form is lethal within the first year of life, while the more common allosomal recessive form has a much better prognosis. In this milder form, in addition to hematopoietic disorders and compression of the cranial nerve by enlarged bone, spinal cord compression may result from vertebral deformities produced by inappropriately remodeled bone (McCleary et al. 1987; Jacques et al. 1975; Klintworth 1963). Bone growth without appropriate remodeling may produce not only spinal stenosis, but also hydrocephalus through narrowing of the cranial openings.

In this group of stenosis caused by systemic diseases, one can also include the genetic osteochondrodystrophies. These tend to produce severe instabilities with significant risk of dislocation that lead to a discrepancy between the spinal cord and the spinal canal that envelops it. Larsen's disease is one of the more common syndromes in which ligamentous instability results from anterior hypoplasia of a vertebral body (Leffort et al. 1983). This group also encompasses Morquio's disease with aplasia of the odontoid process of the axis (Denaro et al. 1973), spondyloepiphyseal dysplasias, and diastrophic dwarfism.

It is important to emphasize that congenital abnormalities of the cervical spine cannot be looked upon as the sole cause or even the immediate cause of cord injury. The malformations act as a predisposing factor, they may present asymptomatic clinical situations until a situation of instability results from normal as well as excessive demands on normal function in adulthood. For example, in adult years the onset of disk degeneration with osteophyte formation in adjacent vertebrae may produce a discrepancy in the cross-sectional area between the cord and the canal that can become clinically symptomatic. It is uncommon for cervical stenoses resulting from malformations to become clinically significant with serious narrowing of the canal since they are rare and not all become sufficiently severe to produce a content to container discrepancy. It is far more common for these malformations to occur without significant morphological deficits in situations that still fall within the category of congenitally narrowed canals. In fact this is the most common group of the category that is met in clinical practice, i.e., the syndromes associated with cervical stenosis of combined pathogenesis; the malformation itself is a predisposing cofactor, while the acquired cofactors are the precipitating cause.

Acquired Stenoses

The discrepancy between the contents and container of the cervical vertebral column in acquired stenoses results from pathological processes that are superimposed on a previously normal spinal column. The etiological factors are multiple and result in the following groups of pathogenetic condition:

1. Degenerative processes are usually slow with gradual protrusion into the canal. Examples would include degenerative disk disease with osteophytes or calcification of the posterior longitudinal ligament.

2. Destructive processes include tumors and infections, i.e., conditions associated with the resorption of bone and the replacement of bone by a softer tissue. Both primary and metastatic tumors are included in this group. These processes act on the integrity of the canal in two manners: directly by inflammatory or neoplastic tissue invading the canal, and indirectly by undermining the stability of osseous structures leading to the collapse of the supporting framework of the osteoligamentous vertebral column. Either method or, more frequently, a combination of the two results in injury to the contents of the spinal canal.

3. Traumatic processes, excluding acute trauma, form a large group of chronic and slowly developing processes that with time produce compression as a result of destabilization of the bony architecture. This can be a consequence of inadequately treated lesions or, in situations of instability, of lesions which have rendered the osteoligamentous structure of the spinal column more susceptible to injury.

4. Arthritic conditions include diseases such as rheumatoid arthritis which in their evolution lead to instability sufficient to produce injury to the cord.

5. Iatrogenic causes may also be responsible for pathological processes. This group includes extensive laminectomy, postoperative fibrosis, and anterior wide decompression without arthrodesis in inherently unstable vertebral columns.

Degenerative Stenosis

Spinal arthrosis (degenerative disk disease) includes the constellation of diseases resulting from functional overload which act not only on cartilage, but also on other articulating constituents of the spine. Relative functional overload may be the result of excessive demands placed on the function of normal cartilage or of a normal load placed on previously altered cartilage. "The final result is a group of lesions that create a vicious circle involving the connective tissue elements including both collagen and proteoglycans. While cellular changes in the pericellular environment diminish the mechanical protection and increase cellular exposure to the effects of mechanical action. Sometimes this can occur even under normal functional load. In response to the degenerative process, chondrocytes and other connective tissue cells respond by increased activity and proliferation in an attempt at repair" (Boni and Denaro 1987). The full expression of the arthroses result in the disorderly and irregular biochemical, morphological, and ultrastructural mixture of these elements. Analogous changes occur in the vertebrae (Boni and Denaro 1982, 1987). Degenerative arthrosis of the vertebral column can affect all three articulating components of the vertebral bodies: the intervertebral disk with the intervertebral articulations (disk arthrosis), the oncovertebral articulations (oncoarthrosis), or the interapophyseal joints (interapophyseal arthrosis). This group includes the cases of organic stenosis resulting from ossification of the posterior longitudinal ligament and those resulting from hypertrophy and thickening of the ligamentum flavum.

In an anatomopathological, radiographic, histologic, and histochemical study of 137 cervical spines undertaken on subjects who had died from a variety of causes and which included a complete review of the clinical status of each patient before death (Boni 1966; Boni and Denaro 1982), it was observed that:

1. The earliest changes ascribed to degenerative disk disease in the cervical spine occur by the third decade (Figs. 2.1–2.2). Hirsch (1967) described fissuring with an irregular pattern and distribution in the intervertebral disk in the 25- to 35-year-old group. These changes appear to

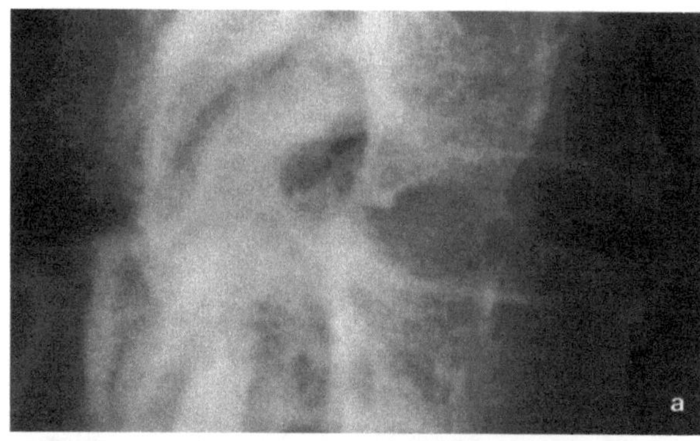

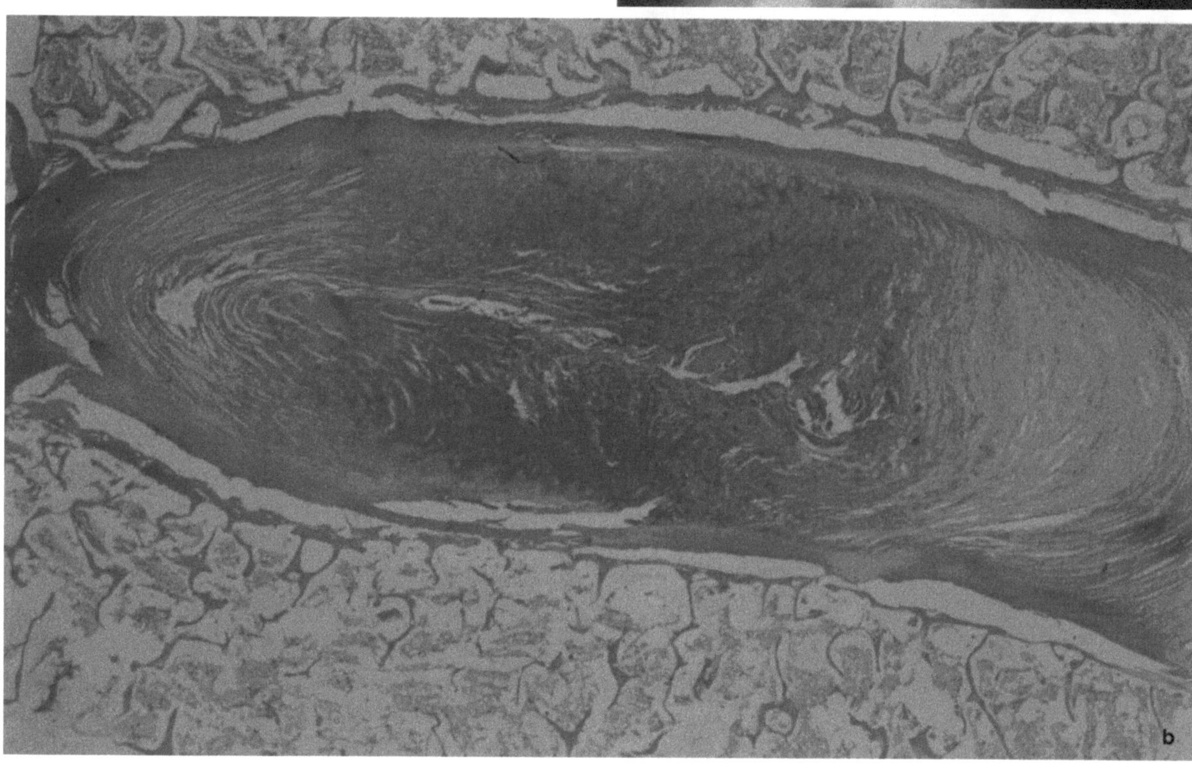

Fig. 2.1 a. Radiograph of C5–C6 segment of the spinal cord in a 33-year-old man. **b** The histologic detail of the C5–C6 disk shows horizontal and longitudinal fissures. (Boni and Denaro 1987). H & E

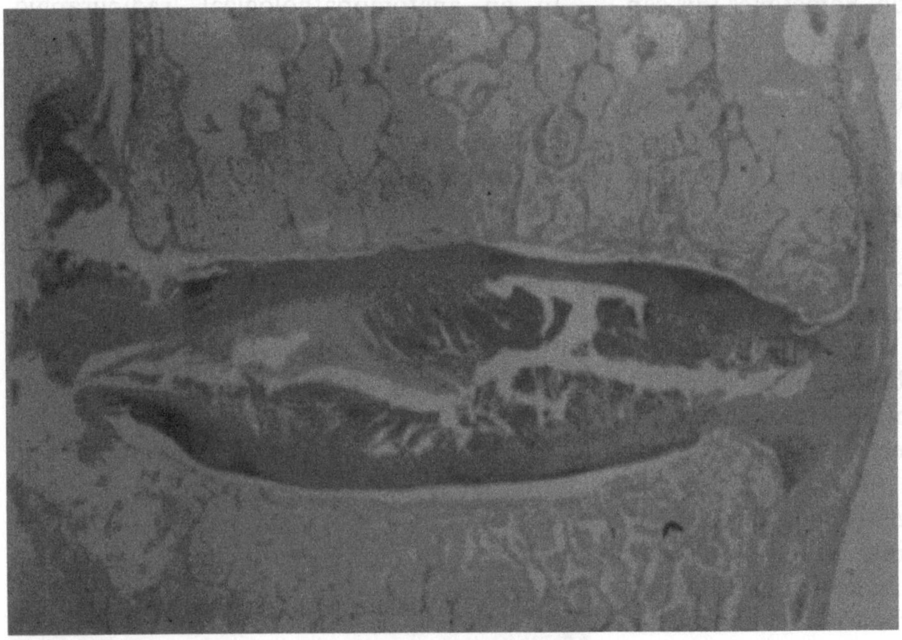

Fig. 2.2. Intervertebral disk in a 61-year-old patient. Note the increased number of fissures, the disorderly array of the disk and the loss of height of the disk space. H & E

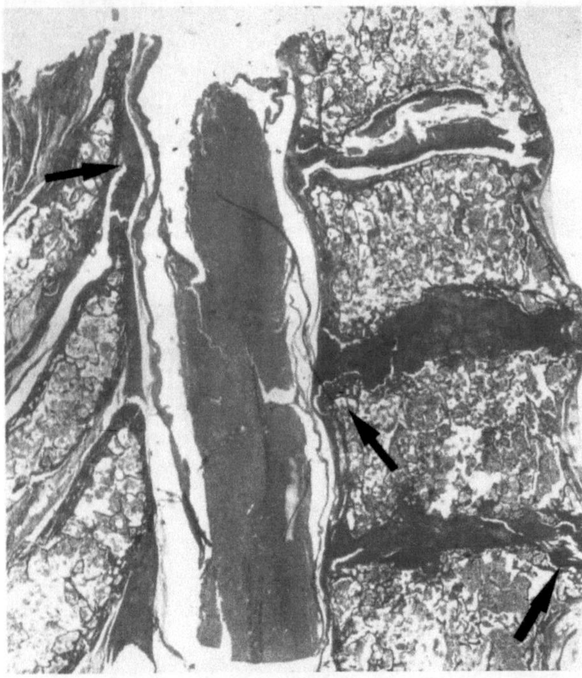

Fig. 2.3. In more advanced degeneration, the bony changes include subchondral sclerosis and both anterior and posterior protrusion by osteophytes (**arrows**). It is the posterior osteophytosis that produces compression with pressure on the posterior longitudinal ligament and hence on the cord and nerve roots. H & E

progress in parallel with the loss of height of the intervertebral disk and while they appear to be primarily concentrated in the nucleus pulposus other changes can be identified involving both the bony and cartilaginous end plates and in the anterior and posterior longitudinal ligaments. Osseous changes tend to be most severe posteriorly and, as they progress, eventually produce radiographically detectable sclerosis and protruding osteophytes, most frequently in the anterior portion (Figs. 2.3–2.4). Even when these anterior osteophytes reach considerable size, they tend to remain asymptomatic; it is extremely rare for them to interfere with swallowing in such a way as to require surgical intervention. Posterior osteophytes are, however, of far greater clinical significance. Herniation and incarceration or sequestering of fragments of a degenerate intervertebral disk posteriorly are not only indications of a decrease in the height of the intervertebral disk, but when posterior osteophytes are also present, protrusion into the canal occurs, leading to the build-up of the posterior longitudinal ligament with a resultant decrease in the anteroposterior diameter of the canal ("hard hernia"; Fig. 2.5). By contrast, acute disk herniation may lead to the escape of intervertebral disk material through the posterior longitudinal ligament and hence into the canal

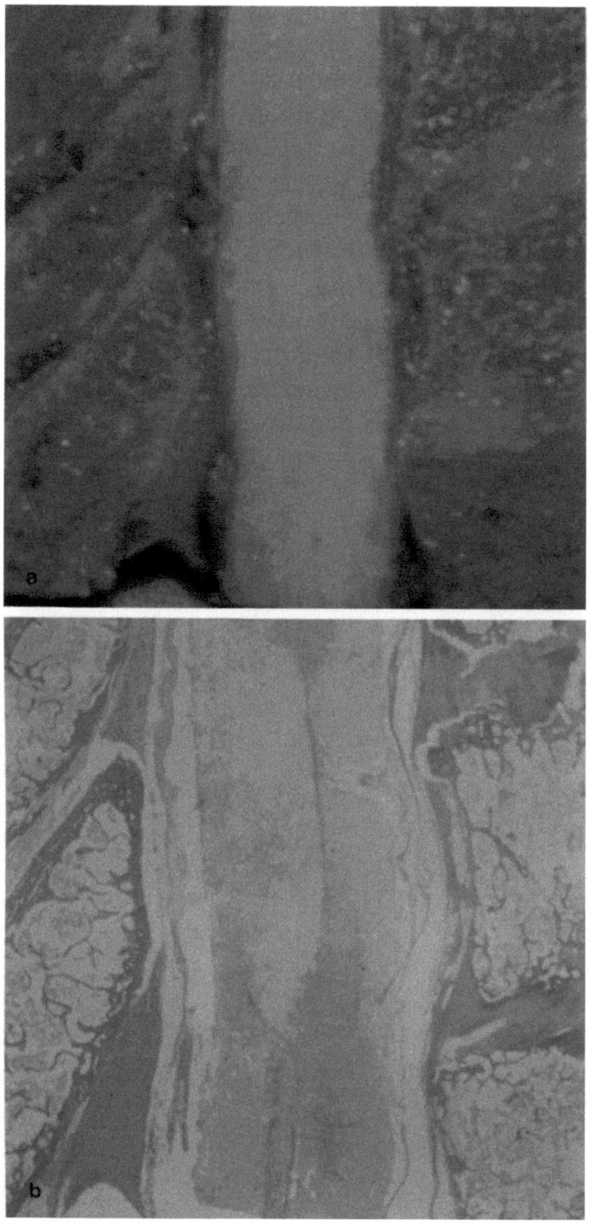

Fig. 2.4 a, b. The macroscopic (a) and microscopic (b) changes which, as a result of the initial osteophytic protrusion into the canal, lead to compression of the spinal cord. H & E

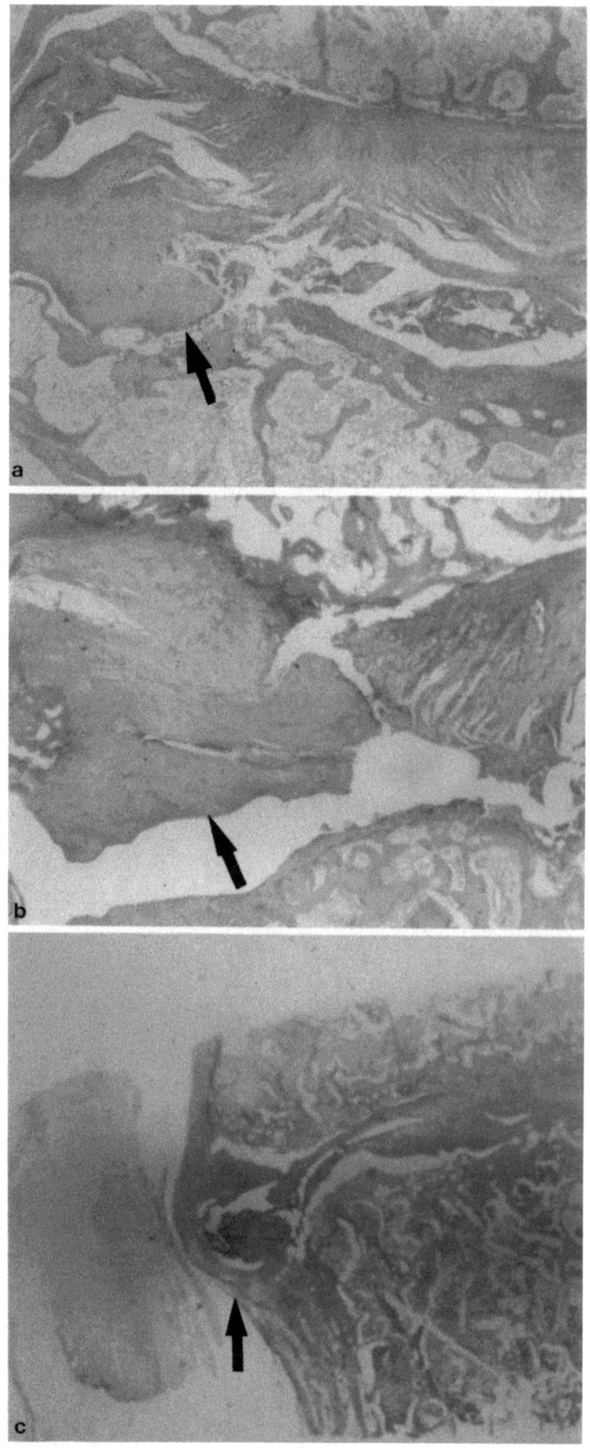

Fig. 2.5 a–c. Histologic appearance of the posterior osteophytes illustrating fragments of the intervertebral disk (a; *arrow*) which are sequestered and pushed posteriorly (b; *arrow*) resulting in the appearance of "hard hernia" (c; *arrow*). H & E

itself ("soft hernia"). This latter tends to occur in younger patients following extremes of loading and stress that result in severe compression of the intervertebral disk. The consequence may be a severe myeloradicular injury, particularly if the situation is compounded by the presence of a congenitally narrowed canal.

2. Intervertebral disk disease is often associated with degeneration of the oncovertebral articulation. The deformity and protrusion of the uncus resulting from this disease can lead to the lateral myeloradicular compression that is part of the complex of diskoarthrotic degeneration usually accompanying oncovertebral degeneration. Narrowing of the intervertebral disk results in approximation of the opposing end plates of the vertebral bodies. Increased density occurs within the bone of the vertebral body and this sets the stage for the development of deformation of the uncus. The lateral protrusion results in the characteristic osteophytes of oncoarthrosis (Figs. 2.6–2.7). It has been said that oncoarthrosis sometimes results in compression of the vertebral artery, with consequent functional disturbances and organic lesions leading to irritation of the perivascular sympathetic plexus. The degenerative anatomical changes seen in advanced age such as shortening of the cervical spine and disk thinning do not correlate with changes in the vertebral artery. On the contrary, certain adaptations such as bone resorption do occur and support continued normal functioning of the vertebral artery. While these may be extreme examples, we are all familiar with the bending that occurs in the second portion of the vertebral artery and which is not known to have pathological significance. In the cases where vertebral artery compression occurs, there may well be deformation of the arterial lumen, but these are the cases with an underlying organic cause which can be easily demonstrated and confirmed by clinical diagnostic imaging.

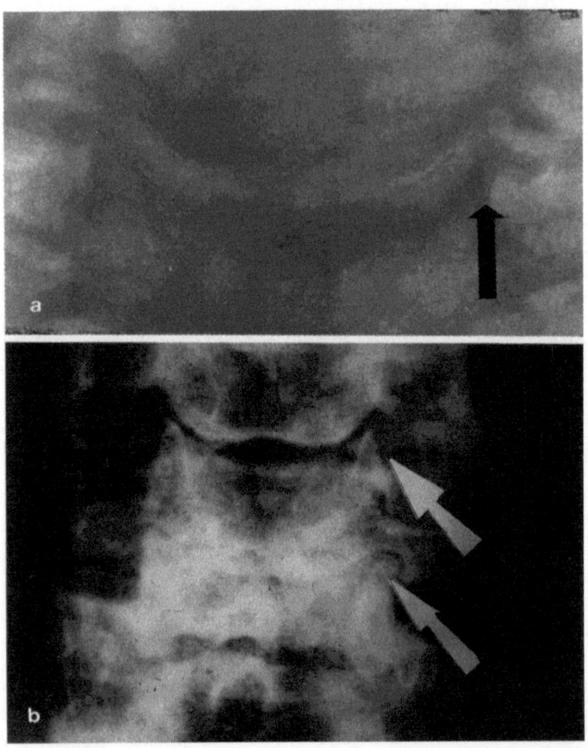

Fig. 2.6 a, b. As the height of the intervertebral disk decreases, the uncus approaches the overlying vertical body. **a** In the cervical spine, this can result in compression of the vertebral artery and of the root canal (*arrow*). **b** Radiograph showing arthritic changes (*arrows*)

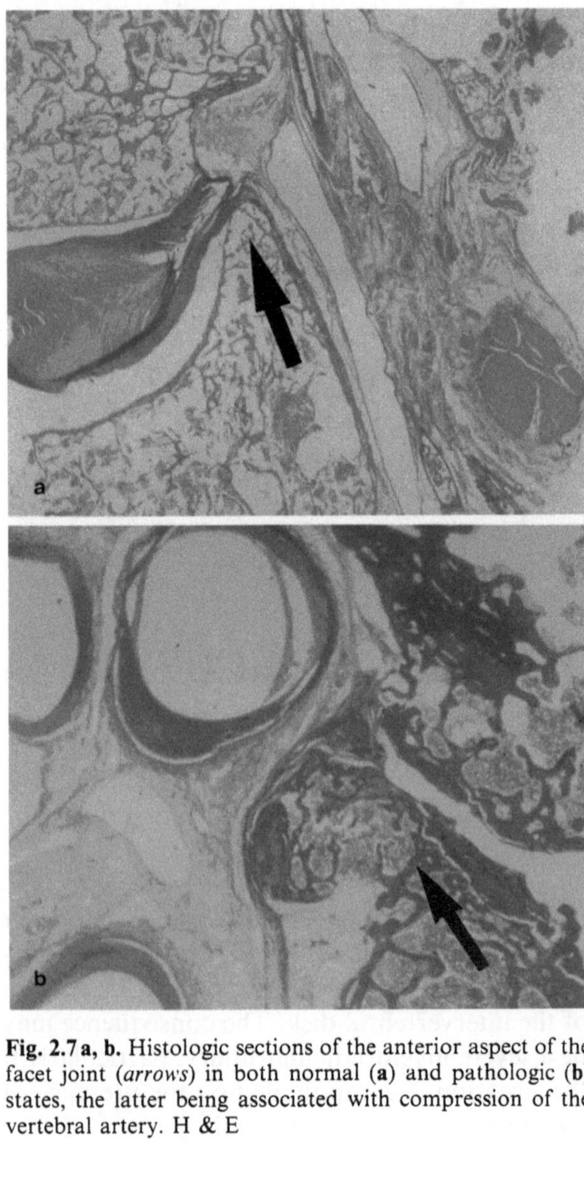

Fig. 2.7 a, b. Histologic sections of the anterior aspect of the facet joint (*arrows*) in both normal (**a**) and pathologic (**b**) states, the latter being associated with compression of the vertebral artery. H & E

3. Arthritic degeneration of the apophyseal joints with hypertrophy of the articulating facets and of the laminae is another cause of cervical spinal stenosis and myeloradicular injury. The interapophyseal joint is a diarthrodial joint subject to cartilaginous degeneration, formation of large osteophytes, and deformation of the articular surface. As such, it is subject to all the changes normally associated with arthritis in other diarthrodial joints. Once the disease is established, the deformed facets protrude anteriorly, restricting the canal, altering the position of the joint capsule and the synovium, and compressing the extrinsic nerve roots. This is often associated with both local and referred pain and, if the nerve roots are involved, there can be cervicobrachialgia and peripheral radicular signs. In spite of the arthritic changes that may occur in the interoapophyseal joint, the vertebral bodies and the intervertebral disks may not be so affected and remain intact and unremarkable. In fact, many authors (Payne and Spillane 1957; Boni 1966; Epstein et al. 1978; Hadley 1957; Holts and Yates 1966; Boni and Denaro 1982) have reported that, in the cervical spine, degenerative arthritic changes may develop contemporaneously in intervertebral disks, but their development and occurrence may be totally independent of the changes in the apophyseal joints (Fig. 2.8). In clinical practice, it is not uncommon to see patients with exclusively posterior stenosis associated with apophyseal joint degeneration and without any degenerative change in the anterior articulations.

4. The ligamentum flavum forms an elastic synostosis as part of the intervertebral articulation. Degeneration of the ligamentum flavum does not occur as part of the degenerative process. The ligamentum flavum, however, has a propensity to hypertrophy, and this enlargement contributes to posterior stenosis of the cervical canal. The bulging of the ligamentum flavum from the posterior wall of the canal may either be the sole cause of stenosis or be a cofactor in the production of stenosis with other changes resulting from spinal arthrosis. The ligamentum flavum is known to lose its elasticity with age and, when this is associated with hypertrophy, the ligament becomes a thicker mass. The ligament inserts on the laminae with a relatively lateral extension that can involve the entire posterior wall of the canal (Mii et al. 1980). In hyperextension, the laminae approximate each other and tend to push forward, and, when a thickened ligamentum flavum is also present, the result is a posterior stenosis in the sagittal plane.

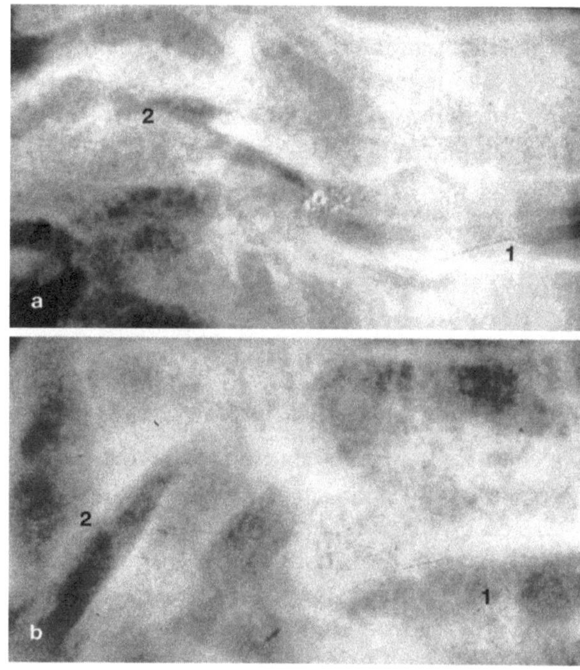

Fig. 2.8 a, b. Radiographs showing that there is no direct correlation between disk degeneration (*1*) and arthrosis of the posterior facet joints (*2*). Frequently one finds a degenerate disk with loss of height in the vertebrae where the posterior facet joints show no evidence of degeneration (Boni and Denaro 1982) H & E

5. In the broad area of proliferative types of stenosis associated with protrusion into the canal, ossification of the posterior longitudinal ligament in the cervical column must be included. It is interesting that this syndrome was first described by Tsukimoto (1960) and Onji et al. (1967) in Japan, where it is far more common than has been reported in caucasian populations. In Eastern Asiatic countries, including Japan, ossification of the posterior longitudinal ligament has been observed in approximately 2%–3% of cervical X-rays. These authors undertook a detailed study in order to define the pathogenesis and management. The etiology and pathogenesis still remain unclear even with the establishment of autosomic dominant hered-

ity (Tsuyama 1984). The observation that there is an increased incidence of diabetes amongst these patients, as reported by the investigation committee on ossification of the posterior longitudinal ligament (1984–1985) certainly brings to mind the possible interrelationship of diabetes with disseminated idiopathic systemic hyperostosis. Ossification of the posterior longitudinal ligament was described before the advent of CT and was classically classified as follows:

- Segmental type (involving individual vertebrae, not only single, but multiple)
- Continuous type (extending to involve several contiguous vertebrae)
- Mixed type (indicating a combination of segmental and continuous types)
- Other types (a group that is impossible to classify into the previous three groups)

Since the introduction of CT, the classification has been based on the pattern of the protrusion of the calcification of the ligament into the canal. This more sophisticated imaging technique has resulted in the identification of three characteristic types: the square type, the "mushroom" type, and the "hill" type.

Several anatomopathological studies from necropsy material (Hashizum et al. 1984; Murakami et al. 1978) have unequivocally demonstrated cord damage caused by stenosis resulting from calcification of the posterior longitudinal ligament. In fact, extensive myelonecrosis involving both the white and the gray matter of the cord, has often been described with a pattern of evolution and damage that is highly suggestive of a vascular pathogenesis. The ossification of the posterior longitudinal ligament begins at the attachment of the fibrous tissue of the ligament to the vertebral body. In the pattern of degenerative enthesial calcification it progresses gradually to the point where it produces a hard mass that bulges into the vertebral canal. It is exactly at this point that ossification plays a role in the modification of the interrelationship between the cord and the canal which is of clinical and pathogenetic significance during movement of the cervical spine, a role which has many similarities with the pathogenetic contribution of degenerative osteophytes. The identification of clinical symptoms and signs that result from combined organic causes of stenosis will depend on the development of the stenosis and the severity of the resulting clinical disease on:

- The structure of the canal – whether normal or congenitally narrowed
- On the type and extent of calcification of the ligament – whether segmental, continuous, or mixed
- On the pattern of the change in luminal diameter – whether it is square, mushroom-shaped, or hill-like

Destructive Stenosis: Stenosis Associated with Neoplasms

Both benign and metastatic tumors have more threatening and serious consequences in the cervical spine than elsewhere in the skeleton. This applies to benign and malignant primary neoplasms as well as to metastases. Depending on the type, grade, and aggressiveness of the tumor, a metastasis in the cervical spine can cause extensive destruction of the vertebral structure. The consequence of this is impingement on the cord. A primary and histologically benign tumor in the cervical spine can, in spite of its benignity in name, destroy enough of the vertebral body to cause as much damage as malignant tumor. Neurological damage can occur:

- Directly, as a result of tumor invasion into the cord and nerve roots with compression or infiltration of these structures.
- Indirectly, as a result of the collapse of a vertebral body leading to compression of the cord and nerve roots. The sudden collapse of a vertebra produces acute and sudden symptoms of cord and nerve root compression. Tumor growth into the canal, particularly if it is slow, produces a more chronic and slowly evolving clinical pattern. In practice, the slowly progressive clinical signs are those which are more likely to raise suspicion of the presence of a neoplasm in these cases (Figs. 9.47 9.51).

An interesting group of diseases with vertebral involvement is the group collectively known as histiocytosis X, which includes eosinophilic granuloma, Hand-Schüller-Christian disease, and Letterer-Siwe disease. These diseases were thought to have histomorphological similarities and to represent a spectrum of diseases with differing clinical patterns of evolution and progression: eosinophilic granuloma was regarded as the solitary from of the disease that characteristically affected bones; Hand-Schüller-Christian disease was felt to primarily involve bone, but also extraskeletal soft tissues, while the Letterer-Siwe-syndrome was thought primarily to affect the soft tissues with very little, if any, bone involvement. The clinical presentations of each of these can be quite different. Eosinophilic granuloma occurs commonly between the ages of 5 and 10 years, but can occur at almost any age. On occasion, the disease presents as a cystic lesion of bone with very little diagnostic or lesional tissue remaining. Hand-Schüller-Christian disease is multifocal and may be associated with exophthalmos and diabetes insipidus as a result of involvement of the cranial bones. By contrast, Letterer-Siwe disease tends to be widely disseminated, often presenting with skin involvement associated with fever and hepatosplenomegaly. The solitary form (eosinophilic granuloma) may also be an incidental finding in radiological imaging taken for unrelated causes. Spinal involvement may produce painful scoliotic deviation and muscular contraction. As long as involvement is limited to the vertebral body, there is less likelihood of serious clinical signs or symptoms occurring. Involvement of the pedicles or articular masses leads to more severe clinical presentations. With the exception of eosinophilic granuloma, which produces the characteristic vertebra plana, spinal involvement usually consists of osteolytic areas of the vertebral body which contain the characteristic proliferation that gives this group of diseases the name reticuloendotheliosis. In this group of diseases, neurological deficits are less common; most cases are devoid of neurological involvement and can be successfully treated in a nonoperative manner with radiation therapy. When neurological deficits occur they are usually the result of vertebral body collapse with impingement on the spinal canal.

Inflammatory Stenosis

In this area of antibiotics, cases of bacterial localization are still encountered all too frequently not only in the spine in general, but specifically in the cervical portion of the spine. Osteomyelitis in the vertebral column is far more serious than elsewhere in the osteoskeletal system. This is a consequence of the early involvement of the cord and related neural tissues. There is a high risk of mortality as a consequence of cervical infection which is the result of multiple factors:

- The virulence and aggressiveness of the bacterial agent
- The difficulty in making an early diagnosis in a complicated clinical presentation
- The need to treat the organisms with a specific antibiotic to which they are susceptible
- The urgent need to decompress the cord by surgical intervention, to perform a debridement before permanent damage has occurred to the neural and vascular structures, and to stabilize and reconstruct the destroyed tissue
- The evolution of organisms that are insensitive to treatment

This last factor may be the most important and often determines the outcome. The incidence of infection in younger patients appears to be increasing. There is a large number of patients with systemic conditions that render them more susceptible to infection such as diabetics, patients with chronic liver disease, and those suffering from the plethora of complications derived from the abuse of drugs (Denaro and Kehr 1990; Fishback et al. 1973). Infection of the spine is also becoming a significant problem in patients with immuno-deficiency syndrome, particularly the acquired form (Denaro 1990).

Under the above circumstances, any organism can settle out in the cervical spine and produce infection. The type of organisms and the patient's ability to respond to the infection are major factors in the clinical outcome of the infection. The infections can be divided into acute and chronic forms as well as into specific and nonspecific variants. *Staphylococcus aureus* is the commonest causative agent of acute infections and *Pseudomonas osteomyelitis* in the cervical spine has also been described in the literature (Holzman and Bishkof 1971). Even in this day and age, mycobacterium tuberculosis is still a common causative agent of chronic infection. Fifty percent of cases of tuberculosis have vertebral involvement (Fig. 9.52).

The pathogenesis and the manner of localization of the infection in the cervical spine has been variously described. In the majority of cases, infection spreads to the spine along the hematogenous pathway, but, particularly in cases of tuberculosis, involvement of lymph nodes adjacent to the vertebral column has been correlated with spread of the infection to the adjacent spine, presumably via the lymphatic pathway (Hodgson and Francis 1960). In a variety of reported circumstances, spread to the spine has occurred from foci in the extraosseous soft tissues adjacent to the bone. This has been known to occur as a complication of penetrating wounds to the neck, as a complication of surgery in the pharynx (Biller et al. 1971) and in the presence of foreign codies in the hypopharynx (Hagadorn et al. 1972). Infection may be of more specific, iatrogenic origin and occur as a complication of surgery of the vertebral body or intervertebral disk to correct such conditions as disk degeneration and herniation, particularly when arthrodesis is performed (Cloward 1958; Denaro and Kehr 1990). The risk of infection is also present in all surgical situations where osseous grafts and internal immobilization are undertaken. Penetrating diagnostic techniques such as diskography also carry a risk of infection that must be recognized.

Infections most commonly occur in the anterior components of the spinal column and are particularly rare in the laminae and the articular facets of the posterior portion of the vertebra. It is important to remember that there are two general patterns of disease. They can be classified according to the virulence of the organism, its sensitivity to therapy, and, of course, the patient's ability to react to the infection.

There are two broad groups of disease:

- The cases where involvement is limited to the body or the disk and which will respond to conservative management.
- The cases where there is a severe, progressive, vertebral body destruction with collapse of the osseous structure and extension of the infection posteriorly into the canal itself and the cord and anteriorly to beyond the vertebral body to involve the soft tissues, forming characteristic paraspinal abscesses. These are the cases where the extent of architectural destruction leads to cord compression with neurological deficits. If inadequately treated, these cases may lead not only to meningeal abscesses, but also to more extensive meningitis that can have a fatal outcome (Forsythe and Rothman 1970).

The importance of the following factors must be emphasized. The inflammatory process not only produces an exudative mass that impinges on the space of the spinal canal but may also cause sufficient damage to the osseous architecture to lead to vertebral collapse. These mechanisms both lead to a discrepancy in the adquacy of the size of the canal to contain the cord. The clinical and pathological features of the disease permit a distinction relative to the location of the lesion:

- High in the cervical spine (the C1/C2 complex; when the C1/C2 complex is affected by a highly virulent and destructive infection it will have severe neurological deficits that can lead to a fatal outcome. In 1930 Grisel described the localization at this level of tuberculosis with a slowly progressive clinical pattern that had been mistaken for a form of wryneck and which became known as Grisel's syndrome (Forsythe and Rothman 1978). In fact what he described was a lateral dislocation of the atlas on the axis resulting in the typical deformity associated with wryneck. When the involvement is between the atlas and the occipital bone, the situation is particularly serious and very frequently associated with a fatal outcome. Fortunately such cases have always been rare and have not been reported in the most recent literature.

- In the lower cervical spine (C3–C7); here one can demonstrate radiologically a full spectrum of severity. Depending on the patient's age and natural defence, involvement can range from a single intervertebral disk, with mild porosity in the adjacent bone, to destruction of one or more vertebral bodies, resulting in severe spinal collapse and instability. One cannot overemphasize the need for immediate and early diagnosis. In addition to careful history and physical examination, radiological imaging and laboratory investigation are crucial. An elevated sedimentation rate and granulocytosis in acute suppurative infection, and eosinophilia in fungal and parasitic infections are characteristic. Radioisotopic scintigraphy is important in determining the localization and the extent of involvement. MRI and CT are not only helpful in defining the site and pattern of involvement, but also permit the use of controlled fine-needle aspiration and biopsy. Open biopsy may, however, be necessary in selected cases. In cases that present with neurological deficits and vertebral body destruction, a broader differential diagnosis that includes neoplasms and trauma must be addressed and assessed on the basis of the clinical findings and the results of the various diagnostic tests described.

Traumatic Stenosis

In this section those clinical situations are discussed in which, as a result of trauma to the cervical spine, there is the risk of an eventual functional or organic stenosis which may progress gradually to produce an imbalance in the relationship between the cord and the cervical spinal canal. Excluded are all cases of recent trauma associated with fracture and dislocation, but injuries that produce no neurological deficit by themselves and those which have been either not treated or inadequately treated because they were missed at the time of the injury are included, as are those cases where inappropriate treatment, missed fractures that did not unite, or malunited fractures have produced a degree of deformity that alters the overal anatomical integrity of the cervical canal. All of these have in common the fact that there are no identifiable neurological deficits at the time of presentation. The best example of this is a fracture or a fracture dislocation that produced no neurological deficits, but which may be associated with the presence of loose osseous fragments within the space of the canal or with a permanent change in the alignment of the vertebral bodies.

We are all too familiar with the events in the Emergency Room where a patient presents following a significant injury, but no neurological abnormality can be identified. As a result, particularly in centers where nonspecialists deal with these cases, there is hesitation in deciding about correct management. Erroneously the attending physician may decide that the danger of complications is too great for an operation that is perceived to have a high risk of iatrogenic injury. The patient is treated and the physician, expectantly awaits that spontaneous stabilization will occur and that, by delaying definitive treatment, spontaneous repair of fracture or reduction in the severity or significance of a subluxation will result. That this is the correct clinical approach could not be further from the truth and the eventual clinical outcome falls into one of the following categories. One possibility is that once the initial symptoms are resolved, the patient does not return for follow-up or is not referred to the appropriate specialist. Once normal activities have been resumed by the patient without the appropriate treatment or precautions, he has an either organic or mechanical predisposition towards the development of stenosis of the canal because of the changes brought about by the injury. Eventually, he will be referred to a specialist when the neurological consequences of this neglected situation have evolved. Management will be far more difficult and will carry greater risks for the patient, and often neurological deficits cannot be reversed. On the other hand, if a patient is referred to a specialist with instability, with or without stabilization and healing of the injured tissues, he is usually referred with the expectation that a reconstructive procedure will stabilize and correct the clinical deficits. The delay between the initial injury and the referral make the surgical management particularly difficult. Bony callus and thick fibrous adhesions make the surgery particularly difficult and lead to secondary vascular problems that can have a direct effect on the adjacent and coinvolved neurological structures. In contrast, early immediate surgery avoids all of these difficulties and their consequences and provides immediate correction of the deficit and instability.

It is important to separate lesions of the upper cervical spine (C1 and C2) from those of the lower cervical spine (C3–C7). In the lower cervical spine (C3–C7) the most frequently encountered lesions are:

- *Fracture dislocation with loose osseous fragments,* particularly so-called "teardrop" fractures. These result from a complex twisting mechanism of the ligamentous structure that unifies the cervical spine into a functional unit. Theoretically, all the posterior elements including interspinal ligament, ligamentum flavum, joint capsules, and, particularly, the posterior longitudinal ligament and the disk articulation can be affected. Radiological imaging demonstrates separation of the anterior margin of the vertebral body (teardrop), while the posterior surface of the vertebral body, which is dislocated by several millimeters posteriorly, protrudes into the canal, thereby decreasing the anteroposterior diameter. The presence of a teardrop fracture indicates a complex mechanical pathogenesis which represents a threat to the cord and requires immediate treatment. When the dislocation is minimal or when the canal is large enough to absorb the change without neurological deficit, it is tempting to choose a nonoperative treatment. If this is selected, the vertebral body remains posteriorly dislocated with consequent narrowing of the canal. Gradually, however, with time neurological signs will appear. The changes may not be detectable early enough, even with careful follow-up, to prevent eventual permanent damage.

  A similar situation can arise from vertebral fractures, with or without disk involvement, which produce dislocation of bone or disk material posteriorly into the canal. Fractures of the margins of the end plates anteriorly can result in a segmental kyphosis which is not reducible. Obviously, "blow-out" fractures of the vertebral body will produce displaced osseous fragments in addition to the more readily apparent structural deformity (Fig. 9.44).
- *Pure dislocations* which are not reduced and which may be associated with dislocations of the apophyseal joints involving one or both sides of the vertebra will result in either symmetrical or asymmetrical deformity of the canal. These dislocations occur when the entire ligamentous structure or functional unit of the cervical spine is involved. Fortunately, in the presence of wide canals and particularly with limited trauma, they may occur without damage to the cord. However, the neural structures may be stretched, forced around sharp angles, or impinged upon by the vertebral body below the dislocated one, while the vertebral arch of the dislocated vertebra compresses it posteriorly. Such cases are subject not only to the spacial imbalance between the cord and the canal, but also to varying degrees of instability that will have serious pathological consequences. Even in cases where the displacement is immediately reduced, there is a risk that the disruption of the ligamentous structure may lead to residual instability.
- *Severe disruption of the spinal cord inferiorly.* This is a group of injuries that are classified as serious because they lead to progressive and extensive neurological deficit. They tend to occur when the mode of injury produces extensive distraction of the ligamentous unit with gradually developing signs and symptoms which are not apparent immediately at the time of injury (a situation that would then be regarded as a dislocation). From the anatomopathological point of view, the entire functional unit is affected, especially the posterior longitudinal ligament at its point of insertion on the vertebrae. These lesions can easily be missed at the time of initial presentation, because any neurological signs may be very slight and easily overlooked. We strongly believe that it is important to have a high index

of suspicion for these lesions when the patient is first examined (Denaro 1987). If, following the initial examination, there are any doubts in the mind of the examining physician, the patient should be closely monitored and dynamic radiological imaging should be performed. The indirect signs of serious disruption can only be detected with X-rays taken at the extremes of movement (e.g., flexion and extension). The signs to look for in the radiological imaging are (Fig. 9.99):

- Anterior segmental kyphosis at the level of the involved disk
- Widening of the spinal apophyses
- Exposure of the apophyseal surfaces
- Anterior dislocation of any vertebral body greater than 3–4 mm

Often the severity of these lesions and, in particular, their instability can be masked by the muscular spasm in the neck when the patient first presents. This dislocation will slowly and insiduously progress to produce a true segmental stenosis with cord damage that will progressively worsen with pain, hypoesthesia, and spastic paresis. These are the signs for which the patient is often referred to a specialist and which are indicative of the presence of cord damage. It is important to remember that the neurological damage develops gradually over time, and it is to be expected that immediate reduction and stabilization of the structural deformity will provide return of function and often complete regression of all signs.

In the upper cervical spine this type of post-traumatic stenoses is far less common, but is of greater clinical and prognostic significance. It is uncommon for the surgeon to see these lesions, because acute lesions in this part of the cervical spine can be lethal: in the literature it is reported that as many as 24% of road accidents with injury at this level are fatal (Alker et al. 1975). The relationship of cord to canal at the C1–C2 level is also far more favorable than in the remaining cervical spine. This suggests that, compared with the lower segments, the post-traumatic deformity and instability are of clinical significance less frequently and with a longer time span. At this level the more common lesions are:

- *Fracture of the atlas,* which is rarely a cause of stenosis and which occurs following a fracture of the lateral masses of this vertebra. The mechanism of injury is usually the downward push of the occipital condyle on the lateral masses against resistance from below by the lateral masses of the axis. This mechanism tends to produce separation with widening of the canal, as is the case in Jefferson fracture. The same occurs in fractures of the posterior arch. Repairing these fractures does not usually cause stenosis, since this would occur only when fragments are displaced medially or posteriorly into the canal such as to impinge on the lumen within the canal. These injuries are more theoretical as they are seldom encountered within the context of post-traumatic stenosis because the mechanisms by which they occur tend to lead to circumstances incompatible with survival.

- *Fractures of the odontoid process,* particularly those of Anderson and d'Alonzo type 2, which tend not to heal and retain varying degrees of instability. The oblique direction of the fracture, which is angled either to the front or to the back, favors abnormal displacement of the occipitoaxis complex with reference to the fractured odontoid process (Fig. 9.95).

- *Post-traumatic atlantoaxial instability.* Dislocation of the atlas on the axis of the plane of instability produces a decrease in the diameter of the spinal canal thereby, compromising the cord. As a result, repeated microtrauma eventually will lead to the clinical onset of a chronic myelopathy, which may have many of the features of amyotrophic lateral sclerosis. Rotatory instability may be very mild and asymptomatic, but when combined with anteroposterior instability does lead to compression and irritation of nerve roots with a severe and progressive myelopathy. The combined instability may initially appear mild and insignificant, but will progress and worsen with time. It is therefore important to carefully investigate these situations right at the time of initial injury. X-rays in the extremes of flexion and extension will be most valuable in identifying this unstable situation, particularly when they show a change in the distance between the arch of the atlas and the odontoid process of the axis greater than 2 mm in adults and more than 3 mm in children. CT undertaken with traction on the head is valuable in detecting the abnormal relationship between the odontoid process and the arch of the atlas; the asymmetry of the lateral masses of the atlas with respect to the axis will be apparent and reliably demonstrated, permitting an accurate diagnosis.

We have discussed the most frequent causes of organic stenoses resulting from trauma and the pathogenetic mechanisms that initiate them. With the exception of those cases where the initial features are not identified, this group of cases is preventable with:

- Early diagnosis [CT, MRI, Somatosensory evoked potential (SEP) monitoring]
- A full understanding of the risk of progression in untreated cases
- The use of good sense in identifying the indications for surgery, once the eventual risk has been recognized.

Overall, organic stenoses comprise a group of clinical situations, in the majority of which one can undertake a program of prevention.

Stenosis in Arthritis

Collagenopathies are known to produce structural and functional changes in joints and, with involvement of the cervical spine, stenosis may result. The most commonly encountered diseases in this group are rheumatoid arthritis and ankylosing spondylitis.

Rheumatoid Arthritis

In the cervical spine, as elsewhere in the skeleton, rheumatoid arthritis presents with a hypertrophic and exudative type of synovitis, followed by involvement of the para-articular ligamentous structure that may be altered, weakened, or even ruptured. There is erosion of the joint cartilage by the pannus that will eventually lead to complete joint destruction. Periarticular osteoporosis is often modified by articular erosions and subchondral cysts. This complex of damage to ligaments, bones, and joints that begins as a synovitis has severe and disrupting consequences for joint function. Purely degenerative changes will be superimposed all of which can lead to varying degrees of joint instability. In addition to the changes brought about by the rheumatoid process and its functional consequences, one must always take into account the effects of therapy and, in particular, the long and often continuous courses of corticosteroids that are used in the management of this disease. The portions of the vertebral column with the greatest mobility are the ones most affected in rheumatoid arthritis and this is most common at the occipitocervical interface. Conlon et al. (1966) reported that 60% of patients with rheumatoid arthritis had symptoms relating to involvement of the cervical spine. The upper (C1 and C2) and lower (C3–C7) levels of the cervical spine will be discussed separately.

Upper Cervical Spine. The atlanto-occipital and the atlantoaxial joints are of particular interest, with special reference to those between the odontoid process and the anterior portion of the arch of the atlas and those between the lateral masses of the atlas and the axis. These joints, once affected, undergo slow, progressive, ligamentous and osteoarticular changes, eventually reaching a point of structural and functional deficit that will have clinical consequences. At the occipito-atlantic articulation between the occipital condyles and the lateral masses of the atlas, the development of instability and articular erosion may reach such a point as to permit the rise of the odontoid process to the level of the foramen magnum. Not only do lesser grades of protrusion of the odontoid process produce a degree of stenosis with cord damage, but the more severe degrees of protrusion can have very serious and even fatal consequences. In order to anticipate the risk involved in rheumatoid disease at this level, it is important that the symptoms and sign be carefully looked for and that the changes be confirmed by traditional and modern imaging (CT, MRI). When the atlantoaxial joints begin to degenerate, they at first show a loss of congruity and there is loss of integrity in the ligamentous structure encompassing the odontoid process and the arch of the atlas. This can result in displacements of 4 to 6 mm. Erosion and instability of the odontoid process can usually be seen in dynamic radiological imaging in the lateral projection. When instability results in displacement of the atlas, the consequences can take two forms. Repeated chronic cord injury may mimic a severe degenerative myelopathy while acute injury may result in sudden death. Mikulowski et al. (1975) reported a 75% incidence of cord damage at autopsy in such cases. Anteroposterior dislocations are never pure because there is extensive ligamentous involvement that results in an accompanying rotatory laxity which can be well demonstrated by CT. Arthritic changes in the atlantoaxial joint may remain neurologically silent for a long time, as they may be partly masked by the associated multilevel ligamentous instability and laxity. Atlantoaxial joint instability may remain asymptomatic even when it is the posterior occipital region in the upper neck. Once the anteroposterior and rotatory instability is associated with protrusion and invagination of the odontoid process, the situation becomes very serious and life-threatening.

Lower cervical spine. At the lower level (C3–C7) the intervertebral, interapophyseal, and uncovertebral joints are involved. There will be capsular, osseous, and cartilage changes with characteristic radiographic features. This degeneration may be associated with erosion of the vertebral body as a result of the instability associated with both anterior and posterior listhesis of the vertebral bodies. The apophyseal joints will show extensive erosion and excess mobility. The interspinous ligaments will show increasing laxity. The uncovertebral joints will show erosion, with narrowing of the joint spaces. In other words, the entire functional unit will go through progressive stages of laxity and incongruity. Symptoms will be less severe and less frequent than in the upper (C1 and C2) levels with a reduced incidence of neurological symptoms. Because of the complexity and variability of involvement, it is impossible to generalize on the clinical findings and prognosis.

Clinical situations in which patients present with early signs and symptoms can, with progression of the disease, quickly develop in severity. Patients who initially present with severe damage may develop neurological signs in a slow and chronic manner. What is important and must always be remembered is that each case must be carefully assessed, particularly for neurological involvement, in order to prevent permanent injury by timely surgical intervention to correct the instability. Neurological symptoms may be masked by muscle atrophy and other functional limitations brought about by the disease process. Only in the advanced cases can clear neurological features be clearly identified. What we do know from experience is that early diagnosis and immediate surgery will control the neurological damage and that 50% of patients with this degree of severity who are not surgically stabilized will rapidly progress to a fatal outcome (Marks and Sharp 1981). The need not only for early but also for accurate and complete assessment of the patient cannot be overemphasized; in addition to cord damage at the cervical level, injury leading to thrombosis of the vertebral arteries can produce cerebellar and brain stem injury.

Ankylosing Spondylitis (Marie-Strümpell spondylitis)

Ankylosing spondylitis is a disease leading to spinal ankylosis in a slow and progressive fashion. Under normal circumstances the cord has ample time to adapt to the changing shape of the spinal canal. However, when only some levels are ankylosed, the nonankylosed levels will be subjected to functional overload as additional demands for movement are made by the now rigid adjacent column. At this point, one should anticipate the onset of instability leading to segmental stenosis that can produce all the clinical signs and symptoms of cord and nerve root impingement (Fig. 9.100).

Iatrogenic Stenosis

Surgery of the neck and spine may be complicated by cervical stenosis. Some effects of surgery such as post-operative fibrosis and scarring are to be expected and are predictable complications which may be difficult to prevent. Other effects such as deformity or instability may result from extensive surgery such as multilevel laminectomy or inadequate or even inappropriate surgery, particularly when osteoarticular structures are removed without appropriate stabilization. These can and should be prevented by correctly selected and applied surgical strategies. In our experience, iatrogenic stenosis may be classified into three categories, as described below.

Instability Resulting from Extensive Laminectomy

In the past, laminectomy was undertaken in order to decompress the cord in traumatic, degenerative, or neoplastic conditions. In the process of widening the canal, the laminae and the ligamentum flavum were widely resected, together with variable portions of the apophyseal joints. When this is done in a rigid spinal column with a posterior stenosis, there are usually no consequences. When, however, there is an inherent spinal instability as a result of a degenerative process or trauma, particularly in young patients, there is a particular propensity for complications due to the instability. When in these cases one removes the posterior wall of the canal where the interspinous ligament, the ligamentum flavum, and the apophyseal joints play an important stabilizing role, then one is in fact producing a deformity with not only morphological and static abnormalities, but also with biomechanical consequences that can lead to neurological injury. These should be prevented by selecting more appropriate and less extensive surgery. If it is necessary to undertake an extensive laminectomy, then it must be associated with simultaneous stabilization of the levels operated upon. If widening of the canal through a posterior approach is deemed necessary, then a nondestabilizing technique must be employed such as the open door type of laminectomy.

Peridural Postoperative Fibrosis

The scarring that follows any surgical procedure involving the uncovering of the meninges may result in stenosis. Usually this is a complication of extensive exposure during very wide laminectomies. This is a well-known problem and there are many recorded methods that have been developed in an attempt to prevent this complication. Massive scarring is usually the result of multiple factors: the patients may have a diathesis towards excessive scarring such as to produce massive fibrosis or even scars of the types that are usually associated with hypertrophic scars and keloids in skin. If intraoperative hemostasis is not carried out with great care, a postoperative hematoma may form, producing large fibrous scars extensive enough to reach out and involve the muscles that surround the spine.

Of the known methods of prevention, some have been adaptations of methods used in the lumbar spine. These include the use of subcutaneous fat as a pad that is placed on the dura mater, but this method has not been successful. It has been reported to produce postoperative compression requiring further surgical intervention to release the resulting cord compression. The use of local corticosteroids directly on the dura mater has not been found to prevent the fibrosis. The use of Gelfilm held great promise since it was found to be very successful in experimental animals. Possibly the best preventive step which a surgeon can take is a careful hemostasis at the completion of the operation, combined with suction drainage in order to prevent the formation of hematoma. Early mobilization of the portion of the column that has been operated on is also helpful (as long as stability is achieved and maintained). Active mobilization at all levels of the cervical column with exercises that stretch the root canals have also been found of value.

Instability Following Anterior Decompression Without Stabilization

In columns that are unstable or actively mobile, instability following anterior decompression without stabilization may occur. Following Cloward or Smith-Robinson operations on one or more vertebral bodies which are not followed by arthrodesis with bone graft or where the graft has been resorbed and therefore does not provide the necessary mechanical stability, a kyphotic deformity may result. This is usually the result of insufficient assessment of the stability (or lack of it) preoperatively, followed by an operation limited to anterior decompression of the cord without arthrodesis. It is not uncommon, under these conditions and following an extensive osseous resection, to have an unstable column. Following the Cloward procedure, if the graft used is such as to be easily resorbed, it will not provide a good supporting arthrodesis (Fig. 9.14, 9.15). This is common when heterologous bone grafts or even autologous bone grafts are used, if they are equal or smaller than the trough prepared for them. It is important that the graft be larger than the defect that it is intended to fill. A graft that is well compacted in its bed becomes well anchored, will have immediate mechanical holding, and will provide better consolidation as healing occurs in both the Cloward or the Smith-Robinson operations. In a personal case, good ankylosis of the spine could be achieved with surgery, but later at the C5–C6 level, a pseudoarthrosis occurred permitting flexion and extension movement. This was associated with progressive degeneration, instability, and stenosis.

Combined Stenoses and Pathogenesis

In the previous section, the organic and functional types of stenosis as well as the more common etiology and pathogenesis were discussed. From this discussion the following conclusions can be derived:

- In clinical practice the most common features are those in which the various pathogenetic factors are combined: by combined we mean that the congenital and acquired morphological features occur in variable combinations with the functional features.
- The mobility of the cervical spine during physiological function, the very extensive articular excursion, and especially the variability in length and diameter of the spinal canal and of its contents are all characteristics that are fundamental to the susceptibility and evolution of clinical symptoms. In the cervical spine, up to 600 physiological motions are possible in the normal range of activity (Jomin 1978). It is, therefore, no wonder that this portion of the spine is so susceptible to overload leading to pathological states. Disease is the result of microtrauma which occurs in this very motile portion of the spine, whether it be normal or congenitally narrowed. In those spines that are congenitally narrowed, there will be a limitation of the extent of movement under physiological conditions, because such spines will be more rigid, almost as if to protect the cord from the greater threat of injury resulting from the extremes of movement, i.e., lower tolerance of otherwise normal movement.
- Cord injury occurs through the combined effect of the pathogenetic mechanisms of the different types of stenosis and the consequences are compounded. The resulting clinical complex can be the result of direct or mechanical factors, depending on the structure of the canal and the type of microtrauma to which it is subjected. The indirect mechanisms are those of vascular origin, resulting from either direct compression of the arteries, venous stasis, or reflex vascular spasms (Fig. 2.9). This is supported by the autopsy studies by Payne and Spillane (1957) and by Waltz (1967), who demonstrated a correlation between neck movement and cord compression. More recent neuroradiological studies by Yu and Jones (1985) provided correlation

of the compression demonstrated by CT and computed tomographic myelography with the clinical findings. There is no doubt that ischemia is a major factor in the development of cord injury. Brain et al. (1952) went so far as to propose that the vascular factors were the cause not just of ischemia but also of edema and venous stasis. Allen (1952) reported pallor, flattening of the cord, and congestion of the venous plexus above and below the levels of osteophytic compression of the cord. Mair and Druckman (1953) described histologic changes that were identical to the lesions known to be produced by ischemia, and suggested that there was a decrease in blood flow in the distribution of the distal portion of the anterior spinal artery. Thrombosis of blood vessels has also been correlated to spondylotic compression by Hughes and Brownell (1964). Taylor (1964) put forth the hypothesis that compression of the radicular arteries at the level of the foramina was the cause of vascular injury to the cord. This theory, however, does not explain how one can have isolated vascular injury to nerve roots without it being associated with cord injury at the same time. Experimentally, Brodkey et al. (1972) were able to demonstrate a reduction in the circulation as a result of cord compression in the cat. Omin (1978) demonstrated reduced blood flow at the compression site of the cord in the dog. He felt that a moderate compression of the cord at what he described as "the maximum tolerance force" produced a reduction in blood flow. He defined maximum tolerance force as that sufficient to cause minimal weakness in one leg.

In their study of stenosis from ossification of the posterior longitudinal ligament, Murakami et al. (1978) identified changes in the gray and white matter of the cord with the pattern of distribution and the characteristics that can only be attained through vascular injury. In addition to the vascular consideration, one must also take into account the importance of the manner by which ischemia develops. If the cases of acute cord compression, as might occur in disk herniation or following severe trauma with instability, are excluded, then the long, slow evolution of

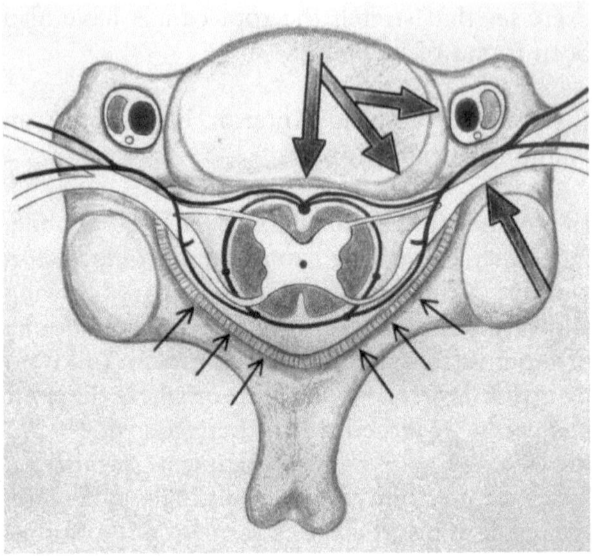

Fig. 2.9. The *arrows* indicate the various methods by which spinal cord and nerve root compression may develop. This may have direct or indirect (i.e., vascular) consequences for the neurological structures of the spinal cord and nerve roots

most of the organic stenosis can be regarded as having two stages. At first microtrauma produces metabolic changes and changes in circulation with local edema and the onset of pain. There then follows a second stage characterized by the onset of paresis. Even at this stage, however, the neurological deficits can be reversed by appropriate conservative management. Lesions may progress to the stage of irreversible stenosis, at which point they can only be corrected by surgical intervention. The early stages represent a stable form of imbalance between cord and canal, which can last for years before progressing to a greater degree of severity. It seems logical to suspect that it is possible for the cord to adapt to changes that develop in the canal in a slow, albeit progressive, manner. Initially, the circulation to the cord may remain adequate, as long as adaptation is possible, and provides sufficient perfusion to the parenchyma; then a critical point is reached in the evolution of the injury beyond which the essential minimum blood supply can no longer be maintained. This must be the mechanism by which adaptation can actually maintain adequate circulatory perfusion, even in cases in which there is a severe degree of stenosis of up to 6 mm, and still maintain normal cord function. If there is a direct relationship between compression and ischemia then the manner in which compression and ischemia occur and their rate of development will be significant factors not only in the severity but also in the timing of the development of the injury.

These observations lead to the conclusion that the pathogenetic factors in the clinical syndromes resulting from stenoses are complex, multiple (both mechanical and vascular), and often act as combined factors with varying degrees of participation.

References

Aboulker J (1965) Les myèlopathies cervicales d'origine rachidienne. Neurochirurgie 11:89-198

Alker G J, Leslie E V, et al. (1975) Post-mortem radiology of head and neck injuries in fatal traffic accidents. Radiology 114:611

Allen K L (1952) Neuropathies caused by bony spurs in the cervical spine with special reference to surgical treatment. J Neurosurg Psychiatry 47:17-20

Babin E (1970) La misure du diamètre sagittal du canal cervical chez l'adulte. Sem Hop Paris 46:2739-2742

Boni M (1966) Considerazioni anatomo-patologiche e cliniche sulle protrusioni del disco nel rachide cervicale. 52st Congress SIOT, Catania

Boni M, Denaro V (1982a) Traitement chirurgical des cervicarthroses. Rev Chir Orthop 68:269-280

Boni M, Denaro V (1982b) The cervical stenosis syndrome. Int Ortho 185-195

Boni M, Denaro V (1987a) Anatomo-clinical correlations in cervical spondylosis. In: Kehr P, Weidner A (eds) Cervical spine I. Springer, Berlin Heidelberg New York

Boni M, Denaro V (1987b) Actualidad en cirurgia cervical. Rev Soc Andaluza Traumatol Ortop 7 (2):133-149

Boni M, Denaro V, Jimenez C, et al. (1984) Tumores primitivos de la columna cervical. Posibilidades diagnosticas y de tratamiento. Rev Soc Andaluza Traumatol Ortop 4 (1):1-42

Biller H F, Ogura J H, Rontal M, Ehrlich C (1971) Cervical osteomyelitis complicating pharyngeal resection. Arch Otolaryongol 94:165-168

Brain W R, Northfield D, Wilkinson M (1952) The neurological manifestation of cervical spondylosis. Brain 75:187-225

Brodkey J S, Richards D E, Blasingame J P, Nulsen F E (1972) Reversible spinal cord trauma in cats: additive effects of direct pressure and ischemia. J Nurosurg 37:591-593

Ceciliani L, Denaro V, Pedrotti L (1985) Cervical spine surgery in children. M. BE. 13:429-442

Cloward R B (1958) The anterior approach for removal of ruptured cervical disks. J Neurosurgery 15:602

Conlon P W, Isdale I C, Rose B S (1966) Rheumatoid arthritis of the cervical spine. Ann Rheum Dis 25:120-126

Cox H E, Bennett W F (1984) Computed tomography of absent cervical pedicle. J Comput Assist Tomogr 8 (3):537-539

Denaro V (1983) Su di un raro caso di spondiloartrite anchilopoietica. Minerva Ortop 34

Denaro V (1987) Il rachide cervicale traumatico: dalla parte dell'ortopedico. Minerva Ortop Traumatol 38 (4):209-224

Denaro V, Kehr P (1990) Infected cervical spine in five cases. In: Louis R, Weidner A (eds) Cervical spine II. Springer, Berlin Heidelberg New York, pp 131-138

Denaro V, Ramaioli F, Cornaglia C (1973) Indicazioni del cloridrato di ketamina nella malattia di Morquio, con aplasia del dente dello epistrofeo. Acta Anaesthesiol 24 (5):539-547

Denaro V, Pedrotti L, Lupo R, Ceciliani L (1985) Eosinophilic granuloma with elective cervical location: clinical and therapeutic aspects. Med Biol Environ 13:537-548

Denaro V, Jelmoni G P, Berzero G F, Centaro G (1986a) Updating on the treatment of limb metastases. Med Biol Environ 14:319-329

Denaro V, Pedrotti L, Lupo R, Barbieri D (1986b) An extremely rare case of bone giant cell tumor involving the upper cervical vertebrae: therapeutic problems. Med Biol Environ 14:333-340

Dubousset J (1986) Torticollis in children caused by congenital anomalies of the atlas. J Bone Joint Surg [Am] 68:178-188

Epstein J A, Epstein N E, Jones M D (1978) Anatomomicroradiological correlations in cervical spine discal disease and stenosis. Clin Neurosurg 25:148-173

Epstein J A, Epstein N E (1989) The cervical spine. 2nd edn. Lippincott, Philadelphia, pp. 625-643

Fardon D F, Fieldin J W (1981) Defects of the pedicle and spondylolisthesis of the second cervical vertebra. J Bone Joint Surg [Br] 63B:526-528

Fishback R S, Rosenblatt J E, Dahlgren J G (1973) Pyogenic vertebral osteomyelitis in heroin addicts. Calif Med 119:1-4

Fornasier V, Horne J (1975) Metastates to the vertebral column. Cancer 36:590

Forsythe M, Rothman R H (1978) New concepts in the diagnosis and treatment of infections of the cervical spine. Orthop Clin North Am 9:1039

Gooding M R, Wilson C B, Hoff J T (1976) Experimental cervical myelopathy: autoradiographic studies of spinal cord blood flow patterns. Surg Neurol 5:233-239

Graaf R (1982) Congenital block vertebrae C2-C3 in patients with cervical myelopathy. Acta Neurol (Napoli) 61:111-126

Hadley L A (1957) The covertebral articulations and cervical foramen encroachment. J Bone Joint Surg [Am] 39A:910-920

Hagadorn B, Smith H W, Rosnagle S (1972) Cervical spine osteomyelitis secondary to a foreign body in the hypopharynx. Arch Otol 95:578-580

Hashizume Y, Lijima S, Kishimoto H, et al. (1984) Pathology of spinal cord lesions caused by ossification of the posterior longitudinal ligament. Acta Neuropathol (Berl) 63:123-130

Henzinger R N (1989) Congenital anomalies of the odontoid (congenital agenesis, hypoplasia and os odontoideum). In: Epstein J A, Epstein N E (eds) The cervical spine. 2nd edn. Lippincott, Philadelphia, pp 248-257

Hirsch C et al. (1967) Structural changes in the cervical spine. Acta Orthop Scand [Suppl] 109

Hodgson A R, Francis E (1960) Anterior spine fusion for the treatment of tuberculosis of the spine. The operative findings and results of treatment in the first one hundred case. J Bone Joint Surg [Am] 42A:295–310

Holt S, Yates P O (1966) Cervical spondylosis and nerve root lesions. Incidence at routine necropsy. J Bone Joint Surg [Br] 48B:407–423

Holtzer H (1952) Experimental analysis of the development of the spinal column: response of precartilage cells to size variations of the spinal cord. Exp Zool 121:121–147

Holzman R S, Bishkof (1971) Osteomyelitis in heroin addicts. Ann Intern Med 75:693

Hughes J T, Brownell B (1964) Cervical spondylosis complicated by anterior spinal artery thrombosis. Neurology (Minneap) 14:1073–1077

Jacques W, Garnet J T, Johnson D, Shelden C H (1975) Osteopetrosis associated with familial paraplegia: report of a family. Paraplegia 13:143–152

Japanese Ministry of Public Health and Welfare (1981–1985) Investigation committee reports on OPLL (Japan). Tokyo

Jomin M (1978) Les myéloradiculopathies par cervicarthrose. Etude clinique et thérapeutique. Lille Med [3e Serie] 23:6

Klintworth G K (1963) The neurologic manifestations of osteopetrosis (Albers-Schonberg disease). Neurology (Minneap) 13:512–519

Leffort G, Mourad H, de Niscault G, Daoud S (1983) Dislocation du rachis cervical supérieur dans le syndrome de Larsen. Chir Pediatr 24:211–212

Mair W G P, Druckman R (1953) The pathology of spinal cord lesions and their relation to the clinical features in protrusion of cervical intervertebral (a report of four cases). Brain 76:70–91

Marks J S, Sharp J (1981) Rheumatoid cervical myelopathy. Q J Med 50:307

McCleary L, Rovit R L, Murali R (1987) Case report: myelopathy secondary to congenital osteopetrosis of the cervical spine. Neurosurgery 20 (3):487–489

Mii K, Ohwada T, Vada K (1980) The role of the ligamenta flava in cervical spondylotic myelopathy. 8th Annual Meeting of the Cervical Spine Research Society, Dec 10–13, Palm Beach

Mikulowski P, Wollheim F A, Rotmil P, Olsen I (1975) Sudden death in rheumatoid arthritis with atlantoaxial dislocation. Acta Med Scand 198:445

Murakami N, Muroga T, Sobue I (1978) Cervical myelopathy due to ossification of the posterior longitudinal ligament. A clinicopathologic study. Arch Neurol 35:33–36

Onji Y, Akiyama H, et al. (1967) Posterior paravertebral ossification causing cervical myelopathy. J Bone Joint Surg [Am] 49A (7):1314–1328.

Payne E, Spillane J D (1957) The cervical spine. An anatomicopathological study of 70 specimens (using a special technique) with particular reference to the problem of cervical spondylosis. Brain 80:571

Prusic V R, Samberg L C, Wesoldwski D P (1985) Klippel Feil syndrome associated with spinal stenosis. J Bone Joint Surg [Am] 67A (1):161–164

Roy-Camille R, Judet T H, Saillant G, Mamondy P, Denaro V (1982) Tumeurs du rachis. In: Encyclopedie Medico-Chirurgicale (Paris), Techniques Chirurgicales, Orthopédie, 44:165, Paris

Taylor A R (1964) Vascular factors in the myelopathy associated with cervical spondylosis. Neurology (Minneap) 14:62–68

Torg J S (1989) Risk factors in congenital stenosis of the cervical spinal canal. In: Epstein J A, Epstein N E (eds) The cervical spine. 2nd edn. Lippincott, Philadelphia, pp 272–285

Tsukimoto H (1960) A case report: autopsy of syndrome of compression of spinal cord owing to ossification within the cervical spine canal. Nippon Geka Hokan 29:1003–1007

Tsuyama N (1984) Ossification of the posterior longitudinal ligament of the spine. Clin Orthop 184:71–84

Vanneuville C, Escande G, Guillot M, Chalaz J, Tanguy A, Bourges M, Verge J, Garret, Deubelle A (1980) 63° Congrès de l'Association des Anatomies, Eléments de biomécanique du rachis 27–31 May. Bloc-Santé, Clermont Ferrand. pp 329–391

Verbiest H (1983) Tumors involving the cervical spine. Benign tumors. In: Cervical Spine Research Society (ed) The cervical spine. Lippincott, Philadelphia, pp 430–477

Waltz T A (1967) Physical factors in the production of the myelopathy of cervical spondylosis. Brain 90:395–404

White A, Southwick W O, Panjabi M (1976) Clinical instability of the lower cervical spine. Spine 1:15–27

Yu YL, Jones S J (1985) Somatosensory evoked potentials in cervical spondylosi: correlation of median, ulnar and posterior tibial nerve responses with clinical and radiological findings. Brain 108:273–300

CHAPTER 3

Anatomy and Anatomical Pathology

J. C. DOSDAT and E. DENARO

The definition and the description of stenosis has shown how the principal causes of the narrowing of the vertebral canal produce a discrepancy in volume between canal and cord which results from the combined effects of both pathological and morphological changes in the anatomical structure of the canal. At this point, it is important to review the various components of the vertebral canal since it is through knowledge of the anatomy that the various forms of cervical stenosis can best be understood (Fig. 3.1). What is proposed is not a discussion of the basic anatomy of the structures that constitute the canal, since this can be found in the classical anatomy textbooks. A review of the anatomy of the cervical canal will be provided by specifically discussing the individual constituents that participate in the pathogenesis through the complex interrelationships with the neurological structures and with particular reference to the vascular components. In order to arrive at the surgical indications and the surgical approaches to be utilized in the decompression of the neurological structures, one must first understand these complex anatomical interrelationships.

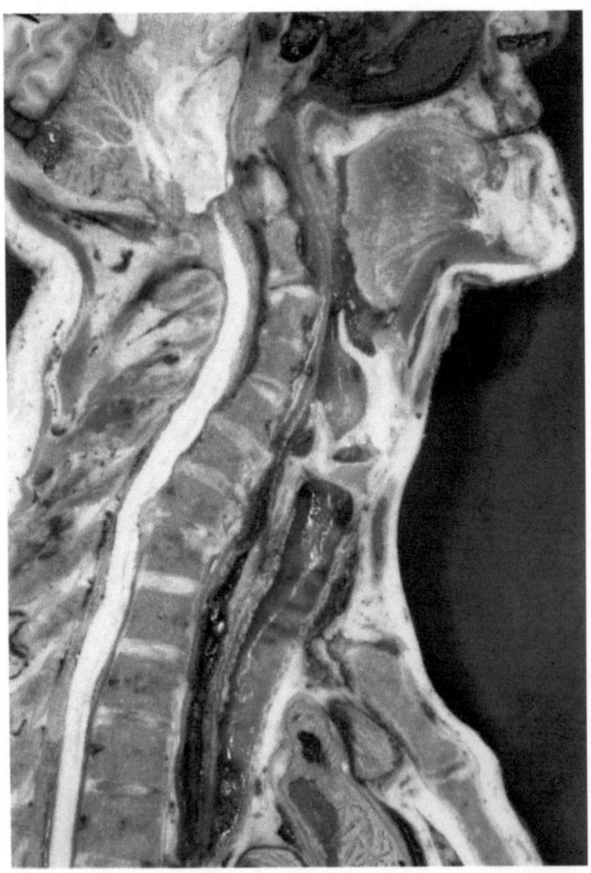

Fig. 3.1. Sagittal midline section through head and neck to show normal structure and anatomy. Note the protrusion of C6–C7 – a common anatomical finding in mature adults which is not of clinical relevance

The Cervical Vertebral Canal

The cervical vertebral canal, like all the spinal segments, is formed by the stacking of the vertebral canals. They are held together into a functional and structural unit by ligamentous and capsular tissues. The diameter of the canal so formed will differ at different levels for it is composed of a total of seven cervical vertebrae with variable anatomical configuration.

Overall, the cervical canal has a triangular outline; the anterior portion is the widest and forms the base along the posterior wall of the vertebral bodies. The anterior wall also includes the interconnecting fibroligamentous structures such as the posterior longitudinal ligament and the posterior margin of the intervertebral disk (Fig. 3.2). The lateral walls are constructed from the vertebral laminae and the powerful ligamentum flavum. The two lateral angles are formed at the anterior margin by the vertebral pedicles. As the vertebrae are stacked one on the other, the pedicles enclose a specific space known as the vertebral canal. The posterolateral wall is formed by the medial side wall of the articular processes. The posterior angle, which is a particularly obtuse angle, is where the laminae join at the midline at the site of the spinous apophysis. The ligamentum flavum binds adjacent vertebrae across the midline of this posterior angle.

In our discussion of the cervical cord, we must remember that there are two sites that are particularly different in their embryologic origins as well as in their structure and function:

- The atlas and the axis (C1 and C2), which form the superior cervical unit
- The remaining five vertebral bodies (C3–C7), which form the lower cervical unit

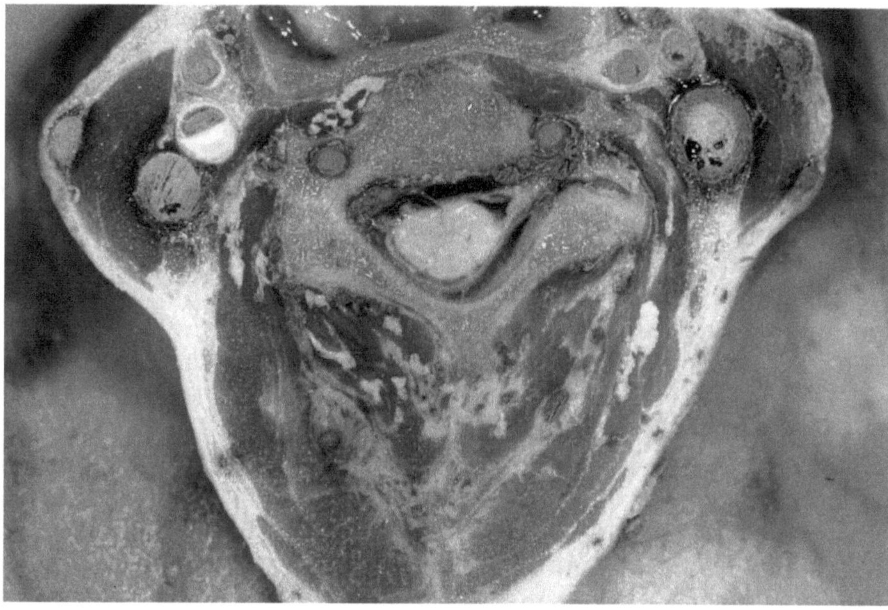

Fig. 3.2. Horizontal transection of neck to show normal interrelationships of bony, ligamentous, neural, and vascular structures (*Top*, anterior aspect; *bottom*, posterior aspect)

The Superior Cervical Unit

At the level of the atlas, the vertebral canal is particularly wide and is shaped like a ring which is anteriorly composed of the anterior arch. The medial surface of the lateral masses protruding from the posterior arch constitute the remaining portion of the ring. This circumferential osseous ring does not define the perimeter of the vertebral canal at this level, however, but is in fact divided into two parts by a thick and wide ligament flattened in the anteroposterior diameter. The ligament is stretched between the two lateral masses on either side of the canal, interfaces on its anterior side with the odontoid process of the axis, and is known as the transverse ligament (Fig. 3.3). At this level, the vertebral canal is divided into two distinct compartments: the anterior portion, which occupies approximately one-third of the area of the canal and which is filled by the odontoid process, and the posterior portion, which occupies approximately two-thirds of the overall area of the canal. It is the posterior portion that actually contains the cord, the epidural spaces, and the intervening spinal fluid. The transverse diameter of this cross-sectional area is greater than that of the lower levels of the cervical spine.

At the level of the axis, the vertebral canal becomes triangular with a wide anterior base. In fact it has a smaller area than the space at the level of the atlas: but this area is, nevertheless, still greater than that of lower cervical vertebrae (Fig. 3.4). The anterior outline corresponds to the posterior wall of the vertebral body of the axis as it rises upward as the posterior surface of the odontoid process. All these surfaces are covered by ligamentous structures, which will be discussed presently (Fig. 3.5). Inferiorly, the body articulates with the inferior cervical unit through the intervertebral disk between C2 and C3. The disk at this level has in part a structure analogous to that of disks at other levels of the vertebral column, but it is, however, characterized on its posterior aspect by an envelope of ligamentous tissue.

The lateral walls of the vertebral canal at the level of the axis are formed by the laminae, which are particularly thick and wide. These are bound superiorly to the posterior portion of the arch of the atlas through a fibrous membrane known as the posterior atlantoaxial ligament. Inferiorly, the laminae are solidly anchored by the first fibers of the ligamentum flavum to the laminae of the lower cervical vertebrae (Fig. 3.4). The lateral angles have very important interrelationships with the adjacent cervical levels. The lateral articulation is a transitional form between the articulation mediated by the atlas with the base of the skull and that of the lower cervical unit. The superior articulating surfaces are in contact with the lateral masses of the atlas and are placed on either side of the odontoid process. The laminae are joined to the body by the isthmus, which at this level is large, thick, and now called the pedicle. These are areas of particular importance in trauma and injury (Fig. 3.4). The joint capsule of the atlantoaxial masses is relatively soft and lax in order to permit a great degree of flexibility at this level. By contrast, the capsule of the posterior articular masses between the axis and C3 is thicker and internally reinforced by large bands of the homologous ligamentum flavum.

The ligamentous structure that is intrinsic to the canal is particularly important and must be discussed in detail. It is a complex structure that is difficult to describe in words. This ligamentous complex covers the anterior portion of the triangular vertebral canal with a deep fibro-osseous unit. The *deep plane* includes layered structures that together form a ligamentous complex reaching from the apex of the odontoid process to the anterior border of the occipital foramen. These layered structures are known as the lateral occipito-odontoid ligaments and are strong, firm bands. They lie in an almost horizontal plane with a frontal direction and for this reason they are also called the alar (wing-like) ligaments. A thinner median bundle is also present and represents an apical component of the alar ligaments (Fig. 3.6). The transverse ligament (described above) is in the posterior plane. It is the thickest and strongest of these ligaments. Anteriorly, it anchors the odontoid process onto the anterior portion of the osseous ring (atlas). Its function is to prevent posterior dislocation under normal function. From its superior margin, there is a supplementary band that reaches to the anterior edge of the occipital foramen. From its inferior edge, however, there is an extension that reaches the posterior aspect of the axis. All these together form the so-called cruciform ligament (Fig. 3.7). The most external division extends from the lateral mass of the atlas to the lateral surface of the body of the axis. It is reinforced by the joint capsule and is also known as Arnold's ligament. The deeper portion joins the lateral margin of the occipital foramen to the same lower insertion, as described above. These two bands are sometimes described as the Y ligament.

The *superficial plane* overlies the previously described ligamentous layers. It is a large fibrous structure extending from the anterior margin of the occipital foramen to the posterior surface of the axis. As it descends towards the axis it narrows forming a fan-like structure. The posterior surface of this layer abuts directly onto the dura mater. In the literature, this fibrous layer, which is quite thick and strong, has also been described as the atlanto-occipital ligament or the tentorial membrane. It is constituted of three bundles: one medial and two lateral. Some authors include in their description a thickening of the posterior longitudinal ligament as it travels along the full length of the vertebral canal, from the occipital foramen and along the posterior aspect of the vertebral body and the intervertebral disk (Fig. 3.8).

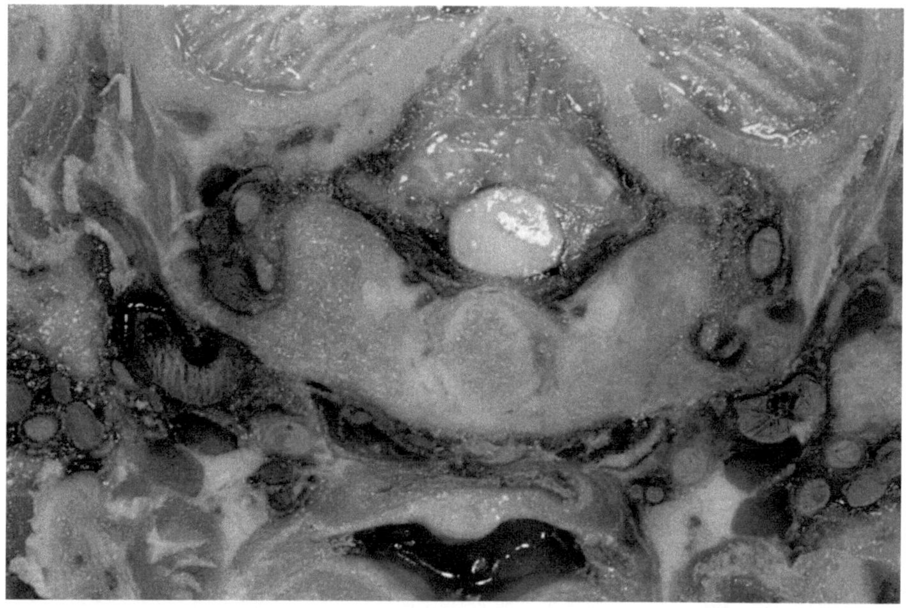

Fig. 3.3. Transverse section of neck at the level of the atlas. Note the transverse ligament between the spinal cord and the odontoid process. This is an oblique plane. The edge of the foramen magnum can be seen at the *top* together with the posterior cranial fossa

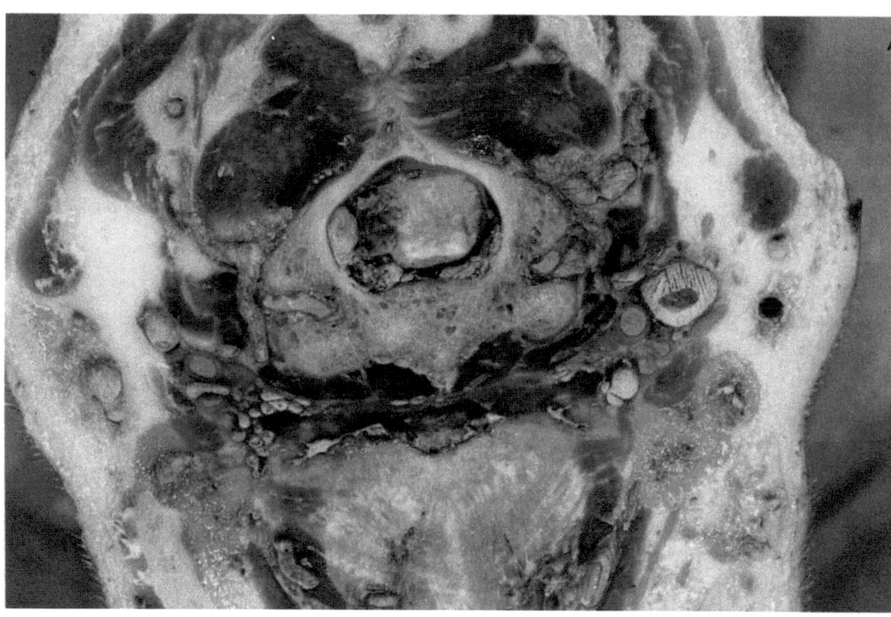

Fig. 3.4. Transverse section at level of axis showing abundant space between the spinal cord and the walls of the vertebral canal

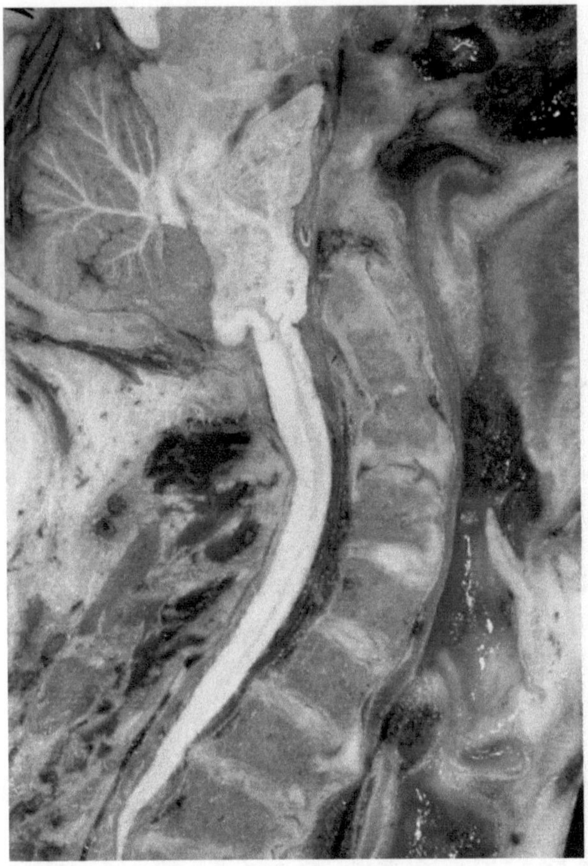

Fig. 3.5. Sagittal midline section through the vertebrae and spinal cord of the neck and the foramen magnum. The cerebellum is at the *top*. Note the decrease in the size of the canal as one proceeds caudad. It is tightest at the C6–C7 levels

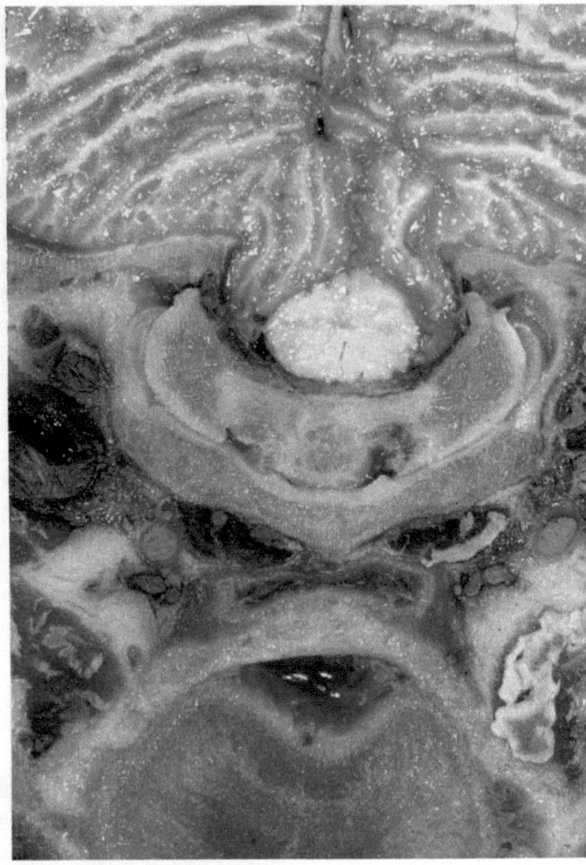

Fig. 3.6. Oblique coronal cross section of neck at the level of the transverse ligament to show its relationship to the odontoid process and the lateral masses of the atlas. The posterior fossa is at the *top* of the figure, together with the cerebellum

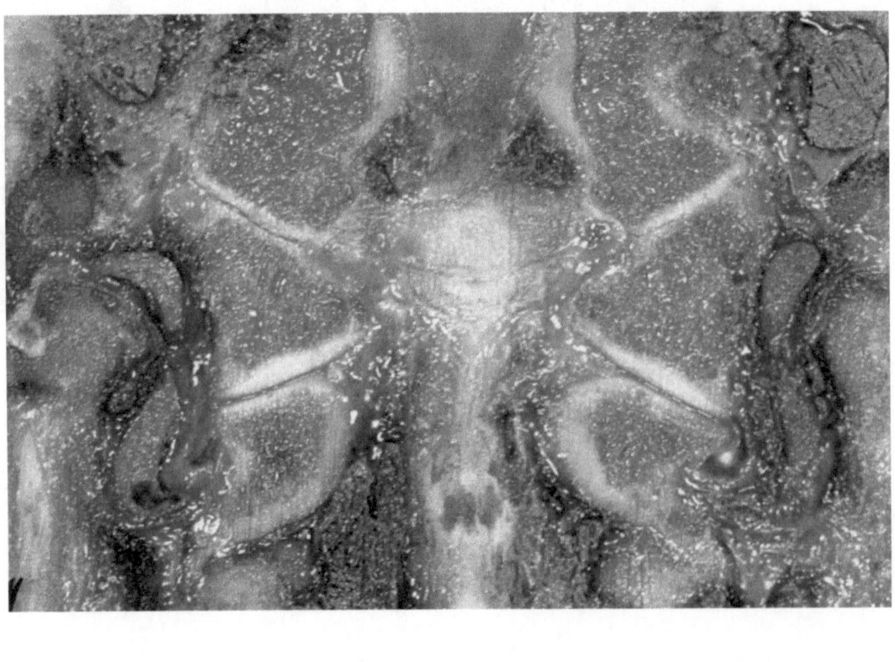

Fig. 3.7. Coronal section anterior to cord showing pattern and extent of cruciform ligament

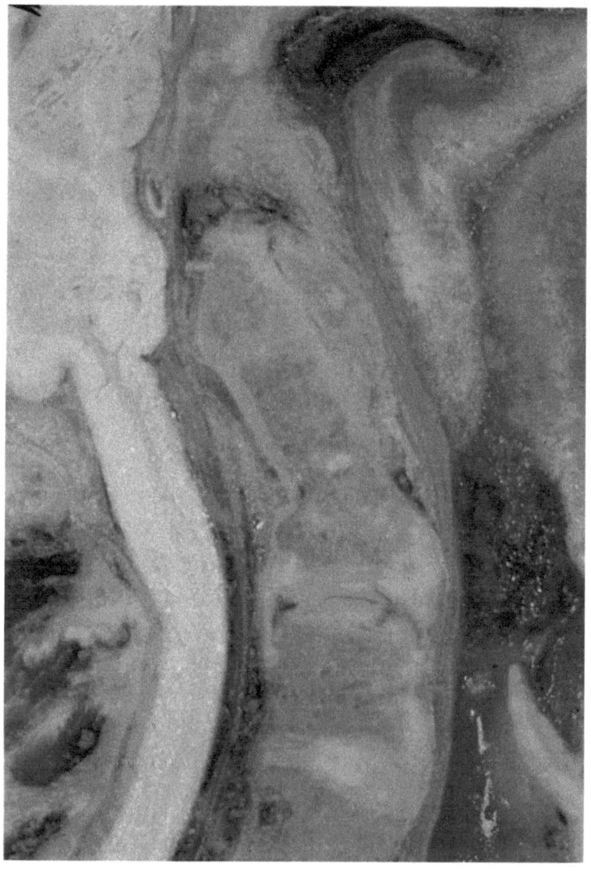

Fig. 3.8. Sagittal section showing the fibrous band that joins the atlanto-occipital ligament lying posterior to the odontoid process between the ligament and the spinal cord

The Inferior Cervical Unit

The structure of the vertebral canal between C3 and C7 is simpler than in the superior cervical unit, and is very similar throughout each of the levels. It is triangular in outline, with the anterior base of the triangle being wider than the two lateral side walls. The posterior surface of the vertebral bodies is covered by the posterior longitudinal ligament; this is a particularly strong continuous ligament. The vertebral bodies are joined by the intervertebral disks. These are all covered by the posterior longitudinal ligament which, at the level of each intervertebral disk, has fibers that interdigitate with the outer margin of the disk (Fig. 3.9). The vertebral pedicles are small and short at this level. By contrast, the joint processes are wide and each overlaps the one below, like the tiles of a roof, thus forming the lateral wall (Figs. 3.10, 3.11). The laminae are thinner than at the level of the axis, but are uniform and symmetrically aligned to each other. They are held together into a functional unit by thick strong ligaments, which are yellow in color, because of the high content of elastic tissue, and which are collectively known as the ligamentum flavum. These ligaments tend to have a rectangular outline. They extend from the anterior surface of the medial portion of the

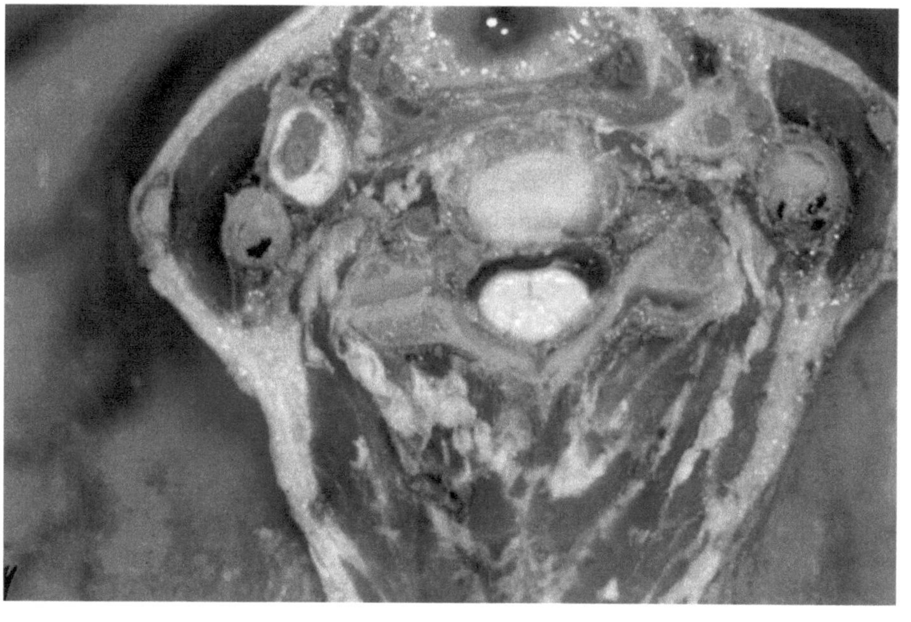

Fig. 3.9. Transverse section of the neck showing the anatomical relationships of the lower cervical spine

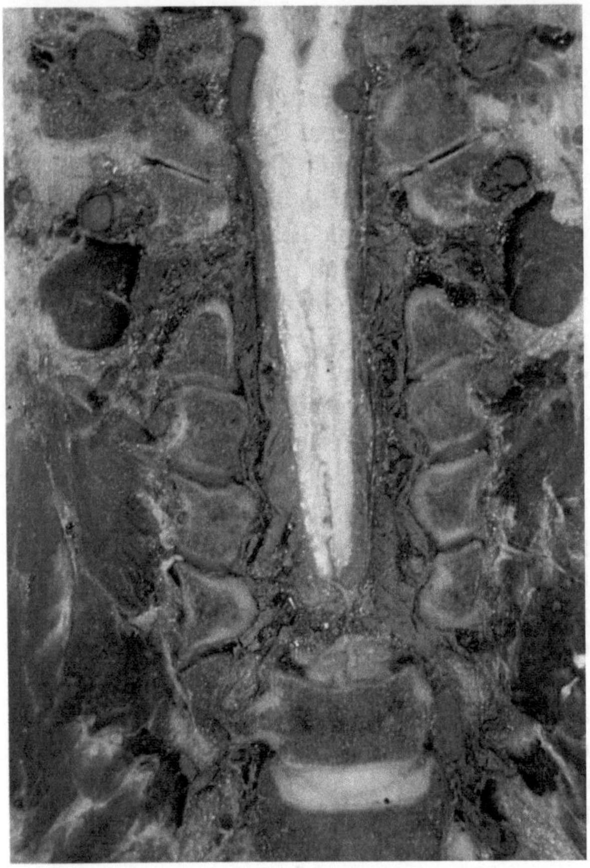

Fig. 3.10. Coronal section of the neck. Note the overlapping of the lateral masses to form the lateral walls of the canal

higher lamina to the superior margin of the lower lamina. The deeper lateral bands of this ligament join and reinforce the joint capsules of the apophseal joints.

In summary, the vertebral canal is formed by a layered structure that includes:

- Osseous elements (the posterior wall of the vertebral body, the pedicles, the joint processes, and the laminae; Fig. 3.12)
- Fibroligamentous elements (intervertebral disk, lateral joints, and ligamentum flavum)

These two elements are generally regarded as responsible for maintaining the stability of the cervical spine and they are divided into two groups; the osseous part is known as the medial vertebral segment, and the fibroligamentous part is known as the neuromobile segment.

The cervical canal has a regular outline (Fig. 3.13). It is wider at its highest level, narrows slightly at the level of the axis, and becomes relatively uniform in size for the length of the remaining inferior portion of the cervical spine. It envelops the cord, to which its configuration is adapted and from which it is separated by the meninges and the cerebrospinal fluid (CSF). Between the meningeal sheath and the fibro-osseous surfaces, there is an epidural space containing the venous plexuses and adipose tissue. Although the appearance of the cervical canal is uniform and fixed anatomically, it is modified during movement of the neck. One cannot ignore the fact that there are anatomical structures which, either through their interrelationships or through pathological changes in the canal, are of particular importance. These include the nerve root canal and the vascular system. In the latter, the vertebral vessels, are of special significance.

The Nerve Root Canal

The root canal opens at the lateral angle of the cervical canal. It is formed between the two overlapping adjacent pedicles, which therefore from the upper and lower margins of the structure. Anteriorly, the margin is formed by the posterolateral edge of the vertebral body below the level of the pedicle and by the adjacent intervertebral disk (Fig. 3.12). The posterior wall is composed of the internal surface of the base of the articulating facets covered by the extension of the ligamentum flavum.

The intervertebral nerve root canal, described above, is a passageway that opens inferiorly, slightly anteriorly, and laterally out of the main spinal canal (Fig. 3.11). In the cervical spine this canal ranges between 6 mm and 8 mm in length and the spinal nerves exit through it. The posterior nerve root first passes through the root ganglion and then fuses with the anterior root to form the exiting spinal nerve. The intervertebral nerve root canal must also encompass the vascular supply. It is apparent that the structures that pass within this intervertebral space are of sufficient volume to completely fill the root canal. Beyond the margin of the canal, the exiting spi-

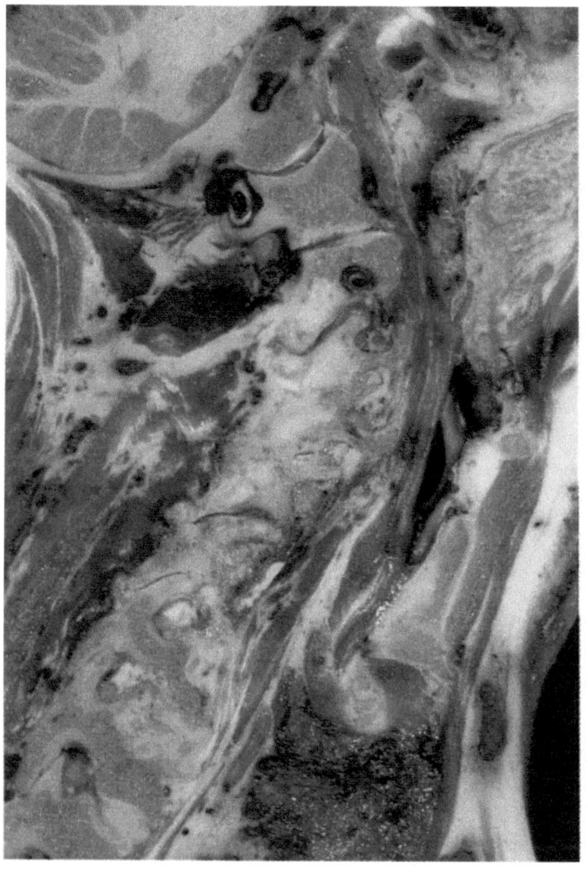

Fig. 3.11. Sagittal section through the neck showing the overlapping pattern of the posterior processes

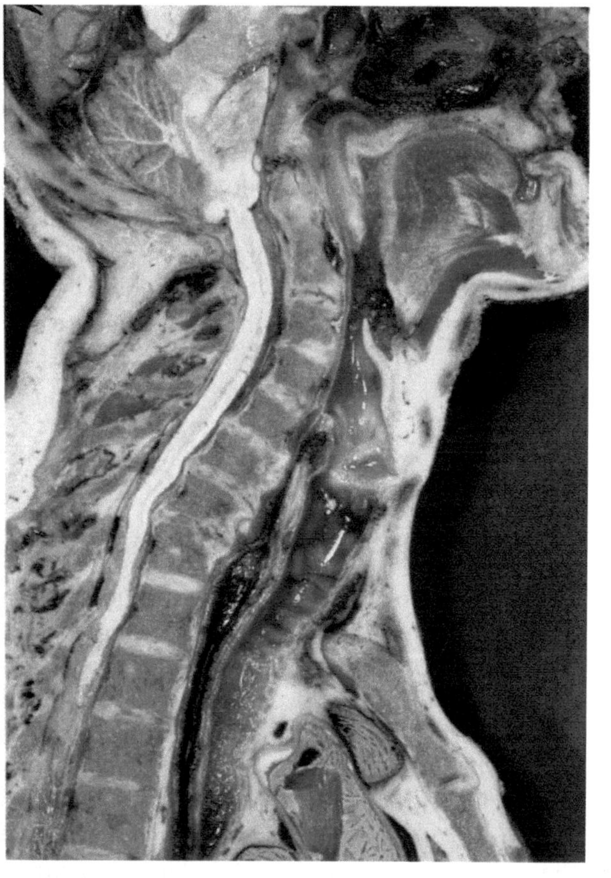

Fig. 3.13. Sagittal section of the head and neck showing the wide canal at the C1 and C2 levels. The canal narrows but remains uniform for the remainder of the cervical spine. Note degenerative changes with osteophytic indentation of the dural space at the lower cervical and at the cervicothoracic levels

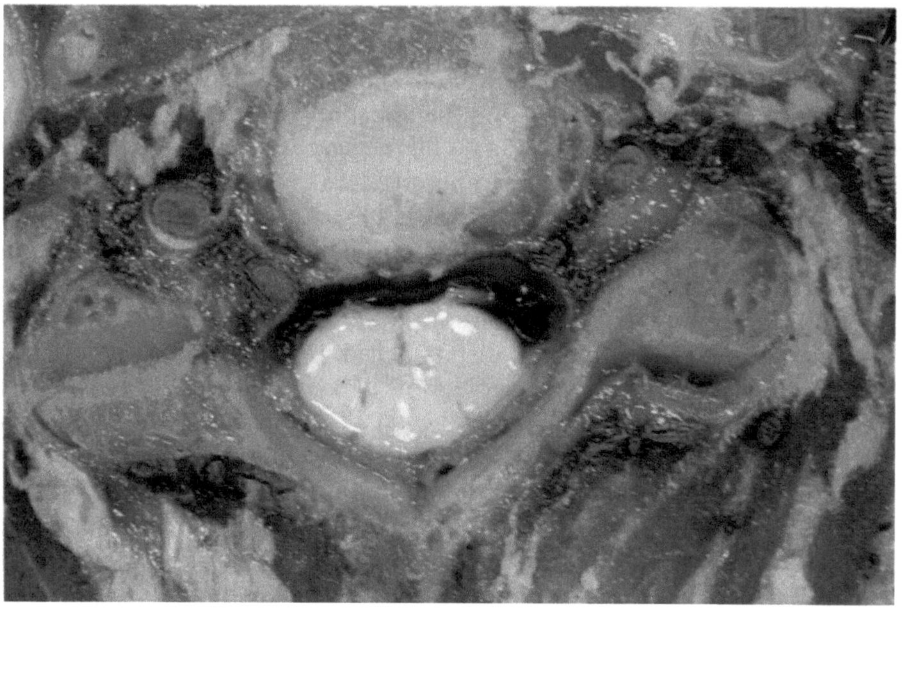

Fig. 3.12. Transverse section showing the osseous constituents of the walls of the vertebral canal.

nal nerve divides into anterior and posterior branches. It is important that the surgeon be able to specifically localize these in the lateral regions. They exit from the cord in a fixed and predictable order and extend within outpouchings of the meninges in between the fibro-osseous units of each vertebral level. The pathway is behind the transverse foramen in association with the vascular bundle which includes the vertebral artery and vein and the perivascular envelope.

The Vascular Supply of the Cervical Spine

The vertebral artery is the first branch of the subclavian artery, arising on its superior surface. Rarely, as a variant of normal, it can arise directly from the aortic arch. Its path is cephalad from its origin to the base of the skull. It travels in a vertical direction between the scalene muscles and the prevertebral muscles. Its path takes it in front of the inferior cervical ganglion and the transverse apophysis of C7. The main carotid artery and the vertebral vein are in front of it at this level. The artery enters the transverse foramen of C6 along with the vertebral sympathetic nerve (Fig. 3.14). It then travels through the intertransverse foramina of all the cervical vertebrae right up to the atlas, where it continues into the occipital foramen above the posterior arch of C1 (Fig. 3.15). The known variants include a lower or a higher entry into the vertebral foramina, ranging from as low as C7 all the way up to C3. As it passes from the transverse foramen of one level to the next, the artery passes between the anterior and posterior small intertransverse muscles. Throughout its path, right up to the axis, the artery is in front of the vertebral vein, from which it must be distinguished. It crosses in front of the cervical nerve roots and is very closely applied to them (Fig. 3.15). The neurovascular bundle that passes through the foramen may adhere to the periosteum and often lies most immediately adjacent to the lateral wall as a result of the elevation produced by the uncus and the uncovertebral joint (Fig. 3.2).

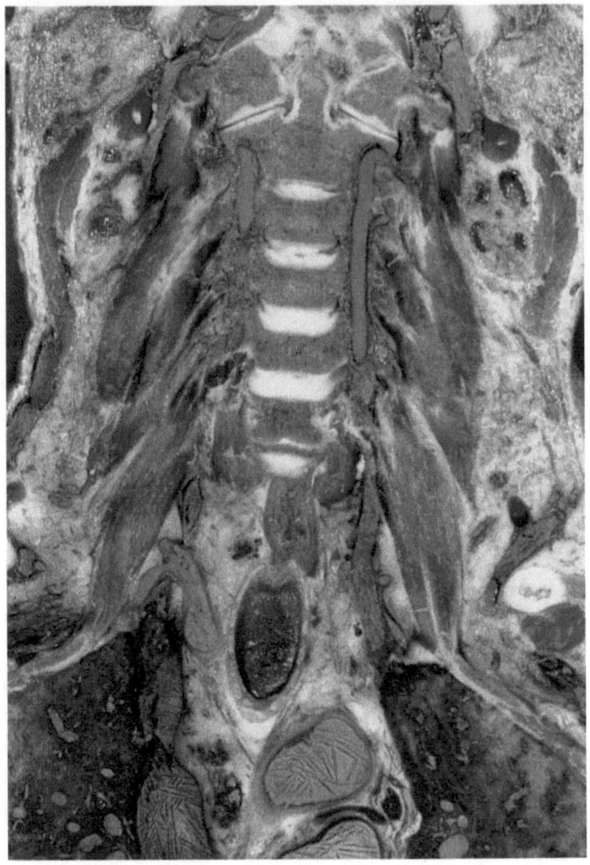

Fig. 3.14. Coronal transection of the neck to show entry of vertebral artery into the transverse foramen of C6 and its further path up the vertebrae that lie more cephalad

It is between the axis and the base of the occiput that the path of the vertebral artery follows an intimate relationship with numerous tissues. The transverse foramen of the atlas is more laterally placed than that of the axis. As a result, the vertebral artery follows a curve, with the concavity being directed anteriorly and outwardly. It then turns towards the occipital foramen in a second more horizontal curve that passes behind the lateral masses of the atlas, producing a depression on the face of the posterior arch. The artery must cross the posterior atlanto-occipital ligament in order to reach the dura mater, which it must also cross (Figs. 3.16–3.19). Its relationship to the vertebrae at this point consists of a close proximity to the pedicle of the axis and then to the lateral and posterior surface of the atlas as it proceeds towards the lateral side of the posterior arch (Fig. 3.4). These anatomical in-

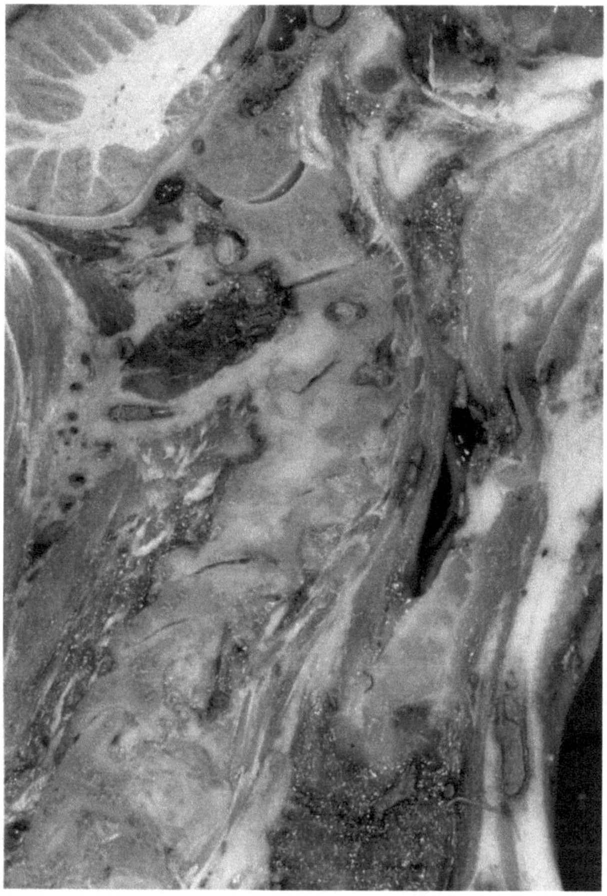

Fig. 3.15. Sagittal transection of the neck showing the path of the vertebral artery in the upper cervical spine. Note the disappearance of the artery at C2 and its reappearance in cross section above the posterior arch of C1

terrelationships must be clearly recognized during surgical dissection. In the classical posterior approach to the posterior arch of the atlas, and in the approach to the lateral processes of the atlas, great care must be taken, regardless of the initial pathway of dissection. In fact, similar care must always be applied in any approach to the transverse foramina at all levels in the cervical spine.

The size of the vertebral arteries is very variable from patient to patient, and frequently there is dominance of one side over the other with regard to the actual blood flow. These arteries pass beside the spinal collaterals at each level as they penetrate the spinal canal through the root canal. These divide into three branches upon passing through the canal: the anterior and posterior branches, which supply the canal itself, and an intramedullary branch, which divides to forms the anterior and posterior radicular arteries, which in turn form the anterior spinal arterial network and the posterolateral arteries, respectively. The radicular arteries have a variable distribution, with some segments being supplied by one radicular artery alone. In addition, there is a complex network of blood supply to the canal, the spinal cord, and the muscles together with all the tissues that surround the column. These include the ascending cervical artery, the deep cervical artery, and the first intercostal arteries.

Venous drainage is achieved by an abundant anastomosis between the subdural and extradural venous plexuses. The intradural venous plexuses form four longitudinal chains that intercommunicate through transverse vessels. These venous chains are placed two on each side, and lie in front of and behind the openings of the spinal root canal. These receive tributaries from the vertebral bodies and from the posterior elements. Through radicular plexuses, they become co-ordinated and form the vertebral veins. The posterior and anterior extradural plexuses then join with the plexus from the root canal to form the principal spinal venous supply.

The posterior extradural plexuses are particularly well developed at the level of the upper cervical cord, where they constitute the occipitovertebral anastomosis. This vascular drainage is of particular importance during surgery. It has a rich anastomotic network with the intradural plexus, the meningeal sinuses, and the subcutaneous vessels. These are the vessels that form the vertebral channels and the posterior jugular veins. It must be remembered that the vertebral venous channels descend in association with the vertebral artery, passing through the root canal of the first six cervical vertebrae. Once this plexus has become the vertebral vein, it can be located on the external surface of the artery. However, on occasion the plexus continues to envelop the artery in an encircling net. Below the sixth root canal, these vessels take on a position more anterior to the artery in order to drain into the brachiocephalic venous trunk, which also receives the spinal veins, the ascending cervical vein, and the deep cervical vein.

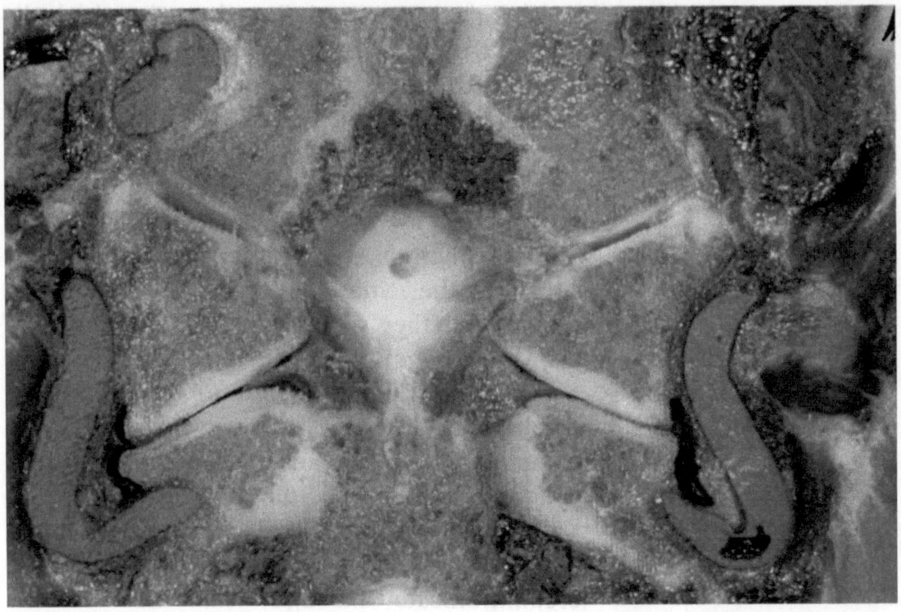

Fig. 3.16. Coronal cross section at the level of C2 (*bottom*) and C1. Note loop of vertebral artery as it exits C2 to proceed around the arch of C1 on its way cephalad to reach the dura mater

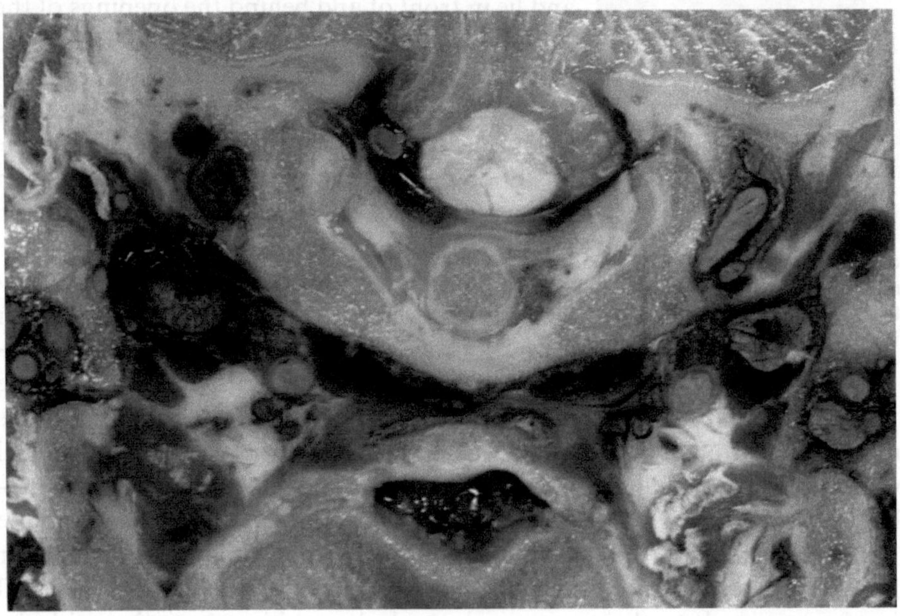

Fig. 3.17. Transverse cross section of neck showing vertebral artery now anterior and posterior to the arch of C1

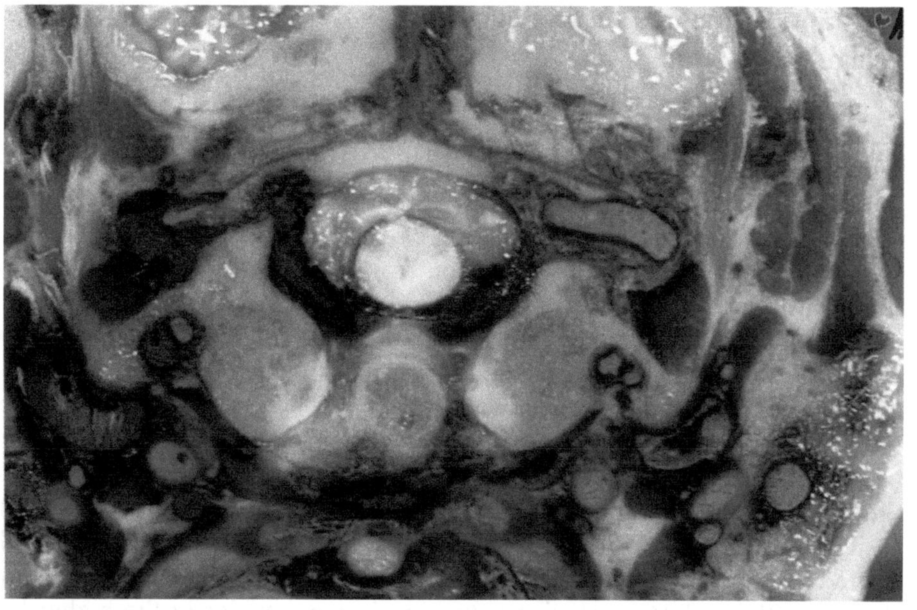

Fig. 3.18. Transverse section of the neck at a level above that shown in Fig. 3.17. Here the vertebral arteries are penetrating the dura mater to proceed into the posterior fossa of the skull

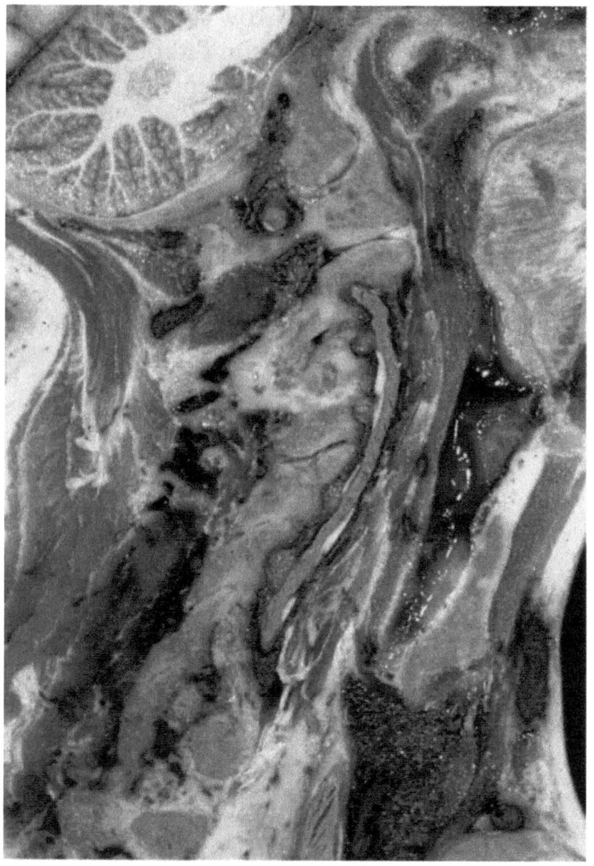

Fig. 3.19. Sagittal transection through the lateral wall of the spinal canal

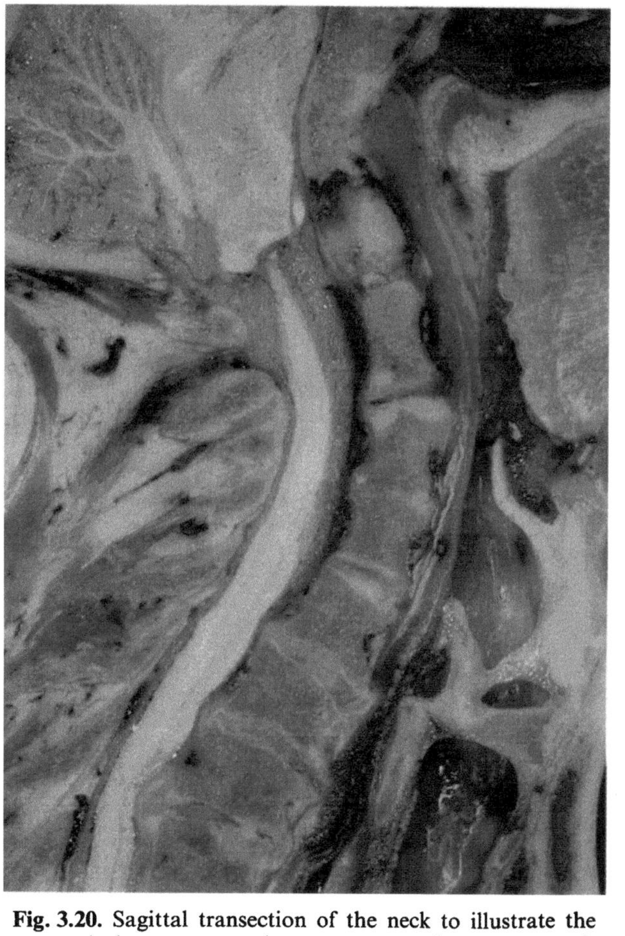

Fig. 3.20. Sagittal transection of the neck to illustrate the anatomical components that are structured so as to permit the laminae (*on the left*) to separate on flexion (limited by the ligamentum flavum at each level)

Dynamic Changes in the Cervical Vertebral Canal

The presence of a fibroligamentous structure between the vertebrae permits changes in the canal during movement of the neck. The width of the canal changes with the flexion and extension movement of the neck. The transition from extension to flexion produces a lengthening of the anterior wall of the canal by between 1.5 cm and 2 cm. This movement involves the intervertebral disk at each level. The posterior wall of the canal stretches even further and can be elongated by as much as 5 cm, as the laminae separate and the ligamentum flavum stretches (Fig. 3.20).

The useable space within the canal is also affected by movement: in flexion it can increase by between 9% and 16%; during extension it can decrease from 11% to 17% (this results from the approximation of adjacent laminae to each other, the bulging of the ligamentum flavum from the posterior surface, and the bulging of the intervertebral disk in front). The spinal cord easily adapts to these changes, undergoing an elastic elongation and contraction during flexion and extension. These mechanisms of change in the canal during flexion and extension could not be demonstrated in a practical and reliable way until very recently when MRI was introduced.

Pathological Anatomy

Verbiest defined stenosis of the vertebral canal as a pathological state resulting from a change in the normal relationship between the walls of the canal and the spinal cord contained therein. In the literature, there has been much discussion of the methods of measurement of the size of the canal. Measurements performed in the sagittal plane with an X-ray taken at 1.83 cm indicate that the anteroposterior diameter is taken to be 13 mm; anything below this value is regarded as a significant narrowing of the canal. In addition, the size of the canal can be measured directly using tomodensitometry. A cut at the pedicles shows that the normal size of the anteroposterior diameter is 14 mm or greater. The canal is wider in the higher levels, and typically a canal that is less than 10 or 11 mm in diameter is classified as a congenitally narrow canal. The significance of smaller diameters in establishing a diagnosis of cervical spinal stenosis has been discussed in previous chapters.

CHAPTER 4

Biomechanics of Spondylotic Cervical Myelopathy

M. M. PANJABI and A. WHITE III

Introduction

Spondylotic cervical myelopahty (SCM) is caused by a compromised spinal canal, leaving less than the necessary space for the cord to function. A certain minimum space is needed, both in neutral position and during physiological movements of the spine, for proper function of the spinal cord. The compromise in the spinal canal size may be partially developmental or primarily due to disk degeneration and osteophytic formations. A narrowed spinal canal may produce mechanical pressure on the spinal cord at one or more levels. The pressure may cause direct neurological damage or produce ischemic changes secondary to canal compromise, which in turn may lead to spinal dysfunction. Physiological movements of the spinal column may further reduce the functional size of the canal. In *extension* of the spinal column, the canal length decreases, thus increasing the cord's cross-sectional area. This is a manifestation of the Poisson's effect, defined as an increase in the cross-sectional area and a decrease in length, whereby the total volume remains the same. In addition, the cord is compressed by posterior protrusion of the annulus fibrosus and buckling of the ligamentum flavum. Another mechanism is active during *flexion* of the spine when the cord tends to stretch. It may be further stretched over an osteophytic spur, producing local compression and bending. In addition, the stretching of the spinal cord may directly reduce its cross-sectional area, in accordance with the principles of elasticity (Poisson's effect).

Although there have been extensive reports on the clinical aspects of SCM, there are relatively few experimental studies in which the effects of chronic compression have been studied. In these animal models, the output of the experiments is monitored by recording electrical potentials, histology of the cord, and sometimes motor dysfunction. Biomechanical aspects are seldom studied. Biomechanical research into the behavior of the spinal cord and nerve roots under loads was pioneered by Alf Brieg. Besides the original research in which he used fresh human cadavers and studied the movements of the cord and nerve roots, he wrote two books detailing his work and ideas concerning the biomechanical effects on the nervous system (Brieg 1960, 1978). Bohlman et al. (1981) conducted experiments using a canine model in which controlled pressures were applied to the spinal cord over a set of time intervals and the functional output of the spinal cord over time was monitored. Unfortunately, the pressures applied to the cord were not quantified. Raynor and Koplik (1985) published a biomechanical analysis of trauma of the spinal cord. They hypothesized that it is the shear stress in the spinal cord, produced by anterior or posterior compression, that results in spinal cord dysfunction. This conceptual engineering analysis correlated nicely with the findings observed clinically and experimentally by Schneider et al. (1955, 1958). Finally, in a series of three papers Tencer and his colleagues presented in vitro experimental results concerning the pressure applied to the spinal cord due to various changes in the spinal column by simulating spinal deformity, canal occlusion, functional postures, and surgical procedures (Tencer et al. (1985a, b, c). These papers have produced reliable, clinically relevant and biomechanically useful data using modern techniques.

This presentation has two purposes: to describe the above-mentioned biomechanics literature in some detail; and, to present a new qualitative biomechanical analysis of stress patterns in the spinal cord relevant to SCM.

Biomechanics of the Spinal Cord and Canal

It is important to analyze the normal functioning of the spinal cord and spinal column before attempting to understand the biomechanics of the pathological conditions of the spinal cord. Brieg (1960, 1978) pioneered this type of research in a series of experiments. He used fresh whole cadavers, appropriately prepared so that the movements and deformations of the spinal cord and the nerve roots could be directly visualized. The movements of the cord were quantified by marking the cord and recording the displacement of the marks. Physiological movements of the spinal column were produced by bending the

spine at different regions and in different planes. Several important findings have come out of these studies. Brieg's work showed that the spinal canal length changes are accompanied by spinal cord length changes without producing any significant stresses in the spinal cord. The mechanism is that of unfolding and folding of the spinal cord, much like an accordion (Fig. 4.1). In *flexion*, the spinal canal increases in length as the centers of rotation of vertebrae are anterior to the canal. There is stretching of the ligamentum flavum. In *extension*, the spinal canal decreases in length. The disk protrudes posteriorly into the canal (Brown et al. 1975), while the ligamentum flavum protrudes anteriorly (Penning 1968). Lesser changes take place during lateral bending and axial rotation. In normal anatomy, these physiological movements of the spinal column do not produce any abnormal stresses and strains in the nerve tissue. In pathological situations, however, such as hypertrophy of the ligament flavum, abnormal disk bulge, osteophytic formations, ossification of posterior longitudinal ligament, and congenital narrow spinal canal, these same functional changes may result in abnormal stresses and strains in the spinal cord leading to neurological problems (Fig. 4.2).

A bulging disk, a hypertrophic ligamentum flavum, and an osteophyte all apply direct compressive forces to the spinal cord in the transverse plane. This results in specific and well-defined stress patterns in the spinal cord. Although the stress patterns are three-dimensional and extremely complex, a simplified biomechanical analysis is still helpful. Raynor and Koplik (1985) conceptualized such a situation in biomechanical terms and provided a qualitative analysis of the stress patterns in the spinal cord caused by direct anterior-posterior compression applied in the transverse plane. Engineering analysis of long structures with elliptical cross sections shows that when a transverse force, also called shear force, is applied to the structure on its flat side, it results in well-defined stress patterns in the structure (stress is defined as force per unit area). These stresses are of the shear type and have a certain distribution in the cross-section: maximum value in the center and along the periphery. Raynor and Koplik (1985) applied this concept to the spinal cord. They argued that the stresses produced in the spinal cord by the application of transverse force adequately explain the neurological dysfunction seen during trauma in which the central areas of the spinal cord are preferentially damaged compared with the peripheral areas. Although the analysis was conducted for trauma of the spinal cord, the results are equally valid for the application of a chronic transverse compressive force, e.g., due to an osteophyte. This subject will be discussed in the next section.

Biomechanics can be helpful in answering several questions of practical and clinical importance concerning the treatment of myelopathy. In a series of experiments, Tencer et al. (1985a, b, c) used fresh cadaveric spines, from occiput to sacrum and including the spinal cord and dura mater. Although the spinal cord and dura mater were severed at the occiput level, the system was sutured closed and pressurized to provide normal cerebrospinal fluid (CSF) pressure. The basic set-up consisted of a specially constructed transverse load applicator and displacement measurement transducer designed respectively to apply force to the spinal cord and continuously monitor the displacement of the anterior and posterior walls of the dura mater. They studied the effects on the spinal cord of several procedures on the spinal column, e.g., flexion angulation, shortening, distraction, laminectomy. One of the interesting results of their study is shown in Fig. 4.3a. The horizontal axis represents the canal occlusion, defined as the ratio of the canal intrusion (by the load applicator) to the canal diameter. On the vertical axis is shown the compression applied. We see that the behavior is nonlinear, i.e., *with increasing* occlusion there is a relatively *greater* increase in the load. Simulating a kyphotic deformity by removing a 75% anterior body wedge or doing a laminectomy did not alter the force-occlusion graph. Shown in Fig. 4.3b is the displacement of the posterior wall of the dura mater as a function of the displacement of the anterior wall of the dura mater. Notice that the posterior wall hardly moves when the anterior wall has been displaced up to 6, 8, or even 10 mm. This supports the

clinical view that the anterior impingement does not significantly affect the posterior wall of the dura mater. Put differently, this implies that posterior decompression, e.g., laminectomy, will have little effect in decreasing the anterior pressure on the cord.

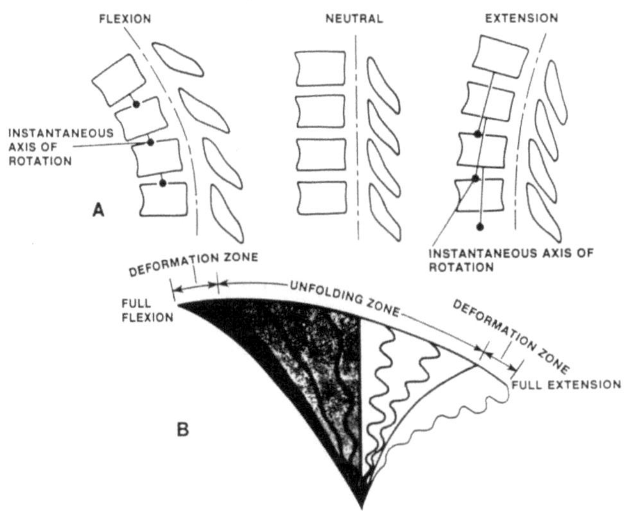

Fig. 4.1 a, b. The spinal canal and cord in flexion and extension. **a** In flexion, the length of the spinal canal increases, compared with its length in neutral position. In extension, the length of the spinal canal decreases. This phenomenon is due to the location of the instantaneous axis of rotation anterior to the spinal canal. **b** The spinal cord is required to follow the changes in length of the spinal canal during physiological motions. This is done through the mechanisms of unfolding/folding and elastic deformation. (Based upon experimental findings of Brieg 1960)

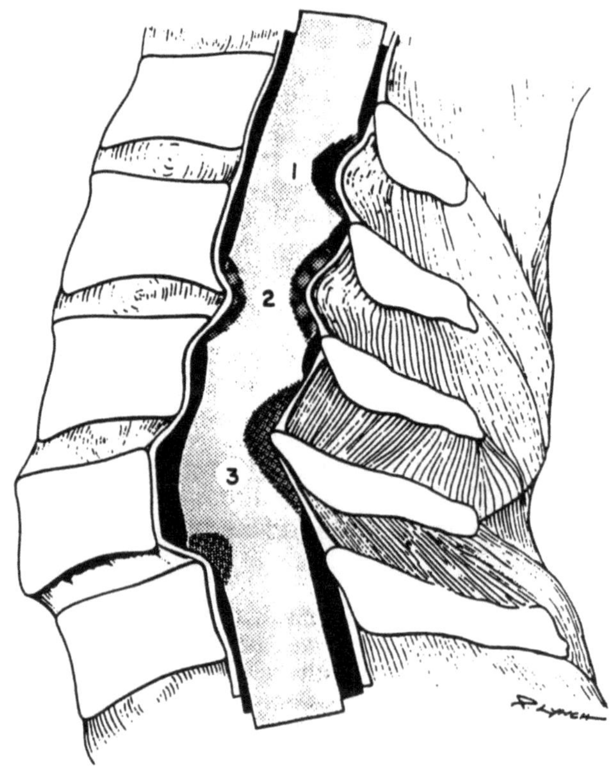

Fig. 4.2. In pathological situations, well-coordinated physiological movements of the spinal canal and the spinal cord may be disturbed, resulting in abnormal stresses and strains in the spinal cord which may lead to neurological problems

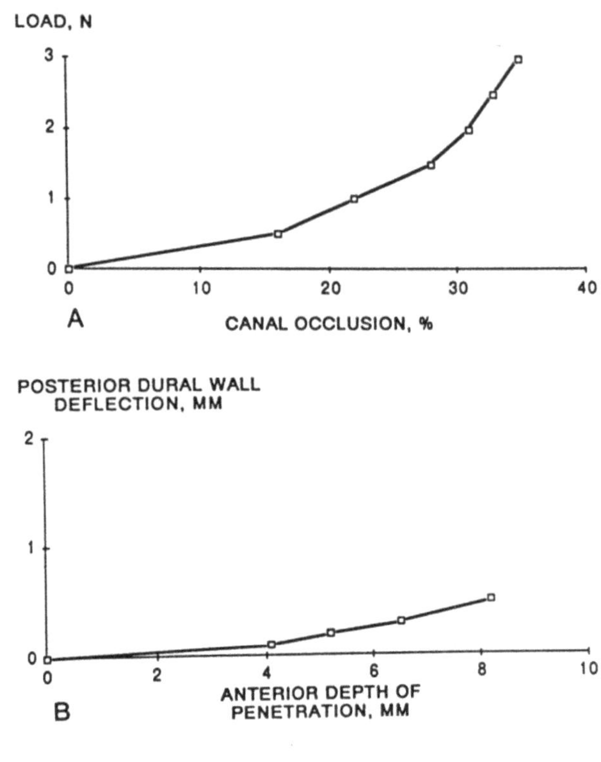

Fig. 4.3. a The relationship between the compression load ▶ applied and the occlusion of the canal. **b** The relationship between the deflection of the posterior wall of the dura mater and the penetration of the spinal canal from the anterior. These results are based upon an experimental study by Tencer et al. (1985a, b, c)

A Qualitative Biomechanical Analysis of Stresses in the Spinal Cord

The purpose of this simple analysis of a complex phenomenon is to look at the qualitative analysis of stress patterns generated in the spinal cord due to a clinically relevant situation, e.g., an impingement of the cord from the anterior, resulting in compression, stretching, and bending of the cord (Fig. 4.4). The analysis builds on the earlier work of Brieg (1960, 1978) and Raynor and Koplik (1985). For our biomechanical analysis, we consider the spinal cord to be a long structure made of a homogeneous material and with an elliptical cross section. Although the term "stress" has been used here throughout, the term "strain" (percentage change in length) is equally valid; because of the qualitative nature of the analysis, both the terms are equivalent. Figure 4.4 depicts a situation which may be seen biomechanically as consisting of three simple loads applied simultaneously to the cord. The loads are the compression load applied by osteophytic impingement, the tensile load due to flexion of the spine, and the bending load due to the change in the direction of the spinal cord over the impingement. We will analyze the stress patterns due to each of the three loads separately and then combine the results. "This implicitly assumes that the system is linear and, therefore, the principle of superposition is vallid."

The first of the three loads considered is the direct compression (impingement) applied on the anterior surface of the cord. This force produces local compressive stresses which decrease in magnitude away from the point of contact (Fig. 4.5a). In addition, such a compression load produces shear stresses that have a zero value at the point of load application, increase towards the middle, and are maximum in the center of the spinal cord (Fig. 4.5b). The compressive and shear stress patterns depicted are in the form of isostress contours, i.e., each contour represents a single constant stress value. This convention is used throughout (Figs. 4.5–4.7). The second load studied is the tensile (tension) load. The tensile load applied to a long structure produces uniform tensile stress across the cross section (Fig. 4.6a). The third load is the bending of the cord over the impingement. When a long structure is bent, differential stresses are produced across the bent cross section. On the concave side of the bent structure compressive stresses develop, while on the convex side there are tensile stresses (Fig. 4.6b). The magnitude of both of these stresses is highest on the outer surface of the structure. The stresses decrease towards the center and reach a zero value in the middle of the structure. The posterior region of the spinal cord is loaded in both tension and compression (also called neutral plane). The tensile forces are exerted in flexion and the compression forces, from invagination of the ligamentum flavum, are exerted during extension. These biomechanical factors may account for the clinical observation of a predominance of posterior spinal cord dysfunction involved in patients with SCM.

The effects of all the three loads acting on the spinal cord may now be combined. This simulates a realistic situation in which, for example, an osteophyte impinges on the spinal cord while the spinal column is flexed, resulting in combined compression, stretching, and bending of the spinal cord. The resulting stress patterns for this situation may be obtained by summation of the stress patterns shown in Figs. 4.5, and 4.6. The compressive and tensile stresses are both normal stresses (i.e., perpendicular to the cross section of the structure) but are opposite in nature (sign). They may be added together to provide a combined distribution of the normal stresses. The resulting stress pattern for the normal stresses is seen in Fig. 4.7a. Starting from the anterior, high compressive stresses decrease towards the center of the cord. A little beyond the center of the cord, the stresses may be nearly zero. Continuing towards the posterior, the stresses again increase, but are now tensile in nature. It may be emphasized that this analysis is only qualitative and, therefore, precise location of the point where the stresses are zero may vary. In addition, there are the shear stresses (Fig. 4.7b; originally shown in Fig. 4.5b), which are maximum in the center of the cross section and decrease towards the periphery. It is interesting to note that the maximum shear stresses occur in the region where the central venulae are

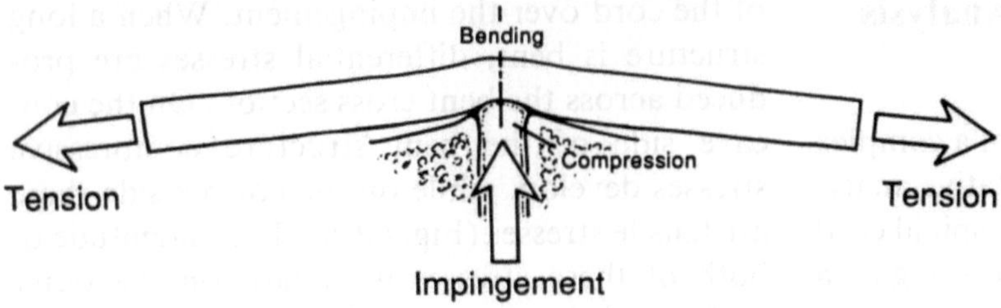

Fig. 4.4. Impingement of the spinal cord from the anterior results in compression, stretching (tension), and bending of the spinal cord

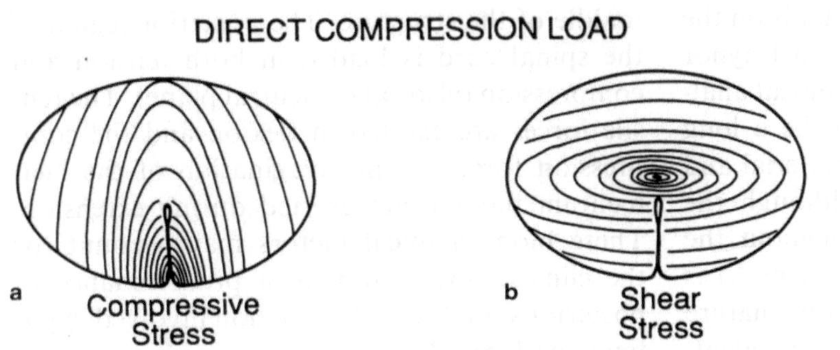

Fig. 4.5. a Direct compression force applied from the anterior produces local compressive stresses which decrease in magnitude away from the point of contact. b In addition, anterior compression also produces shear stresses in the cord that have the maximum value in the center of the cord

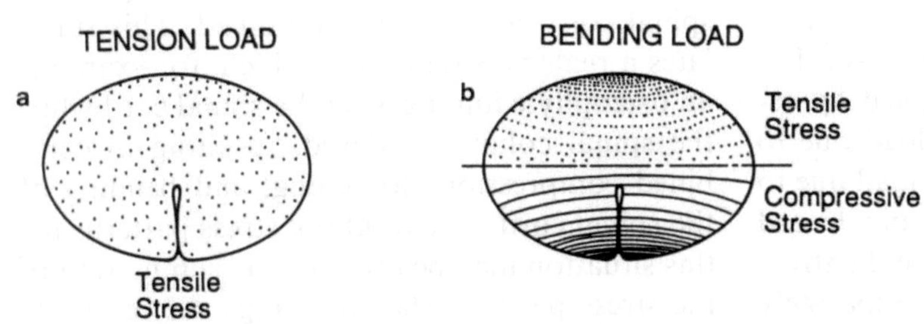

Fig. 4.6. a Tension load applied to the cord produces uniform tensile stresses in the entire cross section of the cord. b Bending of the spinal cord produces compressive stresses on the concave side and tensile stresses on the convex side of the bent spinal cord

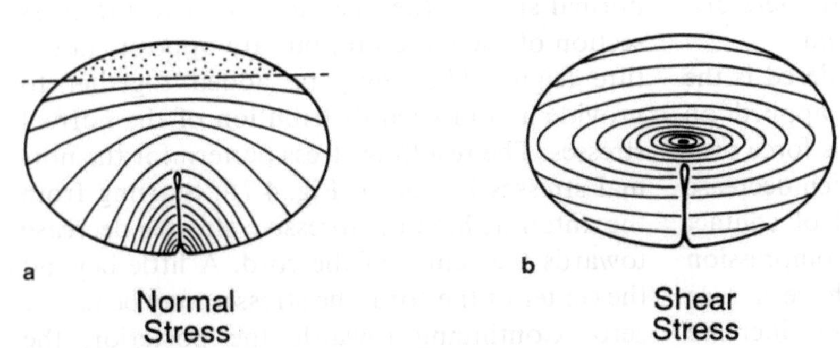

Fig. 4.7 a, b. The stresses due to the combined loads of compression, tension, and bending. a Normal stresses, i.e., stresses that are in the same direction as the length of the spinal cord, are compressive on the anterior side and tensile on the posterior side. b The shear stresses have a maximum value in the middle of the spinal cord and near zero values on the anterior and posterior surfaces of the cord

located. These venulae are thought to be the structures in the spinal cord least resistant to mechanical damage (Dohrmann 1972).

Discussion

A better understanding of SCM can be achieved by using the concepts of biomechanics. When external forces are applied to the spinal cord they result in internal stresses and strains. To determine the basis of neurological dysfunction due to the loads applied to the cord, it is necessary to obtain precise relationships between the anatomical structures of the spinal cord (gray and white matter and blood supply) and the stresses produced in these structures. To obtain such relationships two items are necessary: detailed quantitative anatomy of the spinal cord and spinal column; and the specific stress patterns generated in the spinal cord. To determine the second item, it is necessary to know the physical properties of tissues comprising the spinal cord and dura mater, and then develop mathematical models to simulate the spinal cord structures being subjected to normal and abnormal loads. There are several studies providing descriptive anatomy of the spinal cord and spinal column, but there seems to be a complete lack of detailed quantitative anatomy. Concerning the mechanical properties of the spinal cord and duramater there are only a few studies (Brieg 1960; Sunderland 1978; Tencer AF et al. 1985). All of these biomechanical studies have been conducted by applying tensile forces to the spinal cord specimen. We have seen that the stresses produced in the spinal cord are of three types: shear, compressive, and tensile. Therefore, studies should be conducted to determine, in addition to the tensile properties, the shear and compressive properties of the spinal cord. Such data are presently not available. To our knowledge, there are no mathematical models available that could relate the external loads applied to the cord to the internal stresses produced in it. However, it is quite feasible to develop such models using modern techniques of finite elements.

Finally, experiments using animal models are needed to relate the computed stresses in the spinal cord to the neurological dysfunction. Many in vivo experiments have been conducted in which mechanical pressure or certain compression was applied to the cord. However, the mechanical input was seldom quantified in precise biomechanical terms. These experiments, have contributed significantly to our knowledge about the neurological dysfunction caused by compression, but are not suitable for relating the mechanical input to the neurological dysfunction in a precise manner. New experiments must be designed and conducted. Specifically, one should precisely measure (a) the mechanical input, in the form of the magnitude of cord compresssion or pressure, its distribution on the spinal cord and its rate and duration of application, and (b) the quantitative functional output of the animal.

Sometime in the future, it may be possible using biomechanical techniques, to relate specific bony pathology to internal stresses in the cord. The stresses, in their turn, may be related to the neurological dysfunction using the knowledge gained from quantitative animal experiments. Thus, a predictive algorithm may be developed to relate spinal column pathology to neurological dysfunction.

References

Bohlman HH, Bahniuk E, Fields G, Raskulinecz G (1981) Incomplete cervical spinal cord injury. Spine 6:428–436

Brieg A (1960) Biomechanics of the central nervous system. Almquist and Wicksell, Stockholm

Brieg A (1978) Adverse mechanical tension in the central nervous system. Almquist and Wicksell, Stockholm

Brown T, Hanson R, Yorra A (1975) Some mechanical tests on the lumbosacral spine with particular reference to the intervertebral discs. J Bone Joint Surg [Am] 39:1135.

Dohrmann GJ (1972) Experimental cord trauma – a historical review. Arch Neurol 27:467

Penning L (1968) Functional pathology of cervical spine. Excerpta Medica, Amsterdam

Raynor RB, Koplik B (1985) Cervical cord trauma: the relationship between clinical syndromes and force of injury. Spine 10:193–197

Schneider RC (1955) The syndrome of acute anterior spinal cord injury. J. Neurosurg 12:95–122

Schneider RC, Thompson JM, Bebin J (1958) The syndrome of acute central cervical cord injury. J. Neurol Neurosurg Psychiatry 21:216–227

Sunderland S (1978) Nerve and nerve injuries. Livingstone, New York

Tencer AF, Allen BL, Ferguson RL (1985a) A biomechanical study of thoracolumbar spinal fractures with bone in the canal. III. Mechanical properties of the dura and its tethering ligaments. Spine 10:741–747

Tencer AF, Ferguson RL, Allen BL (1985b) A biomechanical study of thoracolumbar spinal fractures with bone in the canal. II. The effect of flexion angulation, distraction, and shortening of the motion segment. Spine 10: 586–589

Tencer A, Allen B, Ferguson RL (1985c) A biomechanical study of thoracolumbar spinal fractures with bone in the canal. I. The effect of laminectomy. Spine 10:580–585

CHAPTER 5

Imaging

In the investigation of myelopathies resulting from stenosis of the cervical spine, after initial and neurological examination, one should undertake electrophysiologic studies (electromyography, somatosensory evoked potential studies) and then proceed to the more definitive assessment provided by the various types of imaging. In the past 10 years, the scope of radiological assessment has been expanded significantly by new diagnostic modalities such as computed tomography, magnetic resonance imaging, and selective arteriography. Individually and in combination these permit more accurate and more complete diagnosis.

This discussion will be limited to the clinically related aspects of these investigations. The reader seeking a deeper knowledge of the technical and radiological aspects of the techniques should refer to the appropriate textbooks. We will attempt to describe what can be derived from the various types of imaging in the way of clinically useful information. Our assessment of the different procedures will be guided by extensive personal experience.

Traditional or Plain Radiography

Conventional radiography provides a significant amount of information that assists diagnostic assessment.

In the *anteroposterior projection*, one can assess the structure of the vertebral bodies, the outlines of the uncovertebral joints, the posterior apophyseal joints, and, to a lesser degree, the laminae and the spinal apophyses. The two last-named overlap the vertebral bodies. The transoral anteroposterior projection (Fig. 9.47a) allows examination of the odontoid process of the axis, the lateral masses of the atlas and the axis, and the atlantoaxial joints.

The *lateral projection* is used to assess the overall architecture of the cervical spine for accentuation, attenuation, or inversion of the physiological lordosis or segmental kyphosis, all features that raise the suspicion of a pathological state.

Assessment of the vertebral bodies and the intervertebral disk spaces on lateral views helps to detect calcification at the anterior or posterior margin of the intervertebral disk where one will usually find osteophytes. The lateral projection also demonstrates posterior interapophyseal joints, the laminae, the spinal processes, and the vertebral pedicles.

In cases of congenitally derived organic stenosis (or in combined stenoses), plain lateral X-rays of the cervical spine provide a good guide to the causes. Figure 5.1 illustrates a simple and quick method to assess the vertebral canal for stenosis. The shape and size of the vertebral body can be clearly appreciated and measured, and one can trace and cut out an exact outline of the vertebral body which can then be placed over the vertebral canal. Under normal conditions the posterior space between the body and the laminae should be sufficient to extend beyond the limits of the vertebral body (as seen from the cut-out): any indication that the body is wider than this posterior canal space is suggestive of stenosis.

Figures 5.2 and 5.3 illustrate additional features of plain radiography. One can identify structural changes such as "short pedicle" or "hypoplastic lamina", that in combination can produce clinically significant spinal stenosis. The same lateral projection demonstrates the topographical relationship of the occiput, C1 and C2, as well as the overall structural interrelationships of the cervical spine, including displacements, indentations of the odontoid process, and structural deformations of the vertebral canal.

Oblique views, both right and left, are essential in the assessment of the root canals and especially of any uncal disease. They are ideal for the assessment of any changes leading to the narrowing of the root canal, and also enable evaluation of the morphology of the pedicles and the apophyseal joints. Their usefulness in the assessment of the cervical vertebral bodies is limited.

Dynamic views of the cervical spine in the lateral projection at rest, in maximal flexion, and in maximal extension are invaluable in assessment of the stability of the cervical spine, especially in functional stenosis resulting from ligamentous deficiencies or osseoligamentous instability (see section on functional stenoses, Chap. 2, and Figs. 9.95, 9.99).

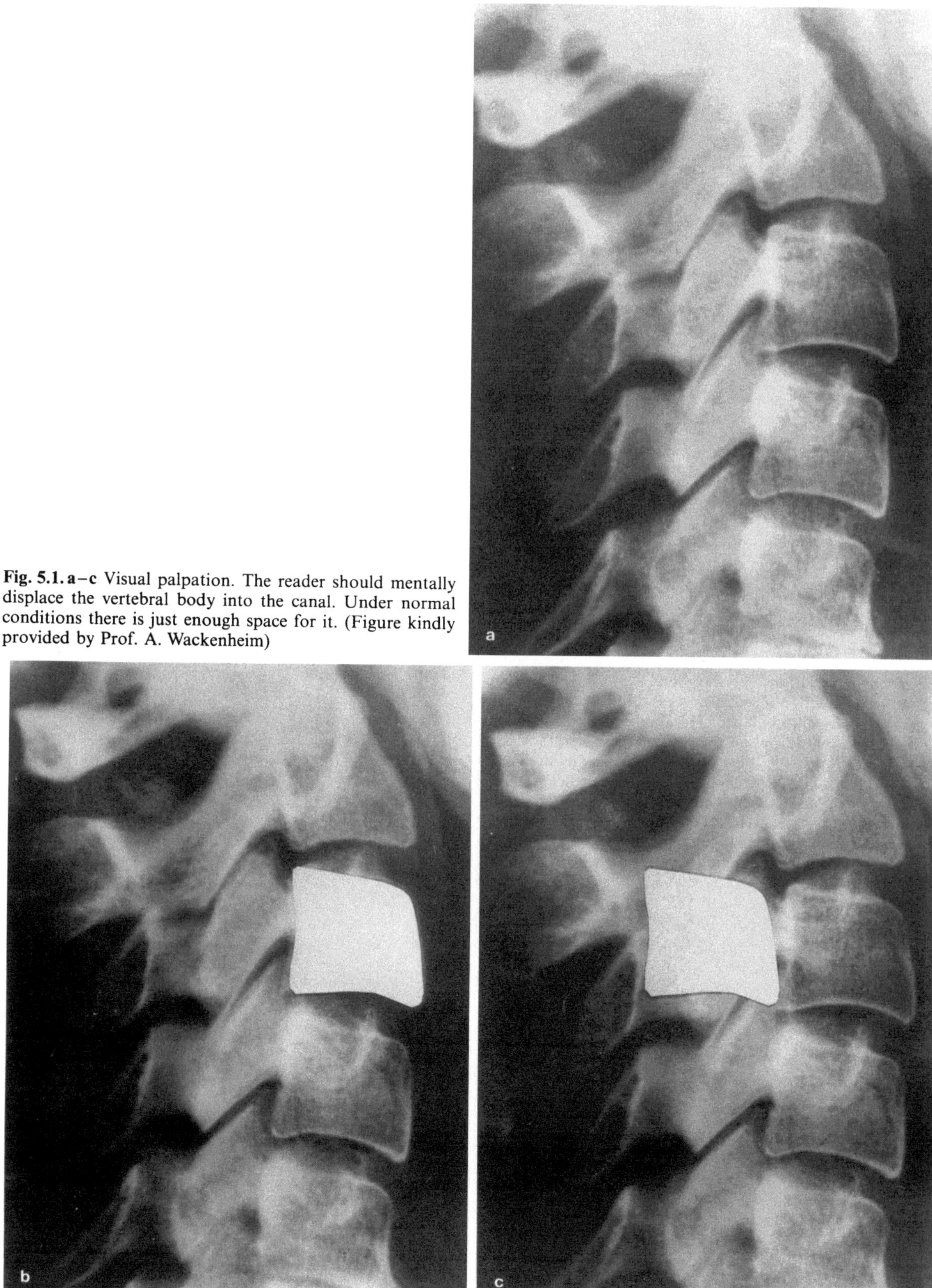

Fig. 5.1. a–c Visual palpation. The reader should mentally displace the vertebral body into the canal. Under normal conditions there is just enough space for it. (Figure kindly provided by Prof. A. Wackenheim)

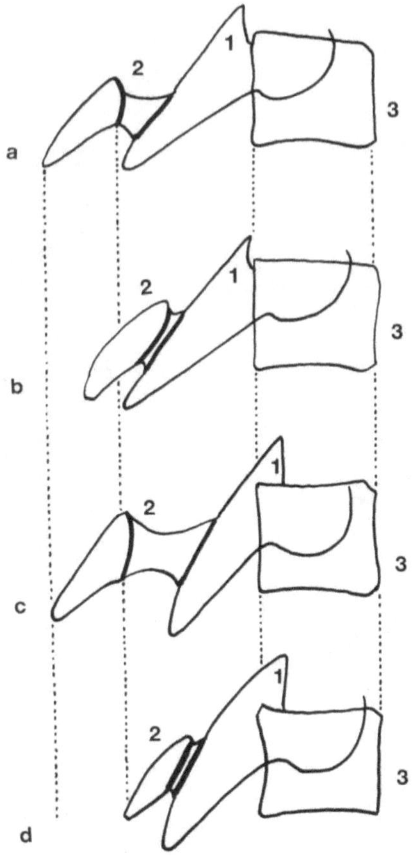

Fig. 5.2 a–d Variations of the cervical canal. **a** Normal conditions: the superior articular process is localized behind the vertebral body (normal pedicle; *1*); the projection of the lamina is normal (*2*); visual palpation demonstrates normal conditions (*3*; see also Fig. 5.10). **b** Hypoplastic lamina (*1*) responsible for canalar stenosis (*2*). **c** Short pedicle (*1*) with anteriorly displaced superior articular process, but without canalar stenosis (*2*). **d** Short pedicle (*1*) with anteriorly displaced superior articular process, short lamina (*2*), and canalar stenosis (*3*). (Figure kindly provided by Prof. A. Wackenheim)

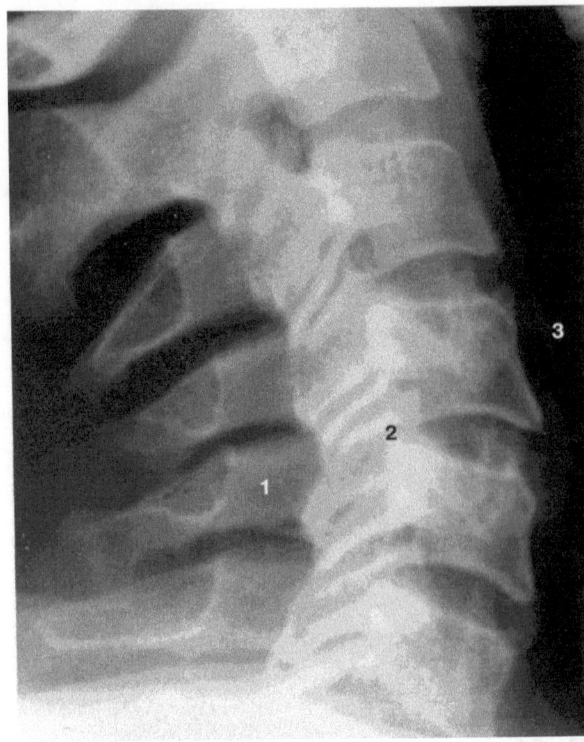

Fig. 5.3. Radiograph of cervical canal which corresponds to Fig. 5.4. The laminae are very long (*1*) so that in spite of the anteriorly displaced articular process (*2*) there is no canalar stenosis (*3*). (Figure kindly provided by Prof. A. Wackenheim)

Computed Tomography

Computed tomography (CT) is one of the essential examinations of the cervical vertebral canal. CT demonstrates to great advantage the structures surrounding the canal, including the laminae, the wall of the bodies, and the lateral recesses, as well as the shape and size of the canal itself, and also provides some information on the contents of the canal. In the cases of very marked stenosis resulting from asymmetrical osteophytic intrusion into the canal, the assessment can be enhanced by the use of contrast media, in the technique called myelo-CT. The resulting images provide specific information on the relations of the contents and the "container", on any actual compression of the cord and of the nerve roots and their relationship to the protruding masses that are causing the stenosis (Figs. 9.108, 9.110). This information is of immense value to the orthopedist in planning both the surgical approach and the procedure of choice for definitive and accurate managment of the true cause of the stenosis. Furthermore, intravenous contrast media are particularly useful in the differential diagnosis of intracanalicular tissues where there may be scarring, as in the case of previous surgery.

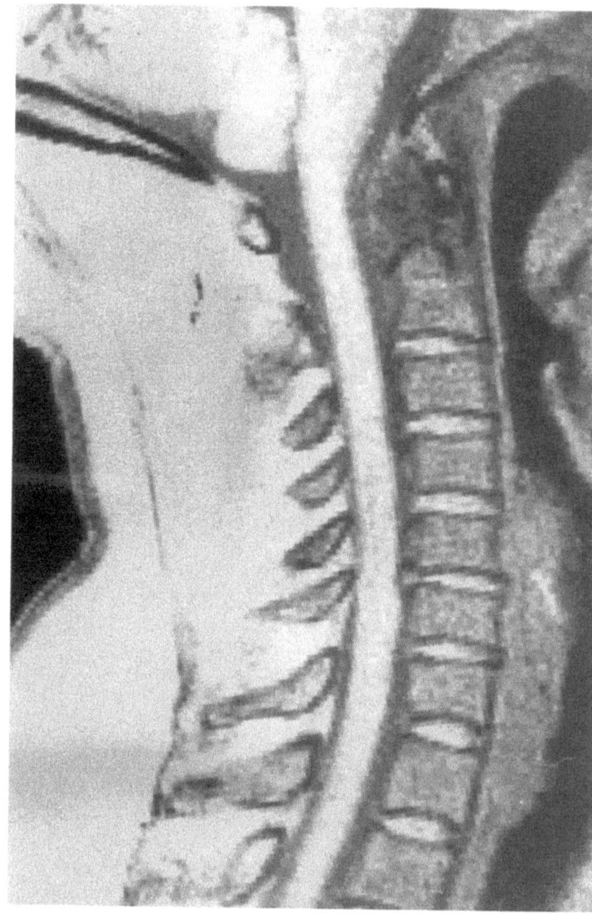

Fig. 5.4. MRI (T1) in a patient with constitutional narrowness of the cervical spinal canal without associated acquired anomaly. Note also the onset of degeneration of the C5/6 disk. (Figure kindly provided by Prof. A. Wackenheim)

Magnetic Resonance Imaging

Magnetic resonance imaging (MRI) provides the best and most complete information with regard to stenosis. It is particularly useful in outlining osteophytes, calcification of the posterior longitudinal ligament, and stenoses due to soft tissues, for example, ligamentum flavum (Figs. 5.4–5.7).

In contradistinction to other radiological methods, including CT, MRI is essential in the visualization and assessment of the spinal cord, the dural and peridural space, and pathological states involving the nerve roots (e.g., enlargement, atrophy, and tumors of the nerve itself).

In other words, MRI not only visualizes the causes of the stenosis but also identifies intrinsic pathology of the spinal cord that clinically mimics spondylitic myelopathies (a good example of this is syringomyelia) (Fig. 5.8). MRI is the method of choice in the assessment of tumors in that it visualizes not only the tumor mass, its extension, its penetration into surrounding structures, and its extension along the vertebral canal, but also its relationship to the cord and the nerve roots, revealing specific changes within the parenchyma of the cord itself (Figs. 9.48–9.50).

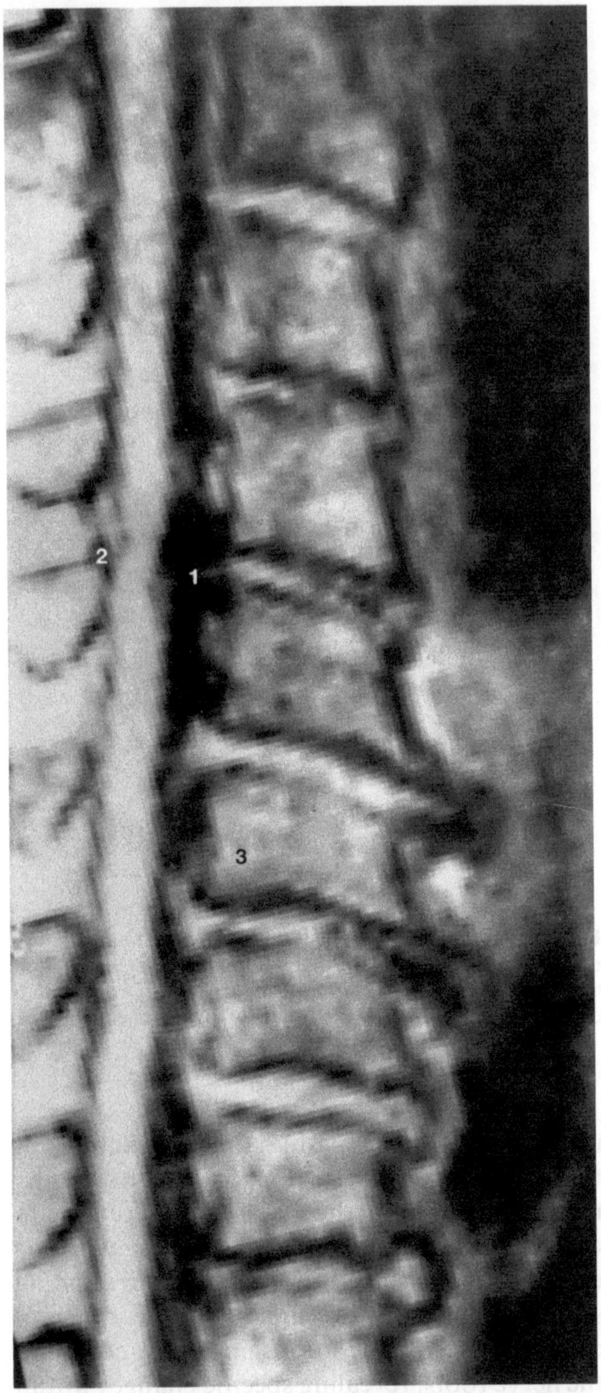

Fig. 5.5. Japanese disease (ossification of the posterior longitudinal ligament) is often associated with cervical canal narrowness. MRI shows the calcifications and ossifications (*1*) as a very dark area of small signal. Spinal cord compression is obvious (*2*). Stenosis is easily recognized with the visual palpation method. (Figure kindly provided by Prof. A. Wackenheim)

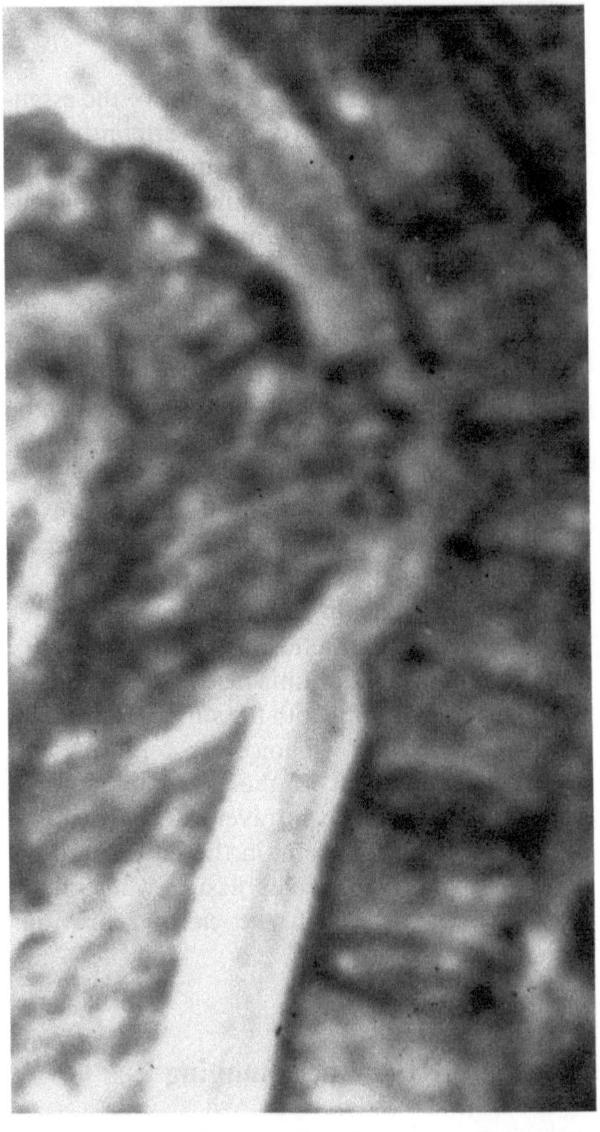

Fig. 5.6. Multiple plications of the ligamentum flavum with severe compression of the spinal cord. (Figure kindly provided by Prof. A. Wackenheim)

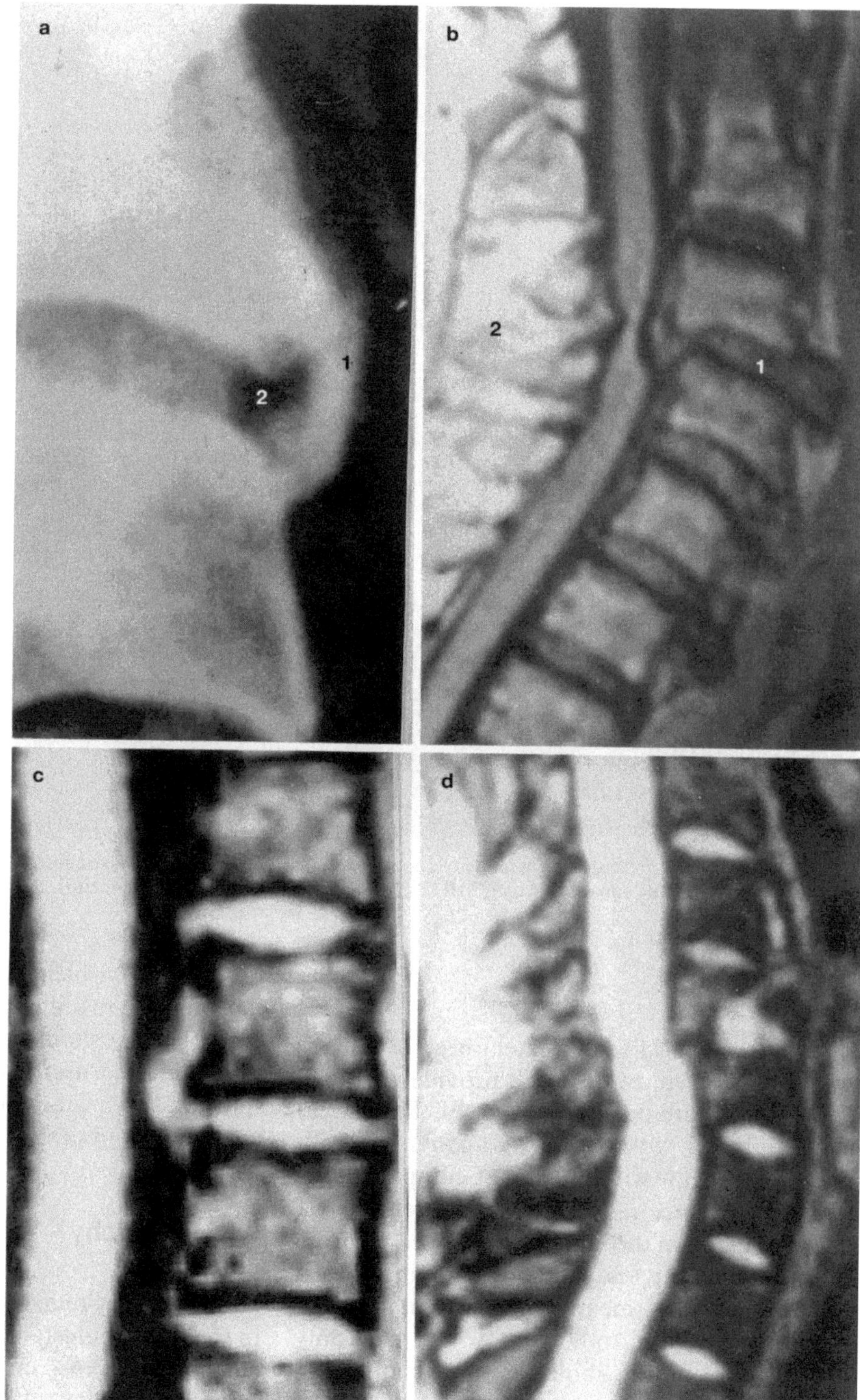

Fig. 5.7. **a** Bony bridge (*1*), demonstrated by conventional imaging, as a sequel of anterior C2/3 disk herniation (*1*) with gas accumulation (*2*). **b** MRI showing spinal cord compression due to a double anomaly at the same level: disk herniation (*1*) and plication of the ligamentum flavum (*2*). **c** Cranially displaced disk herniation. **d** Tear drop fracture with displaces disk herniation. (Figure kindly provided by Prof. A. Wackenheim)

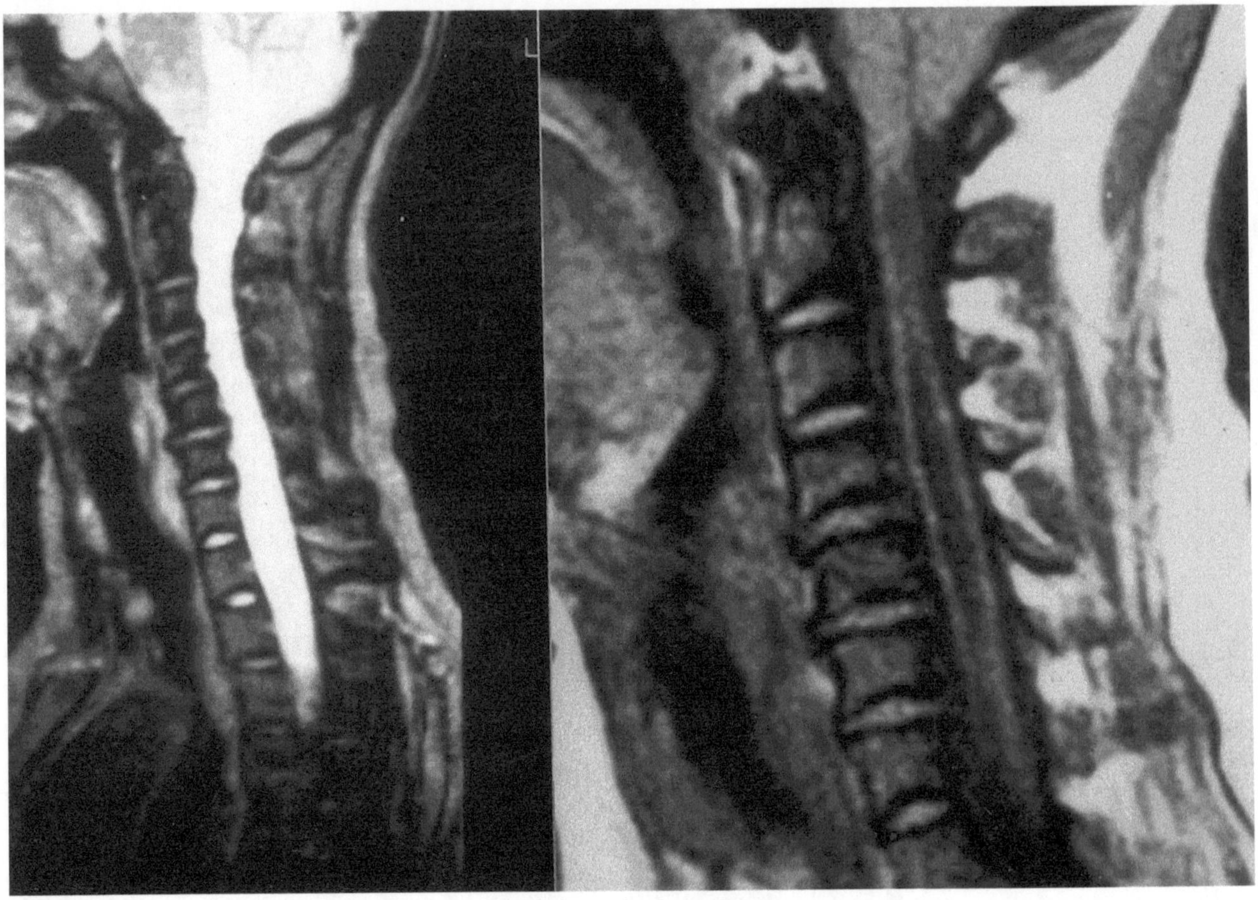

Fig. 5.8. This patient presented a chronic myelopathy which mimics a stenosis of the canal but which MRI clearly identified as due to syringomyelia. (Figure kindly provided by Prof. A. Wackenheim)

Myelography

Myelography has to some extent been overshadowed by MRI and CT, which provide more accurate and more detailed images of the cervical spine and cord. Myelography is an invasive technique that is not without risk of complications, particularly since it involves the injection of a contrast medium through the meninges. However, it remains the one method that can be used for dynamic assessment of the cervical spine, in contrast with CT and MRI, which can only provide information about the static state of the vertebral column.

In certain cases myelography with the appropriate contrast medium can be used through the full range of movement of the neck to identify segmental instability, disk protrusion, and soft tissue impingement (e.g., by ligamentum flavum), which can best be seen in maximal flexion or maximal extension (Fig. 9.36). Myelography should therefore still be regarded as a valid and useful study in selected cases, in spite of the availability of more sophisticated imaging techniques.

Arteriography

Arteriography remains an essential examination in specific circumstances. It is used to investigate clinical syndromes involving vertebrobasilar artery insufficiency with a view to confirming or excluding vascular changes in the differential diagnosis of pathology of the uncus (Fig. 9.58).

Arteriography is particularly valuable in the assessment of tumors. For purposes of diagnosis, it is useful in defining the limits of the tumor and the extent of invasion into surrounding structures. Obviously, it provides information on the extent of vascularization of the neoplasm which is helpful both as a diagnostic characteristic to be compared with other methods of assessment and in planning instrumentation and biopsies (Fig. 9.47). From the therapeutic point of view, in tumors that are large, ill-defined, and richly vascularized one can plan preoperative embolization of the tumor mass with a view to controlling bleeding during the surgical procedure (Fig. 9.44). The skills of a neuroradiologist are required to determine the pathway of the vascular supply of the tumor and distinguish it from the blood supply of the cord. Whether this distinction can or cannot be made determines whether one can achieve total or partial embolization of the tumor. Also, because of the neovascularization associated with tumors, it is important to identify the vascular supply to the cord, in particular the somatic and radicular arterial supply, which must be protected in order to avoid the intraoperative development of ischemia in the cord. This is a risk both during embolization and during the surgical removal of the tumor mass.

Arteriography is therefore essential in planning and carrying out the surgical removal of tumors in the neck because it defines the relationship between the pathological neovascularization and the major blood vessels of the neck. Obviously, it is important in surgery of the cervical spine for the orthopedist to know preoperatively whether or not there is tumor involvement of, for instance, the vertebral artery. If involvement is known preoperatively, then the surgeon can be prepared to deal with the consequences of ligation of the artery during surgery. Unexpected involvement of the vertebral artery found intraoperatively has extremely serious consequences in that it precludes a well-planned procedure.

Scintigraphy

Scintigraphic imaging is useful in the investigation of vertebral osteolysis associated with stenosis, not only to determine the local extent of the bony changes but also from the point of view of assessment of the rest of the skeleton; additional lesions in adjacent bone may lead the surgeon to choose a modified or different surgical procedure.

Conclusions

There are two distinct aspects of the assessment of the value of imaging in the study of the cervical spine.

From the purely *diagnostic* point of view, images are produced which permit the visualization and study of skeletal and soft tissue elements in order to arrive at a specific diagnosis. The pathogenesis of individual types of stenosis may well become apparent. For this purpose, the selection of appropriate imaging modalities should be the domain of a skilled neuroradiologist specializing in this area.

Generally speaking, the examination of the cervical spine for stenosis should begin with traditional or plain radiographs in six projections and positions: anteroposterior, lateral at rest, in maximum flexion, and in maximum extension, and right and left oblique.

The next step should be MRI, which, as stated above, provides the most detailed documentation, of the actual causes of the stenosis, of the size and diameter of the vertebral canal, and of intramedullary and root canal changes. It helps in differential diagnosis, particularly in cases that may feature various types of primary medullary degeneration such as syringomyelia.

If a neoplasm is suspected to be the cause of stenosis or cord compression, one should then undertake arteriography. This may be associated with embolization if deemed clinically essential in the preoperative management of the lesion. Scintigraphy may be necessary to outline the extent of the lesion and thestate of the skeleton overall. If, instead, the problem is an organic stenosis produced by spondyloarthrosis, one may wish to view a horizontal cross section of the bony structure of the canal in order to define its size and shape. For this, CT is most valuable.

In extreme cases, particularly those involving post-traumatic stenosis or instability, there may be a discrepancy between the clinical situation and the findings on initial imaging (including CT and MRI). In such cases it may be essential to obtain a dynamic view of the cervical spine using myelography with or withou myelo-CT.

From the surgeon's point of view, when planning the approach and the surgical procedure, specific information is needed going beyond the determination of the level of involvement and of the pathology present. Information is required that may not necessarily be related to that needed in order to obtain a clear diagnosis. The surgical implications of the lesions are of interest in terms of the technical aspects of planning.

The surgeon needs to know whether a particular space or recess is or is not narrowed and by how much. He must know whether an osteophyte is strictly central, lateral, or posterolateral and at what point and to what extent it impinges on the structures in the space into which it protrudes. It is at this point that one encounters the contrast in concerns between the neuroradiologist, who feels that MRI is sufficient in the assessment of stenosis of the cervical spine, and the surgeon, who requires more detailed and accurate visualization of the bony outlines of the canal in the horizontal plane in order to plan the surgical procedure in detail.

The surgeon must also carefully assess cases in which organic stenosis of the vertebral canal is producing compression at multiple levels, for this has important implications on the choice of surgical management. The extent of the lesion, the level of the abnormality produced, and the state of the disk spaces which may have to be operated on must be ascertained. In fact, patients with diffuse or multiple stenosis have disk spaces (distal or proximal to the level of arthrodesis) that may be in a borderline state of health with varying degrees of narrowing. The surgeon must determine preoperatively the seriousness of these changes and their significance for the choice of operative procedure. These levels above and below the arthrodesis bear the brunt of the rigidity imposed at the operated level or levels. The surgeon must anticipate the consequences of surgery on these altered segments, which may be overloaded and then themselves produce symptoms and signs of extension or recurrence of stenosis with eventual cord compression.

It is for these reasons that the surgeon must undertake dynamic examinations. Myelography will identify the extent of the protrusion and the resulting compression of the sac, but it is also necessary to find out whether the severity of the stenosis can be revealed more clearly by dynamic studies of the spine during function. CT and MRI unfortunately are still purely static examinations and do not yet permit functional evaluation. The selection of appropriate imaging procedures is basic not only to the diagnosis, but also to the planning of the surgical approach and the choice of the appropriate surgical procedure for definitive managment of the cause of the stenosis.

Imaging also has an important part to play in the postoperative assessment of the patient. Appropriately selected examinations need to be performed to confirm that the defect or deformity has been corrected. CT and MRI (as long as no metal implant or stabilizing device has been used) are the postoperative examinations that best assess the success of the surgical procedure. This is an essential step in the final evaluation of cases where cord decompression has been carried out (Figs. 9.36, 9.37, 9.44).

References

Arlet J, Geraud G, Bonafe A, Richaud J (1985) Rachis cervical hyperostosique. Masson, Paris

Czervionke, LF, Daniels DI (1988) Cervical spine anatomy and pathologic processes. Applications of new M.R. imaging techniques. Radiol Clin North Am 26 (5):921–947

Edwards WC, La Rocca H (1983) The developmental sagittal diameter of the cervical spinal canal in patients with cervical spondylosis. Spine 1:20–27

Harsh GR, Sypert GW, Weinstein PR, Ross DA, Wilson CB (1987) Cervical spine stenosis secondary to ossification of the posterior longitudinal ligament. J Neurosurg 67 (3):349–357

Hinck VC, Sachdev NS (1968) Developmental stenosis of the cervical canal. Brain 89:27–36

Kehr P, Jung FM (1976) Pathologie et chirurgie de l'artère vertébrale. Expansion Scientifique Française Strasbourg

Nurick S (1972) The pathogenesis of the spinal cord disorder associated with cervical spondylosis. Brain 95:87–100, 101–108

Pavlow H, Torg JS, Robie B, Jahre C (1987) Cervical spinal stenosis: determination with vertebral body ratio method. Radiology 164 (3): 771–775

Pelissier J, Privat JM, Leroux JL (1985) La myélopathie cervicarthrosique. Masson, Paris

Privat JM (1985) Myélopathies cervicarthrosiques, intérêt et indications du double abord chirurgical. Masson, Paris

Roy-Camille R et al. (1979) Journées d'orthopédie de la Pitié, series 1. Masson, Paries (Series 5: 1986; series 6: 1988)

Senegas J (1985) Chirurgie des complications radiculo-médullaires de la cervicarthrose. Expansion Scientifique Française, Strasbourg (Cahiers d'enseignement de la SOFCOT, no. 23)

Verbiest H (1955). Further experiences on the pathologic influence of a developmental narrowness of the bony lumbar vertebral canal. J Bone J Surg 37 (B): 576

CHAPTER 6

Clinical Aspects of Cervical Stenosis

E. DENARO, A. GRASSO, and
F. D'ALPA

Cervical stenosis afflicts men more often than women (60% and 40% respectively). It is most common in middle age; the average age of 50% of patients is between 40 and 50 years, while up to 80% of patients have an average age of 60 years. Spondylotic cervical myelopathy has long been regarded as a consequence of intervertebral disk degeneration, on the basis that it produces narrowing of the diameter of the spinal canal in the adult. The same can occur as a consequence both of congenital and of acquired stenosis (e.g., hypertrophy of the laminae or of the ligamentum flavum or malformation of the pedicles). In the development of neurological disorders, mechanical factors (e.g., direct compression, instability, excessive tension on the neural structure) are as important as the vascular factors that produce injury by ischemia. The part that each of these plays in the development of the pathology is incompletely understood. In up to 60% of cases, definable neurological deficits occur as a result of spinal cord injury (pure myelopathy). In the remaining cases there is an associated injury to the nerve roots (myeloradiculopathy).

Clinical Presentations

A great variety of clinical presentations exist, which occur as a result of the variable patterns of neurological injuries. Tables 6.1 and 6.2 indicate how these can be classified into clinically specific groups. In the majority of cases, the presenting symptoms are not preceded by neck stiffness or pain. It is most common for patients who present with a very clear history of injury to the cervical spine to be in the fourth decade, with a decreased incidence in later years. It is not uncommon for the symptoms to begin following a general anesthetic; the patient may have been positioned without appropriate support of the head and neck or, while fully anesthetized and with completely relaxed neck muscles, was moved without appropriate precautions (such as head and neck support). Some of the earliest presenting symptoms occur following heavy weight lifting or prolonged hyperextension and rotation of the head. First symptoms may have an acute onset or be chronic. The progression is always slow, insidious, and continuous. Thus a full spectrum of clinical presentations should be expected.

Occasionally, the presence of a pre-existing cervical stenosis can be brought to clinical attention by trauma, where the combination of these two factors can produce either a paraplegia or a tetraplegia. In such cases the only distinguishing feature is that the clinical deficit has resulted from a disproportionately slight trauma, which would not be expected to produce such severe damage were the spine is normal. In our experience, in between 70% and as many 90% of cases, the first symptoms relate to the legs. Later, sensory or motor deficits may appear in the arms. We have been surprised by patients who presented with urinary difficulties and were referred for neurological assessment by the urologist who could not explain the clinical findings. In the majority of cases, however, it is the orthopedic surgeon who is asked to review these patients because the symptoms and signs of lower limb deficits are frequently attributed to lumbosacral arthropathies. Only careful history and physical examination may lead one to suspect that the clinical findings are due to disease of the cervical spine. In fact, it is not uncommon for the patient to complain of disturbances in walking, with stiffness and cramps in one or both legs, and a feeling of heaviness or tightness which makes the patient unable to move his legs or control their movement. Pain may stimulate sciatica, especially when the patient describes pain in the knee or numbness in the leg. There is no doubt that these symptoms are the result of cord irritation at the cervical level where the superficial sensory tracts are injured or compressed. As the afferent nerves join the cord, they are placed in appositional layers at each level (like onion skins). As a result, the long fibers for the legs are external to those for more proximal levels (Fig. 6.1).

The difficulty in interpreting these neurological findings may be also compounded by myotactic reflexes, particularly when the posterior tracts of the spinal cord are the affected ones. Lasègue's sign may also be misleading: extension of the legs may lead to an immediate flexion

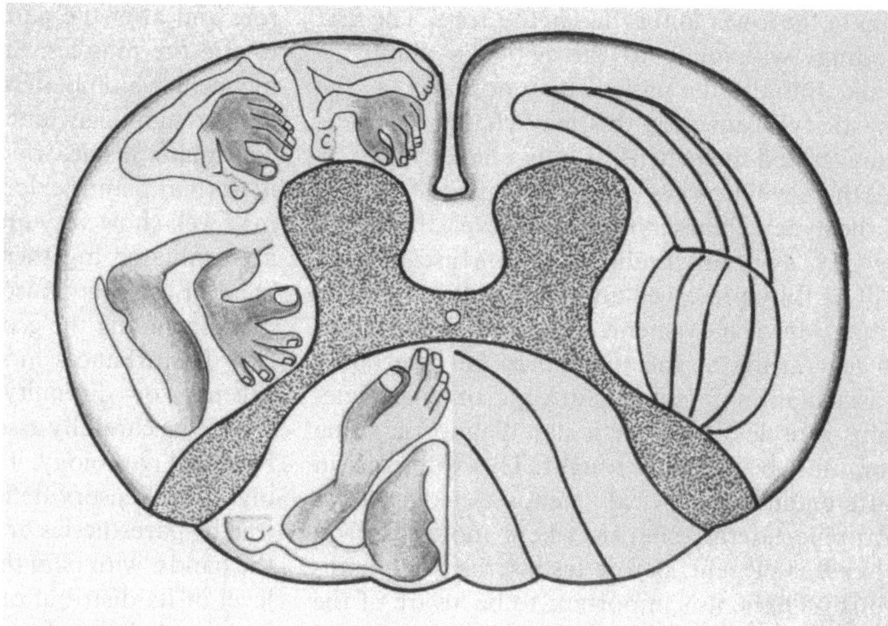

Fig. 6.1. The sensory pathway of the spinothalamic tract joins the cord in layers. The outer layers are those that supply the more distal portions of the lower limbs, the inner ones the more proximal. Any impingement on the spinothalamic tract in the cervical region will, therefore, at first involve sensation, particularly pain sensation in the lower limbs

because of the hypertonia in the femoral biceps muscle.

The symptoms in the arms include first of all paraesthesias that seem to be worse at night and quite disturbing to the patients, who undertake a variety of maneuvers as a result. Some patients continuously rub their hands and soak them in water at varying temperatures. No improvement results from these steps, however, and even rest in the supine position may not be sufficient to relieve the symptoms in some cases. These patients will only be relieved by resting in the lateral decubitus position or by bending forward as in a fetal position.

Patients may present with intermittent spinal claudication in the legs. They complain of stiffness and easy fatigability of the legs after short walks. This forces the patients to repeatedly stop after short distances for a period of rest before continuing. Pain is not a severe problem, a feature that helps to distinguish these patients from those with symptoms resulting from arterial disease, which is characterized by a very severe pain in the calf. The arms may also present similar symptoms of muscle stiffness and easy fatigability that resemble a form of claudication. This is usually precipitated by slow and repeated flexion and extension of the head, which produces compression of the anterior spinal artery and, hence, the symptoms. In addition, anoxic cervical spinal cord injury may occur, which is characterized by spasticity of the upper limbs. This is typical of the tetraparesis associated with cervical spondylosis. Lhermitte's sign has similar implications; it induces a sensation of tingling or of the passage of an electric current along the back in patients with cervical stenosis as a result of irritation of the descending tracts of the spine. Hyperflexion of the head may produce this to a greater degree than hyperextension. Pain of sympathetic origin or brachial causalgia are symptoms of ischemia in the intermediolateral area of the medullary gray matter.

Clinical Features

As we have seen, neurological assessment of the patient in the early stages will provide more findings in the lower limbs than in the arms. The first findings will relate to the patient's ability to walk. Initially the patient may hop and, as the spasticity progresses, this may change to a less exaggerated movement. If only one leg is affected, there will be a sweeping movement of the leg. If the hypertonia is minimal, however, there may be very few if any findings at all. Muscle power will be fully preserved and there will not be any limitation of movement. Only a mild limitation to leg raising at the thigh may be detectable. Fasciculation in the quadriceps or gastrocnemius muscles is of particular diagnostic value and must be carefully sought. This will assist in differentiating cervical stenosis from amyotrophic lateral sclerosis where motor neuron disease is present. Before testing the osteotendinous reflexes, it is important to be aware of the patient's condition. The patient may be tired and his muscles fatigued and these are factors that will influence his responses and hence the assessment of the pyramidal tracts. A patient who is well rested will not display the same signs as after a period of activity.

Osteotendinous hyperreflexia in one or both legs can be elicited in a high proportion of patients (up to 90%). In the early and acute forms, there may be a threshold to the reflex and, therefore, one must always compare the intensity of the response to the firmness of the tap with the reflex hammer; firm or strong taps may not bring out slight differences in the reflexes between the two sides. Obviously one is not going to depend entirely on the findings from testing one reflex in diagnosing pyramidal deficits. These can only be identified by taking the sum of all the clinical findings. Diffusion of the response to testing a reflex will occur if there is spasticity. This can be seen in the reflexes of the fingers as well as in the legs. In the lower limbs there may be contraction of the adductor muscles in the thigh, with an extensor reaction when the opposite side is tested.

Very slight symptoms that in themselves do not appear to have any clinical significance may, however, contribute to the overall pattern that leads to the identification of abnormalities of pyramidal origin; tests for the Barrés pyramidal and Mingazzini signs should be carried out before and after the patient has exercised enough to tire the muscles. Similarly, a nonspecific or inconclusive omolateral plantar reflex may not appear significant until it is compared with the contralateral side, which gives a more completely normal plantiflexion. The abdominal reflexes may well show very little abnormality until they are evaluated together, with a complete assessment of the deep muscular reflexes of the abdomen, including the costal insertions of the muscles. Disturbances in sphincter control such as urgency or difficulty in initiating urination should be carefully assessed as indicators of neurological pathology. The motor tracts are rarely involved. Sensory deficits tend to be characterized by paresthesias or numbness, particularly of the hands, with pain that involves a specific root level in its distribution and, hence, tends to be unilateral. Loss of specific sensation may take the form of astereognosis, i.e., the patient may be unable to identify the shapes or the nature of objects. This may also be combined with athetosis-like movement of the fingers as part of the involvement of deep sensory involvement. One should always suspect involvement of a cervical nerve when either pain or paresthesia can be elicited through pressure over Erb's point. The test for Spurling sign is said to elicit root pain following the application of pressure on a hyperextended head which is bent towards the side of the pain; it is very difficult to interpret this, except where there is a soft or recent hernia in cases of cervical spondylosis; traction of the head should produce symptomatic relief of the pain, confirming the mechanism of injury at the root level. When this same maneuver brings on dizziness or vertigo, it is known as the De Klein test and is indicative of vertebral artery compression; this supports the opinion that a high proportion of patients have cervical spine pathology that is related to vertebro-basilar arterial deficit.

It must be emphasized that sensory deficits do not follow a specific pattern. The level of involvement will be found to be quite variable, even within one patient, and often it extends far lower than expected (it may extend down as low as T4 with only cervical level pathology). There may be unilateral, contralateral, or bilateral involvement of the pyramidal tract, and the sensory deficits can be extremely variable in degree. In addition to involvement of the pyramidal tracts, a Brown-Séquard syndrome, a spinal syndrome (if both motor and sensory deficits are found in the same side), or a funicular myelosis (with hypopallesthesia and posterior cord deficits on the same side as the pyramidal loss) will sometimes be found. The combinations are many, variable, and unpredictable. It is always important to establish the presence or absence of sensory losses, particularly since they tend to be absent when there is motor neuron involvement.

In the upper limbs one of the most important observations in terms of differential diagnosis is the presence of fasciculations; in spondylomyelopathies these are rarely observed, even if the frequency of discharge, severity, and distribution point towards motor neuron disease. Muscle fasciculation, even in anatomical sites that appear removed from the levels of the cervical spine (for example, on the inner aspect of the thigh or in the calf), should always suggest that the principal disease is a motor neuron disease. Atrophy of muscles in the arms is not a common occurrence in spondylomyelopathies, where it is detectable in no more than 15% of cases. By contrast, spasticity particularly of the forearm and hand is much more common. This results from involvement of the pyramidal tracts and is expressed as the Hoffmann sign (also known as Trömner sign). In these cases flexion of the fingers and thumb results from the sudden release of forced flexion of the index finger. Lessening or complete absence of a muscle reflex is, however, a far more precise indicator of the level of involvement. Muscle power is not always affected. When it is affected, patients may complain of loss of ability to undertake specific activities. This is often first noted in the hands, when a patient becomes unable to carry out some undertaking which he was able to carry out in the past (such as open a bottle).

One of the ways in which movement or activity precipitates clinically detectable symptoms or signs is a ride in an automobile. A long trip on rough roads may produce irritation of cord, nerve roots, or blood vessels, particularly in the presence of bony osteophytes that may compress the soft tissues such as nerve roots and vertebral arteries which are fixed in a rigid passageway.

Cervical tract involvement may be associated with very complex and confusing symptoms and signs. This results from the complex anatomical and functional distribution of both the neurological and vascular supplies. For example, injury to the anterior spinal artery or vertebral arteries may produce symptoms that suggest involvement of the upper cervical levels and even the cranial nerves. This can lead to great difficulty in interpreting poorly developed symptoms that are difficult to confirm, elicit, reproduce, or evaluate; these may include paraesthesias, nystagmus, and cranial nerve deficits. Careful assessment of cranial nerve function will provide useful information that may help to distinguish cervical from intracranial disease.

We are here attempting to point out the variability in clinical presentations, symptoms, and

Table 6.1. Clinicoanatomical features

Central compression
Pyramidal signs in all four limbs
Superficial sensory changes (most common in the superior limbs)
Deep sensory changes (particularly involving the lower limbs)
Root signs
Changes in urinary bladder function
Unilateral lateral compression
Root signs
Pyramidal signs (rare)
Bilateral lateral compression
Root signs
Pyramidal signs (more common than in the unilateral form)
Urinary bladder function changes (more frequent than in the unilateral form)
Multiple compressions[a]
Pyramidal signs
Sensory changes
Changes in urinary bladder function

[a] The clinical signs and symptoms are usually more severe than in cases of simple medial protrusion

Table 6.2. Common clinical pictures

Brachialgia (predominant symptom)
Polyradiculopathy-like syndrome
Progressive diffuse cervical myelopathy with para- or tetraparesis
Acute cervical transverse myelopathy (mainly C5–C6)
Brown-Séquard myelopathy
Findings simulating acute traumatic para- or tetraparesis

signs in spondylotic cervical myelopathies; these will run the full gamut from a Brown Séquard syndrome to hemiplegia, paraspasticity, amyotrophy, myelomalacia, syringomyelia, and many others (Table 6.3). In patients aged over 50 years, one must be cautious in interpreting the results of computed tomographic (CT) studies. There may well be evidence of spondyloarthrosis with osteophytosis, but this may not mecessarily be fully or even partly causally related to the clinical presentation or findings in a patient. This is comparable to the absence of clinical evidence of a deficit of any kind in patients with CT evidence of cerebrocortical atrophy.

Table 6.3. Clinical signs

- Radicular signs
  - Sensory signs of irritation
    - Pain
    - Paraesthesias (brachialgia or root symptoms)
  - Sensory signs with deficits
    - Hypoesthesias
  - Motor signs of irritation
    - Contractures
    - Torticollis
    - Fasciculations
  - Signs of motor deficits
    - Muscle weakness
    - Muscle atrophy
    - Hyperreflexia
- Signs of myelopathy
  - Sensory signs of irritation
    - Root signs
    - Lhermitte's sign
  - Signs of sensory deficit including:
    - Loss of pinprick discrimination
    - Loss of touch sensation
    - Loss of proprioception
    - Loss of sensitivity to heat and cold
    - Hypopallesthesia
    - Root signs
  - Motor signs in upper extremities
    - Fasciculation
    - Tetraplegia
    - Weakness
  - Motor signs in lower extremities
    - Paraplegia
    - Gait disturbances
    - Weakness and hypoesthesia of the legs
    - Spinal claudication
  - Long tract signs
    - Loss of abdominal reflexes
    - Disturbances of bowel function
    - Disturbances of urinary bladder function (neurogenic bladder)
    - Recurrent urinary infections
  - Vegetative signs (cervicosympathetic)
    - Pain of sympathetic origin
    - Brachial causalgia
  - Unusual supraspinal signs
    - Nystagmus
    - Lower cranial nerve palsy
    - Facial paresthesias

Differential Diagnosis

Differential diagnosis can be particularly difficult and varied and must take into account the following situations or conditions (Table 6.4):

Hypertrophic cervical dural meningitis is a condition of unknown etiology, although in the past it was attributed to syphilis. It is characterized by a process of fibrosis that thickens the internal layers of the duramater within the spinal canal, which eventually form a thick inelastic cylinder about the cord. Before the introduction of modern imaging, this could only be identified intraoperatively.

Our understanding of *syringomyelia* has undergone significant changes with the introduction of modern imaging. Clinicopathological correlation has been redefined, so that the rare incidence of sensory deficits is now understood. The identification of small or multiple syringomyelic cysts is no longer surprising; these can be clearly identified with magnetic resonance imaging (MRI), but with CT they may have been misinterpreted as a spondylitic myelopathy or a post-traumatic cystic myelopathy.

In *degenerative vascular diseases*, the cortical-subcortical involvement is known to produce cranial nerve deficits. CT is regarded in such cases as essential to the diagnosis, in order to exclude extraspinal diseases such as a meningioma of the falx as well as pathology of the blood vessels, as noted above. MRI is most helpful, in our experience, in differentiating syringomyelia from the more rare demyelinizing diseases such as multiple sclerosis or pontine myelolysis.

Amyotrophic lateral sclerosis presents with the typical muscle fasciculation and distal muscular atrophy associated with hyperreflexia of the arms, absence of changes in sphincter control, and sensory losses; these features may be of critical importance in differential diagnosis. In pa-

Table 6.4 Differential diagnosis

Spinal pathology
Acute disk herniation
Hypertrophic cervical dural meningitis
Syringomyelia
Amyotrophic lateral sclerosis
Spinal muscle atrophy
Extramedullary tumors
Intramedullary tumors
Multiple sclerosis (particularly the spinal progressive type)
Nerve entrapment syndromes (carpal tunnel and thoracic outlet)
Spastic spinal paraparesis
Neuralgic amyotrophy (Parsonage-Turner syndrome)
Funicular myelosis
Paraneoplastic myelopathy
Acute traumatic myelopathy (centro-medullary syndrome)
Lumbosacral myelopathy
Friedrich syndrome
Posterior cervicosympathetic syndrome
Supraspinal (central) pathology
Cerebral tumors
Cortical atrophy
Psychoneurosis ("the great imitator")

tients with stenosis of the upper cervical canal, it is not infrequent to find fasciculation in the quadriceps muscle through involvement of the reticulospinal pathways. In the pseudopolyneuritic form of amyotrophic lateral sclerosis, it must be pointed out that there can be sensory involvement that is both symmetrical and distal in distribution. In such cases, one must depend on specific neurophysiological tests for identification.

In the investigation of *intra- or extramedullary tumors*, the characteristic diagnostic features include a relatively rapid and progressive worsening of symptoms, characteristic changes in the cerebrospinal fluid (CSF), and night pains which are not relieved by rest. The use of CT and MRI is most helpful in the delineation of the involvement and in the identification of the etiology in these cases.

Multiple sclerosis can mimic almost any neurological pathology. This explains why it may be easily confused in terms of clinical symptoms and findings with spondylotic cervical myelopathy. The features to be kept in mind are that it occurs in young patients, it will progress in stages, there will be typical immunoelectrophoretic monoclonal bands, peak expiratory velocity (PEV) and brain stem auditory evoked potentials (BAEP) will often show typical changes, and imaging will identify often asymptomatic, but demonstrable, areas of periventricular demyelination; these features are characteristic enough to establish a diagnosis.

In the initial stages of *carpal tunnel syndrome*, there will be complaints of pain in the arms and paresthesias, particularly at night. The symptoms may involve one or both arms and may extend right up to the shoulder, characteristically with paresthesias of the hands which are very difficult for the patient to specifically define or describe. In such cases one should carefully confirm whether the paresthesias also involved the ulnar side of the ring and little fingers. Positive Tinel and Phalen signs (pain on flexion or forced extension of the wrist) are characteristic; tests of median nerve motor and sensory conduction are usually required to establish this diagnosis. However, one must remember that median nerve entrapment at the carpus may occur simultaneously with cervical spondylosis and, before considering any surgical procedure, one must confirm the cause of the patient's problem.

Differentiating *familial spastic spinal paraparesis* (Strümpell-Lorrain syndrome) from the chronic vascular myelopathy that occurs in the mature adult can be particularly difficult. This syndrome is the result of degenerative changes below the pyramidal crossing of the lateral tracts, and only rarely of the anterior tracts. SEP monitoring is the one helpful test in differentiating these two entities.

Pain and weakness in both upper limbs may follow a flu-like illness in *acute neuralgic amyotrophy* or Parsonage-Turner syndrome. The involvement tends not to be symmetrical, and there may be muscle fasciculations without any signs of nerve root involvement, since the symptoms are not brought on by straining or coughing.

In the psychoneurotic patient the presence of cervical arthrosis may be exaggerated or imitated, resulting in *emotionally induced hyperreflexia* with magnification of minimal true sensory symptoms. Often investigations such as MRI and SEP do identify spinal changes, but there is a significant discrepancy between the patient's symptoms and the objective observations that can be made at physical examination. Often the best solution in such cases is to follow the patient for a sufficiently long period of time to establish whether objective signs develop or whether the symptoms change or disappear.

Finally, brief mention should be made of clinical situations that are particularly rare or that usually have very little bearing on the differential diagnosis of spondylotic cervical myelopathy. These include hand-shoulder syndrome, vertebro basilar syndrome, and supraclavicular fossa syndrome. In these, clinical presentation indicates cervical sympathetic irritation with subjective complaints suggestive of a myelopathy. Other rare conditions include posterior spinal artery syndrome, which is more common that the anterior variant, funicular myelosis, paraneoplastic myelopathy, and neoplastic involvement of the parietal lobe.

CHAPTER 7

Neurophysiological Studies in Cervical Stenosis

In the investigation of cervical stenosis, neurological assessment must always be regarded as fundamental. The types of tests that are routinely performed include electromyography (EMG) nerve conduction velocity (NCV) tests, and sensory and motor evoked potential studies. The purpose of these is to evaluate the extent of the myeloradicular compromise, define the type of neuropathological process, help establish the differential diagnosis, predict the probable results of surgery, and monitor the status of medullary function in both surgical and nonoperative treatment. EMG studies are usually undertaken first, as part of any extensive and complete laboratory assessment but only somatostensory evoked potential (SEP) studies can assess cord function.

EMG and NCV Findings

Introduction

The basic functional unit of the peripheral motor nerve system is called the motor unit. A number of motor neurons are present in the gray matter of the spinal ventral horn. A peripheral extension of a single spinal motor nerve cell forms the axon that exits the spine and goes to form the peripheral nerve which eventually will innervate a number of muscle fibers within skeletal muscle. Each muscle receives axons from motor nerves that arise at more than one spinal level and which therefore come from different cervical roots. Inversely, every spinal root contributes to more than one nerve and hence to more than one muscle. Activation of the motor neuron produces a synchronized signal or discharge in all dependent muscle fibers. The electrical activity related to the muscle contraction can be detected by means of a needle, usually placed in the muscle, or on the surface by skin electrodes applied over the muscle. The discharge of a single motor unit is identified and recorded as a motor unit potential. The different motor units within the same muscle are physiologically discharged synchronously, so that the strength of a contraction is uniform for its duration (the refractory periods of different motor units are temporally distributed). When all the motor units of one muscle are activated synchronously by electrically stimulating the peripheral nerve that supplies that muscle, the result is the evoked compound muscle action potential.

The activity of sensory fibers can be detected throughout the course of nerves as nerve potential. Various EMG techniques that are useful in assessing spinal cord and peripheral nerve function are discussed below. Pathology in the cervical spine may affect the nerve system within the spinal cord (causing spinal nerve or spinal tract damage) or outside the cord at the cervical nerve roots (causing peripheral nerve damage). Primary or secondary vascular insufficiency and direct compression of the spinal gray matter may result in anatomical and functional loss of spinal neurons. As the number of neurons decreases, so does the number of active motor units and this will affect one or more muscles in the distribution of that nerve. With time this progresses to degeneration of the axons and consequent atrophy of the muscle fibers in their distribution. There will be some regeneration of axon dendrites from the remaining intact motor units to the denervated fibers. These expanded motor units will have an increased muscle fiber density and increased innervation ratio.

Traditional EMG

Activity at Rest. The main sign of denervation is the presence of fibrillation potentials. Unfortunately, these can only be detected between 1 and 6 months after the onset of denervation and they are rarely present after this period of time. In chronic denervation, as in the case of chronic spondylitic myelopathy, pseudomyotonic discharges do sometimes occur and can be detected. From our discussion it is apparent that the presence of fibrillation potentials is a definite sign of (recent) denervation, while its absence is not necessarily a sign of the contrary.

Maximal Effort EMG Pattern. An interference pattern at clinical maximal effort indicates a normal discharge of all motor neurons innervating that muscle with normal function of the supplying peripheral nerve. A reduction in the number of functioning motor neurons or axons causes a reduced effort pattern (intermediate or single oscillation patterns) and the active motor units discharge at increased frequency.

Morphology of Motor Unit Potentials. Normal motor units are detected by means of needle electrodes mainly as bi- or triphasic potentials. The proportion of polyphasic (more than three phases) potentials is quite low. Axonal derangements cause a dispersion of motor conduction velocity in the intramuscular nerve endings so that fibers within the same motor unit discharge asynchronously. The resulting compound motor unit potential shows an increased number of phases; the higher the proportion of polyphasic motor unit potentials is, the greater the significance in acute myelopathy. In chronic myelopathy, the presence of giant motor unit potentials (resulting from increased density of motor unit fibers) is a more common finding. A reduction in the proportion of polyphasic motor unit potentials may be seen in the recovery phase from an acute myelopathy with normalization of the trophic properties of the axons. Giant motor unit potentials are of greater significance in chronic myelopathy where the number of motor units can not return to the original state.

Reflex Response Studies

H Reflex. A reflex contraction of muscle fibers can be obtained by stimulating muscle spindle afferents that centrally activate motor neurons, only some of which discharge at every stimulus. The result is small compound muscle action potential, the latency of which depends on the peripheral, root and medullary conduction velocities and on the central synaptic delay. In neuropathies, the H reflex is of reduced amplitude or is delayed. In the case of a radiculopathy, a segmental myelopathy, or a myeloradiculopathy, the abnormalities occur only in the muscles dependent on that root (Ioku et al. 1988). With the exception of the cases in which a latency delay is the only sign of compression, the incidence of abnormalities and the accuracy of diagnosis of this test is less than that of the effort pattern. Furthermore, H reflexes in the upper limbs are not constant in normal subjects and they are enhanced in spastic limbs (Ioku 1984).

Motor Conduction Studies

As stated above, one of the signs of axonopathy is a reduction in the conduction velocity of the intramuscular nerve distribution. In more severe cases, the conduction velocity may also be reduced along the major part of the nerve. A reduced maximal motor conduction velocity is an electrophysiological sign of myelopathy. This finding can be differentiated from peripheral mono- or polyneuropathies, of which the most common is the coexistence of a median or ulnar nerve entrapment.

F Response. A contraction of some of the muscle fibers evoked by stimulating motor axons resulting in antidromical activation of a few motor neurons is represented by the F response. A radiculopathy may delay or reduce the F response in a manner comparable to the H reflex.

Computerized EMG. Automatic frequency analysis has been recently introduced as part of the current interest for increasing computer-assisted evaluation in the hope that a significant modification of maximal effort pattern can automatically be detected. At the present time this is experimental and not a routine test with established patterns of response; its clinical application must yet be established.

Guidelines for Diagnosis

The diagnosis of the level of a radiculopathy is based on knowledge of the normal pattern of muscle innervation. There have been many excellent studies of this subject, but no definite formula has been established to take into account the high degree of interindividual variability. For this reason, the identification of the level is based on the characterization of EMG abnormalities in all (or nearly all) muscles supplied from one root, and the lack of abnormalities in muscles supplied from adjacent roots. Root disease can be differentiated from peripheral nerve trunk disease in that root involvement is associated with EMG changes in the paraspinal muscle, while in peripheral nerve involvement the paraspinal or proximally innervated muscle will show no EMG changes.

Differentiating peripheral nerve involvement from root involvement and myelopathy can sometimes be difficult. Certain featues, however, may be helpful. In myelopathy, peripheral sensory nerve axons should not be involved and motor denervation can be identified without any associated sensory loss, since the cells of sensory neurons are located outside the spinal cord. The relation between dorsal root ganglia and intervertebral foramina is less precise. Reduction in the diameter of the root canal may cause nerve compression either proximally or distally to the dorsal ganglia, or at a combination of both sites, so that differentiation may be particularly difficult. If radicular compression is the cause of sensory nerve damage, then the study of peripheral SEP may show isolated reduction or actual loss of sensation in the first, third, or fifth fingers in the case of compression of the C6, C7, and C8 nerve roots, respectively[1].

Spondylotic cervical myelopathy affects mainly the sixth and seventh decades of life. In this age group, amyotrophic lateral sclerosis is the main differential diagnosis. Neurophysiological tests tend to be specifically diagnostic in these cases.

Somatosensory Evoked Potential

Principles of Analysis

Electrodes placed at selected sites can detect impulses travelling along the central nervous system. The action potential is recorded as a distant potential. Averaging of some hundred monitored impulses gives a typical waveform for every recording. The recording of SEP is a technique of growing interest in both preoperative (D'Alpa et al. 1985; El Negamy and Sedgwick 1978; Ganes 1980; Sivola et al. 1981; Stohr et al. 1982; Drechsler 1985) and intraoperative (Brown et al. 1984; Lesser et al. 1981) evaluation of cervical spinal cord function in patients suffering from spondylotic cervical myelopathies or cervical spinal stenosis. SEP monitoring permits the assessment of the extent and gravity of the spinal dysfunction (Hattori et al. 1979) and prediction of the outcome of treatment.

Cervical Response Waveform

SEP is recorded by means of a noninvasive technique with the same instrumentation as conventional EMG. In cervical pathology, the nerves that are stimulated are mainly the median, radial, or ulnar nerves at the wrist. Only in selected studies are the musculocutaneous nerves or the digital nerves of the hands selectively activated to test root afferents (C6 for the first, C7 for the third, and C8 for the fifth finger, Eisen and Elleker 1980; Jorg et al. 1982; La Joie and Melvin 1983; Louis et al. 1985; D'Alpa et al. 1986). Responses of the cervical cord are detected by means of surface electrodes placed on the spinal processes generally at the level of the C2 and C7 vertebrae.

Two types of reference electrode placement have been generally utilized. In the first, the reference electrode is placed on the scalp, while in the second the reference is a noncephalic electrode in the contralateral shoulder, arm, or hand. While some authors have expressed a preference for the second choice (Desmedt and Cheran 1980), the cephalic reference is the one most commonly used in routine clinical examination. An invasive technique has been described by some laboratories with needle electrodes inserted posteriorly. In our laboratory, the technique consists of two-channel recording. Standard placements are at C'_3 $(C'_4)-C_2$ and C'_3 $(C'_4)-C_7$, where C'_3 and C'_4 designate the location according to the 10–20 international EEG system. SEP consists of a series of positive-negative deflections, which have been designated (with respect to mean latency for medial nerve SEP) as P9, P11, P13, and P14 followed by a negative complex N18. For the purposes of the current discussion, these denominations will be used for SEP of other nerves or dermatomes, regardless of their absolute latencies.

P9 reflects the activity of the peripheral volley between the axilla and plexus; it precedes the P10 waves originating from the plexus. P11 is a composite potential reflecting the activity of both roots and cervical cord (Desmedt and Cheron 1980; Anziska and Cracco 1980; Yamada et al. 1980). Our studies (D'Alpa 1984) suggest that there are at least two different P11 components: the first (P11A) was best detected at the C7 level while the second (P11B) was best detected at the C2 level.

P13 potential is almost the same in recordings at the C2 and C7 levels. Many authors consider this a spinal cord response generated at the level of the dorsal horn neurons (Desmedt and Cheron 1981), but in our experience we have found that it is related to the brainstem activity (as seen in scalp-spine recordings). P14 (brain stem and/or thalamus) and N18 (thalamus and/or cortex) are supraspinal or central events.

Analysis of Responses

Figure 7.1 shows the typical SEP for median, radial, and ulnar nerve stimulation. In our laboratory, latencies are measured at the onset of P11 and P13 and at the peak of P14 and N18. The P11 onset is regarded as the latency of the sensory volley of the spinal entry (Desmedt and Cheron 1980). We consider the latency of the P13 onset to be the onset of supraspinal (medullary) activity, regardless of the fact that it may or may not be related to a specific low brain stem origin with entry as low as the occipital foramen. We consider the P11–P13 onset interval as an approximate measure of the spinal cord transit time from the spinal entry level to the cerebrum. This interval is different for median (1.87 ± 0.15 m), ulnar (2.26 ± 0.16 m), and radial (1.87 ± 0.17 m) nerves (D'Alpa 1985), reflecting the different length of the respective pathways from the spinal entry at the highest root level of each nerve (C6 for median and radial, and C8 for ulnar) to the brain stem. The difference between the P11–P13 onset intervals of the ulnar and median nerves reflects the transit time in the lower cervical cord (C8–C6). When the P11–P13 onset interval is prolonged, the two major components of the P11 potential are differently affected.

We first measure the interval between P11A onset and P11B peak; this hybrid measurement gives us precise information about the conduction time of the spinal cord level at the point of entry of the afferent nerve to an approximate spinal level of C2–C3. Another hybrid measurement of the interval between P11B peak and P13 onset gives us information on the transit time from the C2–C3 level to the brain stem. It is important to underline that the P11B peak–P13 onset interval is independent of the nerve stimulated, as one would predict for spinal pathways of equal length, while the P11A–P11B peak intervals show the same changes in the median, radial, and ulnar nerves as do the P11-P13 onset interval changes.

SEP in Myelopathies

Demyelation of the central nervous system produces a slowing of spinal conduction, i.e., a prolonged P11–P13 onset interval. With regards to root innervation, the P11–P13 onset interval increases for the median, radial and ulnar nerves generally in the cases of pathology in the upper cervical cord down to the C5–C6 nerve level. The interval is prolonged only for the ulnar nerve in the case of compromise in the lower cervical cord. Slowing of conduction is invariably greater for the ulnar nerve than the median nerve, as is to be expected from the longer spinal tract of the ulnar nerve. In the same manner, the distortion of the waveform is generally greater for the ulnar nerve. Some patients show more pronounced abnormalities of the median nerve than the ulnar nerve in their SEP. In such cases, we believe that a significant radiculopathy of the median nerve is contemporaneously present. Usually spinal stenosis due to ossification of the posterior longitudinal ligament is associated with greater SEP abnormalities (Yu et al. 1988).

Pattern of Response

Typical patterns of responses that can be diagnostic have been described. Median nerve SEP are normal in myelopathies at the C7–C8 level while ulnar nerve SEP show a reduced amplitude in P11 potential and/or an increase in P11–P13 onset interval (Figs. 7.2–7.3). In more severe cases, P13 potential may be of reduced amplitude and have a distorted waveform, and the supraspinal response may be dispersed or absent.

Median nerve SEP in myelopathies at the C3–C5 levels show changes similar to those described above for ulnar nerve SEP in myelopathies at the C7–C8 level. Ulnar nerve abnormalities may parallel those of the median nerve, but sometimes they are more pronounced if the myelopathy extends to the lower cervical levels (Fig. 7.3). Median nerve abnormalities in myelopathies at the C6 level may be the same as in myelopathies at the C3–C5 level, but in some cases only ulnar nerve SEP may show pathological changes. Myelopathies above the C3 level will show prolongation (generally to the same degree) of the P11–P13 onset interval in both median and ulnar nerve SEP, and changes in the P11B peak–P13 onset intervals may be also detectable. SEP of the radial nerve in myelopathies will vary in the same manner as the median nerve.

Differentiation of Myelopathies from Radiculopathies

The abnormalities described above are those which are typical of pure spinal pathology. If a radiculopathy is also present, an increased variability of the responses will result. The P11A potential will appear reduced in amplitude, particularly if all roots of the nerve are compressed. If only the C6, C7, or C8 roots are involved, median and ulnar nerve P11 may or may not show any abnormality. These patients may show changes in the P11 responses obtained from single dermatome stimulation.

It is sometimes possible to differentiate a myelopathy from a radiculopathy using SEP. This is possible when the P11–P13 onset interval shows very little or no prolongation, but the P11 amplitude is markedly reduced, with asymmetry between the two sides.

Clinical Correlation

Patients with cervical myelopathies are known to have either sensory or motor signs, or both. The frequency and severity of the SEP abnormalities are greatest in the presence of pain, paresthesias, or sensory defects (Ganes 1980). Patients with only motor signs generally show mild and less developed changes. Furthermore, patients with clinical impairment of the cervical cord may not show any SEP abnormalities (El Negamy and Sedgwick 1978; Ganes 1980). False positive results may occur in patient in whom no clinical or radiological signs of cord damage are evident and in whom the SEP may suggest unilateral or bilateral spinal involvement.

SEP does not distinguish cervical spondylosis from other cervical lesions because the changes in waveform or latency are similar in nature and degree, regardless of the underlying pathology. In our experience, we have found that responses are characteristic only in cases of multiple sclerosis; in these a reduction in the amplitude of P3 is seen, while in cervical spondylosis the commonest abnormalities are a reduction in the amplitude or delay in the latency of P11. Some patients with multiple sclerosis may show a distinct variability of response waveform during the course of one SEP examination.

SEP abnormalities are maximal in severe radiculopathies, giving severely distorted responses, while a definite P11 cannot be detected (El Negamy and Sedgwick 1979). Clinically, the most important differential question is whether a patient has a radiculopathy or a myeloradiculopathy, particularly in patients in whom clinical examination shows no definite evidence of

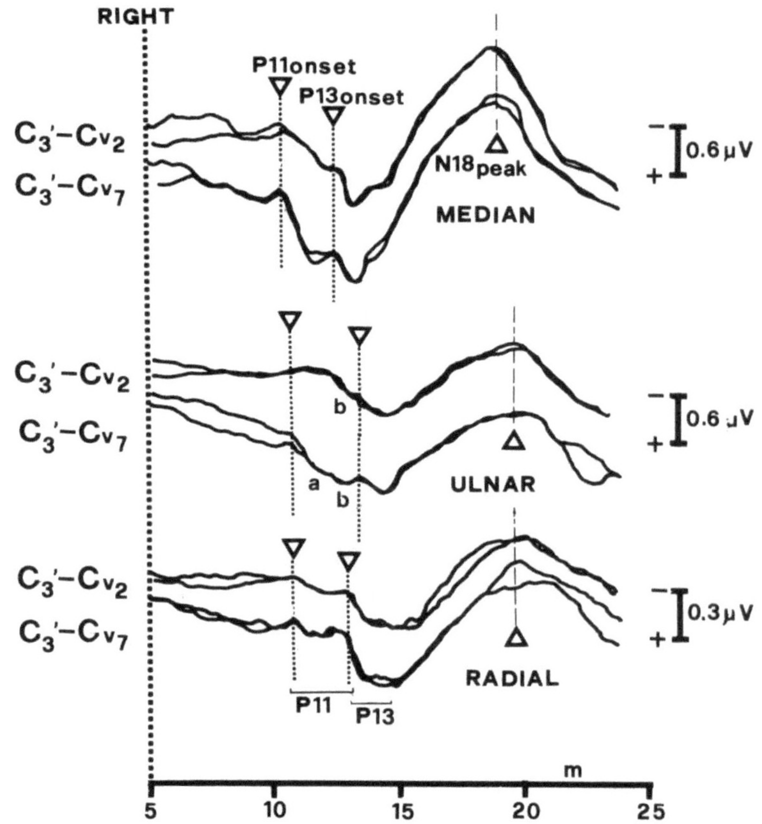

Fig. 7.1. SEP from median, ulnar, and radial nerves in a healthy subject. The P11–P13 onset interval is the time of conduction along the cervical spine. The difference in waveforms in the different nerves is related to a better resolution of the P11A and P11B peaks in the case of ulnar and radial nerves. The supraspinal response (N18) is similar for all nerves. Electrode placement was at the parietal location (C_3') and on the cervical vertebrae C2 and C7

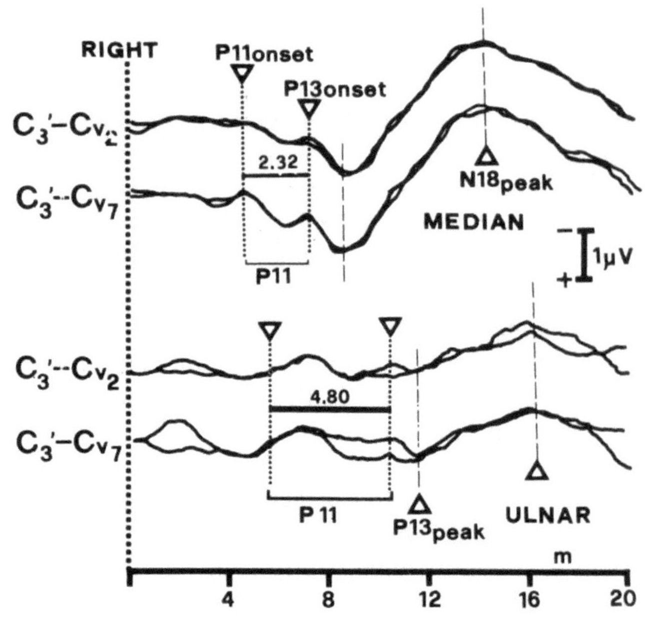

Fig. 7.2. Abnormal SEP in a patient with spinal stenosis at the C6–C7 level. The P11–P13 onset interval of the median nerve is normal, while that of ulnar nerve is markedly prolonged. The supraspinal conduction time (P13 onset–N18 peak) is similar for both nerves. Electrode placement was at the parietal location (C_3') and on the cervical vertebrae C2 and C7

myelopathy. SEP monitoring permits the examination of many nerves and nerve levels which may be essential in the investigation of a difficult clinical diagnostic problem. P11 abnormalities have been described as more severe in radiculopathies (Sivola et al. 1981) than in myelopathies. This has also been our experience. In many cases we have been able to distinguish a radiculopathy from a myelopathy on the basis of SEP alone. If the P11–P13 onset interval is modified only for the median or radial nerves and not for the ulnar nerve, we have found this to be a sign of the absence of definite myelopathy. Furthermore, a reduction in the amplitude of P11 without prolongation of the P11–P13 onset interval is almost invariably a sign of radiculopathy rather than a myelopathy. Prolongation of the P11–P13 onset interval without changes in P11 amplitude is almost invariably a sign of a myelopathy.

Preoperative Assessment

The main purposes of the neurophysiological assessment of patients with myelopathies are as follows:

To establish the extent of cervical stenosis induced damage. The extent of spinal damage can be approximately evaluated by observing the type of abnormal response and the number of involved nerves. Based on median nerve and ulnar nerve SEP, it is our policy to examine at least three segments of the cord: C8–C6, C5–C3, and C2–brain stem (the rationale for this has been discussed above). A detailed analysis may be necessary in some cases and then SEP is carried out at each spinal level; the P11–P13 onset intervals are determined for each root and for each spinal segment. If more than one functional segment is involved, then a diffuse myelopathy is diagnosed.

To assess the severity of the neurological disorder. The degree of SEP abnormality does not necessarily reflect the gravity of spinal damage. Generally the severity of SEP changes parallel the extent and severity of the spinal damage and the involvement of the dorsal tracts. Abnormalities in waveform and a reduction in amplitude associated with increased intervals are more significant than increased intervals alone.

To indicate prognosis. Our experience indicates that minimal SEP changes are associated with better postoperative recovery of function. More severe SEP distortion is associated with improvement or recovery only in a small proportion of cases and, if there is improvement, the degree of recovery of normal function is less.

In the early preoperative assessment of patients, SEP monitoring can be advantageous. Myelopathy is commonly associated with cervical trauma. In patients with a fracture and/or dislocation of one or more vertebrae, one must suspect vascular and/or compressive spinal cord damage. In patients in whom there is no apparent clinical motor damage, it is important to establish if there is any subclinical compromise as early as possible. Repeated examinations may be necessary if there is any evidence of possible spinal injury that is not otherwise identifiable clinically. One must also determine at what point surgical treatment must be undertaken. SEP can objectively and accurately evaluate the progression of a patient during conservative nonoperative treatment (halo jacket or collar), and if a deterioration of spinal function is detected by assessing spinal conduction, the decision for intervention can be undertaken at a much earlier point.

Intraoperative Monitoring

The maneuvers used to achieve reduction of vertebral fractures or dislocations may cause transitory dysfunction of the spinal cord. Intraoperative monitoring using the P11–P13 onset intervals together with the spinal and cortical waveform and amplitude response may detect any changes during manipulation, thus warning the surgeon that a spinal dysfunction has been induced (Grundy 1982; Dinner et al. 1986). This

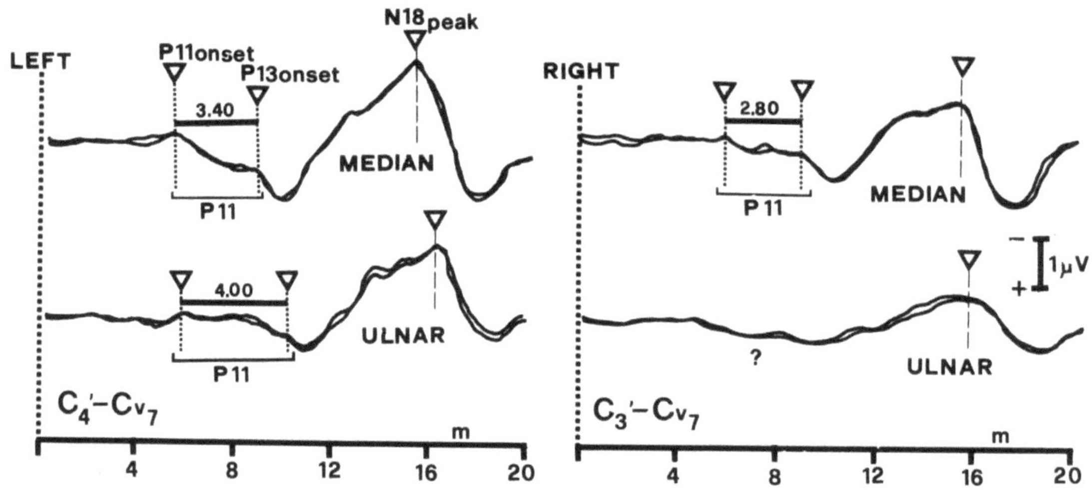

Fig. 7.3. Abnormal SEP in a patient with listhesis at the C5–C6 level. The P11–P13 onset intervals of the median and ulnar nerves are prolonged by approximately the same extent. This confirms normal spinal conduction below the level of compression. Electrode placement was at the parietal location C_3' and on the cervical vertebra C7 during stimulation of the right median and ulnar nerves. The parietal location C_4' was used during stimulation of the left median and ulnar nerves

is of particular value in posterior approaches when attempting to reduce joint dislocation. In such cases, if the SEP alteration is not reversed within a few minutes, the vertebral bodies should be relaxed and it may be necessary to undertake a large decompression of neurological structures before returning to the manipulation for reduction, fixation, and stabilization of the vertebral bodies; this may now require a combined anterior and posterior approach. In some cases, while attempting reduction of vertebral bodies, posterior prolapse of the intervertebral disk may be associated with SEP improvement, as confirmed by intraoperative myelography.

Motor Evoked Potentials

The usefulness of the SEP is limited by its being entirely dependent on the integrity of the function of the dorsal column, regardless of the status of the motor tract and of the spinal gray matter (Cusick et al. 1978). Direct electrical or magnetic stimulation of the central motor tract (through the scalp or the neck) can now be performed easily and safely (Merton et al. 1982; Marsden et al. 1982). A conduction block or a slowing of conduction along the cervical cord can be detected by stimulating above and below the compressed level of the spinal cord (Rossini et al. 1985; Mills and Murray 1986). Monitoring during vertebral column surgery has also been described.

Conclusion

The accuracy of preoperative assessment of cervical myelopathy may be increased by adding SEP to EMG studies. The localization, severity, and extent of spinal involvement can be assessed accurately by analyzing cervical evoked responses.

References

Anziska B, Cracco RO (1980) Short latency somatosensory evoked potentials: studies in patients with focal neurological disease. Electroencephalogr Clin Neurophysiol 49:227–239

Brown RH, Nash CL, Berilla JA, Amaddio MD (1984) Cortical evoked potential monitoring. A system for intraoperative monitoring of spinal cord function. Spine 9:256–261

Cusick JF, Myklebust J, Larson SJ, Sances A Jr (1978) Spinal evoked potentials in the primate: neural substrates. J Neurosurg 49:551–557

D'Alpa F, Russo P, Bonfiglio G, Pero G, Grasso A (1985) Assessment of spinal cord function in cervical myelopathies by spinal stenosis or herniated disc. Acta Neurol (Napoli) 40:394–398

D'Alpa F (1984) An analysis of spinal (median nerve) SEPs components in healthy subjects. Acta Neurol (Napoli) 39; 413–417

D'Alpa F (1985) Comparison of cervical SEPs on median, radial and ulnar nerve stimulation. Ital J Neurol Sci 6:177–183

D'Alpa F, Sallemi G, Triffiletti L, Grasso A (1986) A Cervical SEPs from radicular (digital) upper limb nerves stimulation. Acta Neurol (Napoli) 41:602–609

Desmedt JE, Cheron G (1980) Central somatosensory conduction in man: neural generators and interpeak latencies of the far-field components recorded from neck and right or left scalp and earlobes. Electoencephalogr Clin Neurophysiol 50:382–403

Desmedt JF, Cheron G (1981) Paravertebral (oesophageal) recording of subcortical somatosensory evoked potential in man: the spinal P13 component and the dual nature of the spinal generators. Electroencephalogr Clin Neurophysiol 52:257–275

Dinner DS, Lueders H, Lesser RP, et al. (1986) Intraoperative spinal somatosensory evoked potential monitoring. J Neurosurg 65:807–814

Drechsler F (1985) Short latency SEP to median nerve stimulation: recording methods, origin of components and clinical application. Electromyogr Clin Neurophysiol 25:115–134

Eisen A, Ellfker G (1980) Sensory nerve stimulation and evoked cerebral potentials. Neurology (NY) 30:1097–1105

El Negamy E, Sedgwick NJ (1978) Delayed cervical somatosensory potentials in cervical spondylosis. J Neurol Neurosurg Psychiatry 42:238–241

Ganes T (1980) Somatosensory conduction times and peripheral, cervical and cortical evoked potentials in patients with cervical spondylosis. J Neurol Neurosurg Psychiatry 43:683–689

Grundy BL (1982) Monitoring of sensory evoked potentials during neurosurgical operations: methods and applications. Neurosurgery 11:556–575

Hattori S, Saiki K, Kawai S (1979) Diagnosis of the level and severity of cord lesion in cervical spondylotic myelopathy. Spinal evoked potentials. Spine 4:478–485

Ioku M (1984) Hand H-reflex demonstrated in patient with central nervous system disorders. Electromyogr Clin Neurophysiol 24:331–339

Ioku M, Otsu T, Akizuki S (1988) Hand H-reflex and short latency somatosensory evoked potentials (SSEPs): clinical evaluation in patients with cervical cord lesions. Electromyogr Clin Neurophysiol 28:295–300

Jorg J, Dullberg W, Koeppen S (1982) Diagnostic value of segmental somatosensory evoked potentials in cases with chronic progressive para or tetra spastic syndrome. Adv Neurol 12

Kubota S, Nagashima C, Ohmori S (1988) Segmental spinal somatosensory evoked potentials in cervical myelopathies due to spondylosis, ossification of the posterior longitudinal ligament and developmental cervical stenosis. Neurorthopedics 5:25–35

La Joie WJ, Melvin JL (1983) Somatosensory evoked potentials elicited from individual cervical dermatomes represented by different fingers. Electromyogr Clin Neurophysiol 23:403–411

Lesser RP, Lueders H, Hahn J, Klem G (1981) Early somatosensory potentials evoked by median nerve stimulation: intraoperative monitoring. Neurology (N4) 31:1519–1523

Louis AA; Gupta P, Perkash I (1985) Localization of sensory levels in traumatic quadriplegia by segmental somatosensory evoked potentials. Electroencephalogr Clin Neurophysiol 62:313–316

Marsden CD, Merton PA, Morton HB (1982) Percutaneous stimulation of spinal cord and brain: pyramidal tract conduction velocities in man. J Physiol (Lond) 328:6P

Merton PA, Morton HB, Hill DK, Marsden CD (1982) Scope of a technique for electrical stimulation of human brain, spinal cord and muscle. Lancet 2:597–600

Mills KR, Murray NMF (1986) Electrical stimulation of the human vertebral column: which neural elements are excited? Electroencephalogr Clin Neurophysiol 63:582–589

Rossini PM, di Stefano F, Stanzione P (1985) Nerve impulse propagation along central and peripheral fast conducting motor and sensory pathways in man. Electroencephalogr Clin Neurophysiol 60:320–334

Siivola J, Sulg I, Heiskari M (1981) Somatosensory evoked potentials in diagnostics of cervical spondylosis and herniated disc. Electroencephalogr Clin Neurophysiol 52:276–282

Stohr M, Buettner UW, Riffel B (1982) Spinal somatosensory evoked potentials in cervical cord lesions. Electroencephalogr Clin Neurophysiol 54:257–265

Yamada T, Kimura J, Nitz DM (1980) Short latency somatosensory evoked potentials following median nerve stimulation in man. Electroencephalogr Clin Neurophysiol 48:367–376

Yu YL, Leong CY, Fang D, Woo E, Huang CY, Lau HK (1988) Cervical myelopathy due to ossification of the posterior longitudinal ligament. Brain 111:769–783

CHAPTER 8

Surgical Approaches

Recent decades have seen great advances that have resulted not only in the improvement of surgical techniques, but also in a better understanding of disease processes and more precise preoperative investigation. Increased knowledge of normal function and of disease of the cervical spine means that the criteria for surgical intervention are now better defined and the most appropriate surgical approach in each patent may be selected more rationally. The purpose of any surgical intervention must be the removal of the cause of the disease; in the case of the cervical spine this means the cause of the stenosis. In order to achieve this, it may often be necessary to use a combination of standard surgical approaches, which may be successfully employed in one operation or staged over an appropriate period of time.

The indications for surgery prescribe the pathway to be used. The indications depend first of all on the level of cervical spine to be operated upon; i.e., the cervico-occipital level, the upper cervical spine (C1–C2), or the lower cervical spine. They depend secondly on the pathological process causing the stenosis, of which there are a variety and among which the most important are:

- Localized compression such as may occur anteriorly from degenerative disk disease or posteriorly from diseases of the laminae or of the ligamentum flavum
- Global stenosis such as may occur as a result of invasion by tumor

It is therefore important to separate the surgical approaches into anterior, posterior, or combined forms for the upper cervical spine and cervico-occipital levels as opposed to lower cervical spine (C3–C7) including the cervical thoracic junction.

Anterior Approaches

Transoral Approach

The transoral approach permits the best access to the anterior arch of the atlas, the base of the odontoid process, and the body of the axis, laterally as far as the atlantoaxial articulation to the C2–C3 disk and the more cranial part of the body of C3. In effect, the posterior wall of the pharynx is the only structure present in front of these vertebral structures. Because of its softness and thinness, it permits easy access to the examining finger allowing palpation of the arch of the axis and its anterior tubercle, to which the long muscles of the neck are inserted, as well as to the body of the axis and to the C2–C3 intervertebral space, where the disk usually bulges anteriorly from the bodies. The posterior wall of the pharynx, composed of mucosa, a thin layer of constrictor muscles, and the buccal fascia, sits immediately in front of the anterior longitudinal ligament. Crowne and Jansen (cf. Southwick and Robinson 1957) were the first to remove an osteoma through this approach in 1944. In 1962, Fang and Ong described using the transoral approach in treating six cases of C1–C2 instability following trauma and were the first to emphasize the intraoperative and postoperative complications. These were further discussed by Verbiest in his report on neoplasms of this area. Because of the records of complications associated with this approach, there was a flurry of interest in extrapharyngeal approaches that provided greater exposure and greater flexibility in the choice of surgery that could be carried out (Southwik and Robinson 1957; Hodgson and Francis 1960; De Andrade and MacNab 1969; Whiteside and Kelly 1966). In spite of all this negative experience, the transoral approach is still valuable today. Not only personal experience but also many reports indicate that the transoral approach can be used very successfully in treating stenosis associated with malformation, neoplasms, and trauma in the high levels of the cervical spine. It is obvious that strict adherence to the principles leading to avoidance of the reported consequences is necessary. Of these the most important are patient selection and modifications of the surgical technique that make the approach simpler and avoid extended operating time.

Technique

In preparing the patient for surgery, the first step is to administer prophylactic antibiotics for a period of at least 24 hours preoperatively. If the patient has any history of previous infection or is known to have had a susceptibility to infection, then it is advisable to undertake a carefull assment of the bacterial flora of the pharynx and to develop an appropriate preoperative antibiotic program. Once in the operating room, the patient is placed in the supine position. The head is in slight hyperextension and is fixed and held in position by an elastic band attached to the table. The neck is supported by a soft pad. Should the patient be in a halojacket, the ring can be used to manipulate the head into the position of mild hyperextension; the head can then be anchored. The operating table should be placed in the Trendelenburg position, which allows better visibility of the operative site for the surgeon and better control of bleeding in that any dependent drainage remains in the operative site and does not seep caudally (Fig. 8.1).

One of the difficulties often encountered is inadequate illumination of the operative site even when converging lights are used. If the surgeon is provided with a head lamp which today can be a fiber-optic system, the light can shine directly into the pharynx and illuminate the depths of the operative site. Some authors have recommended the use of an operative microscope, particularly when operating deep in the canal. I and my collegues do not routinely perform tracheotomy, since we have found that any respiratory problems or postoperative edema can be dealt with successfully without it. Transoral intubation is used for anesthesia, with the reinforced tube placed in the groove of the tongue retractor. After preoperative cleansing, the upper teeth are protected and a tongue retractor with an appropriate groove to hold the transoral intubation tube is secured over the mandible and tongue externally. The base of the tongue, the pharynx, and the soft palate can be displaced with packing. When the soft palate is fixed in this position, the availability of light in the operative site is limited, particularly superiorly. The retractor we use has a double hook with tapered tips. As this is inserted below the soft palate, it retracts it posteriorly. In spite of their softness, the soft palate and the uvula are not injured by the retractor, which is anchored externally with only sufficient tension to maintain it in the position desired by the surgeon. The use of this type of retractor avoids the problems associated with self-retaining retractors which may decrease the amount of light that reaches the depths of the operative site and may even interfere with access to the operative site through the mouth (Figs. 8.2–8.4). Occasionally, we have resorted to suture retraction of the uvula and soft palate in order to obtain better exposure. We have found it best to pass the free ends of these sutures out through the nose and to fix them externally. They must be used with great care since excessive traction will tear the tissues, leading to loss of retraction, of exposure, and to tissue damage. In order to achieve sufficient exposure to reach the base of the skull and the clivus, the soft palate may be split longitudinally and the hard palate may even be resected posteriorly in order to obtain unobstructed access to the clivus. If this resection is necessary in order to obtain adequate exposure, then the portion of the hard palate removed can be regrafted back into position at the end of the procedure. In order to flush the operative site, a soft tube is placed on the lateral aspect of the operative field. We use a double suction apparatus, a coarser or larger one for flushing and a smaller one to aspirate the deeper regions of the operative site (Fig. 8.5).

Once the area is prepared and retractors are in place, a midline incision is made in the posterior pharyngeal wall, cutting the full thickness of the mucosa right down to the anterior longitudinal ligament of the spine (Figs. 8.6, 8.7). Hemostasis must be very carefully obtained immediately. Lateral widening of the incision is possible. Any bleeding is controlled and gently packed with Surgicel (Fig. 8.8). Once the incision has been made in the pharyngeal wall, retraction is necessary in order to provide adequate exposure. Self-retaining retractors tend to block access to the operative site, and for this reason we prefer to use silk sutures that evert the pharyngeal margins and which can be anchored to the lateral wall on the lateral pillars (Fig. 8.9). Once this has been done, the anterior longitudinal ligament can be inspected and split longitudinally, obtaining access to the anterior surface of the vertebrae (Fig. 8.10). At this point the actual surgical procedure can be carried out (Fig. 8.11).

At the end of the procedure, drainage must be provided (Fig. 8.12) and usually the drain is fixed through sutures that are passed to the outside via the nose and anchored externally. Drainage is crucial only when a particularly large cavitiy has been created, with incomplete debridement, or where there is a question of possible oozing of blood in spite of overall adequate hemostasis.

Care must be taken when large grafts are used that they do not protrude beyond the limits of the host bone. If they do, they will make closure of soft tissues over them difficult, will have a tendency to produce dehiscence of tissue, and may be the cause of swallowing dysfunction postoperatively. Closure of the pharyngeal wall should be full thickness with individual sutures, preferably made of reabsorbable material. On occasion we have used silk sutures, these are not reabsorbable and will eventually fall out. When using this approach, there may be considerable difficulty in suturing an incision that reaches the C3 vertebral level or below. The pharyngeal wall is particularly thin in this lower part, and this can create significant difficulties in obtaining adequate closure. If widely separated surgical margins are left in the pharyngeal wall, it may be necessary to release the lateral portions of the pharynx in order to permit approximation of the wound immediately. Practically speaking, if the underlying bony structure is intact, one can obtain adequate healing even if the surgical edges are not perfectly approximated and sutured.

After the packing has been removed, a final rinse out of the area is carried out in order to permit an accurate and complete inspection of the area for hemostasis. At this point a nasogastric tube is introduced under direct vision and left in place for at least 24 hours in order to avoid vomiting and the possibility of an aspiration pneumonitis.

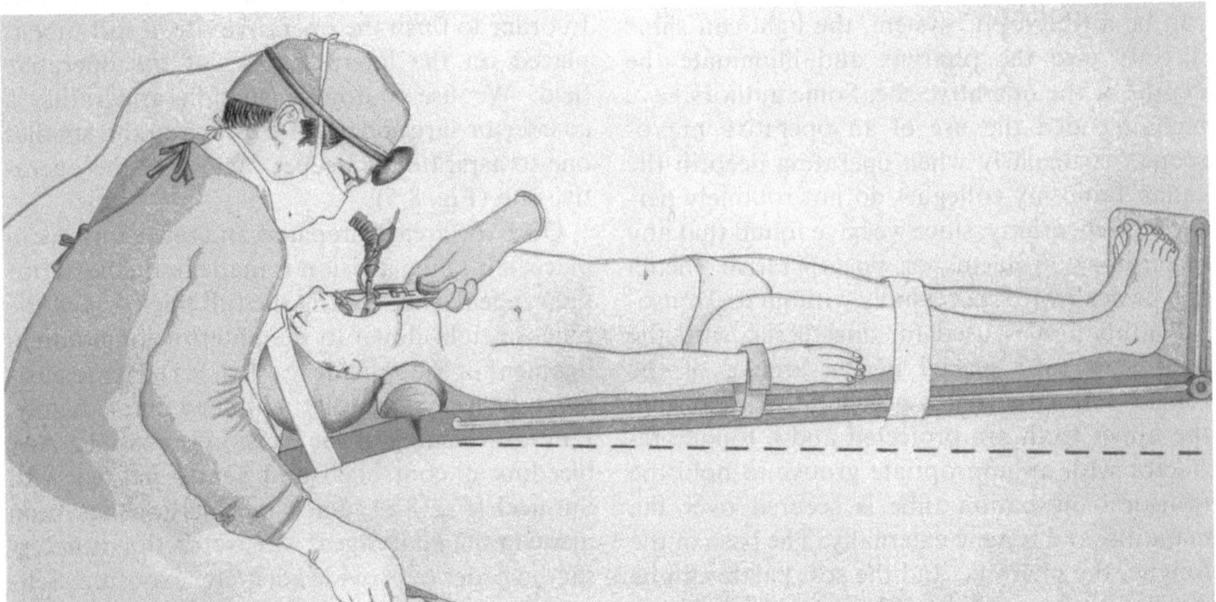

Fig. 8.1. The patient is positioned on the operating table. The neck rests on a rigid support and the head is fixed with tapes. The anesthetic intubation is placed in the distal portion of the mouth, and the surgeon operates in a sitting position, illuminating the operative site with a head lamp

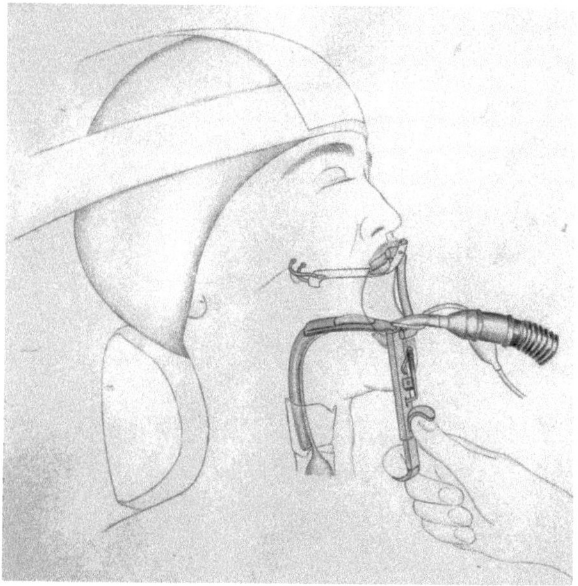

Fig. 8.2. Orotracheal intubation with a rigid tube that sits in a groove in the lingual portion of the special mouth retractor. The degree of retraction of the mandible that can be achieved will vary in each patient

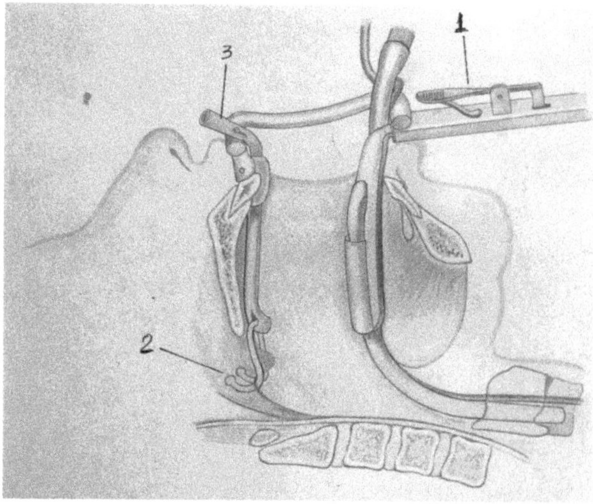

Fig. 8.3. Sagittal view showing details of the oral retractor (*1*). The semi-rigid orotracheal tube for anesthesia is out of the operative field, but is actually protected by the retractor itself. Note the special instrument used to raise the uvula and broaden the field of view in the operative site (*2*). It is constructed with a double hook with blunted ends that latches onto and raises by retracting the soft palate. An elastic band maintains the traction on this specially designed hook and can be anchored onto the superior arm of the oral retractor (*3*)

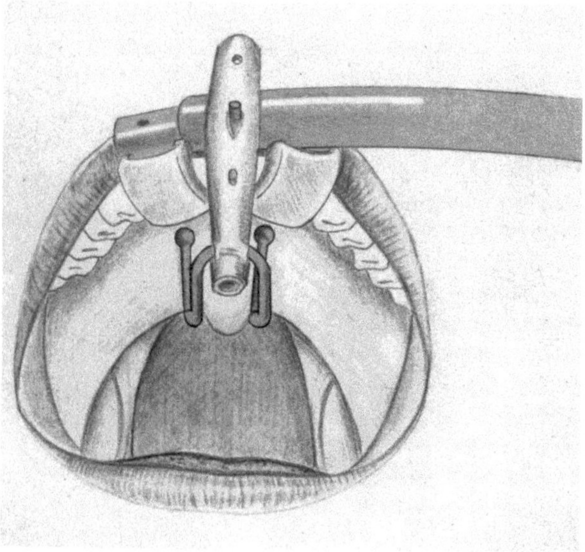

Fig. 8.4. Detail of the soft palate retractor showing its tip and external anchoring

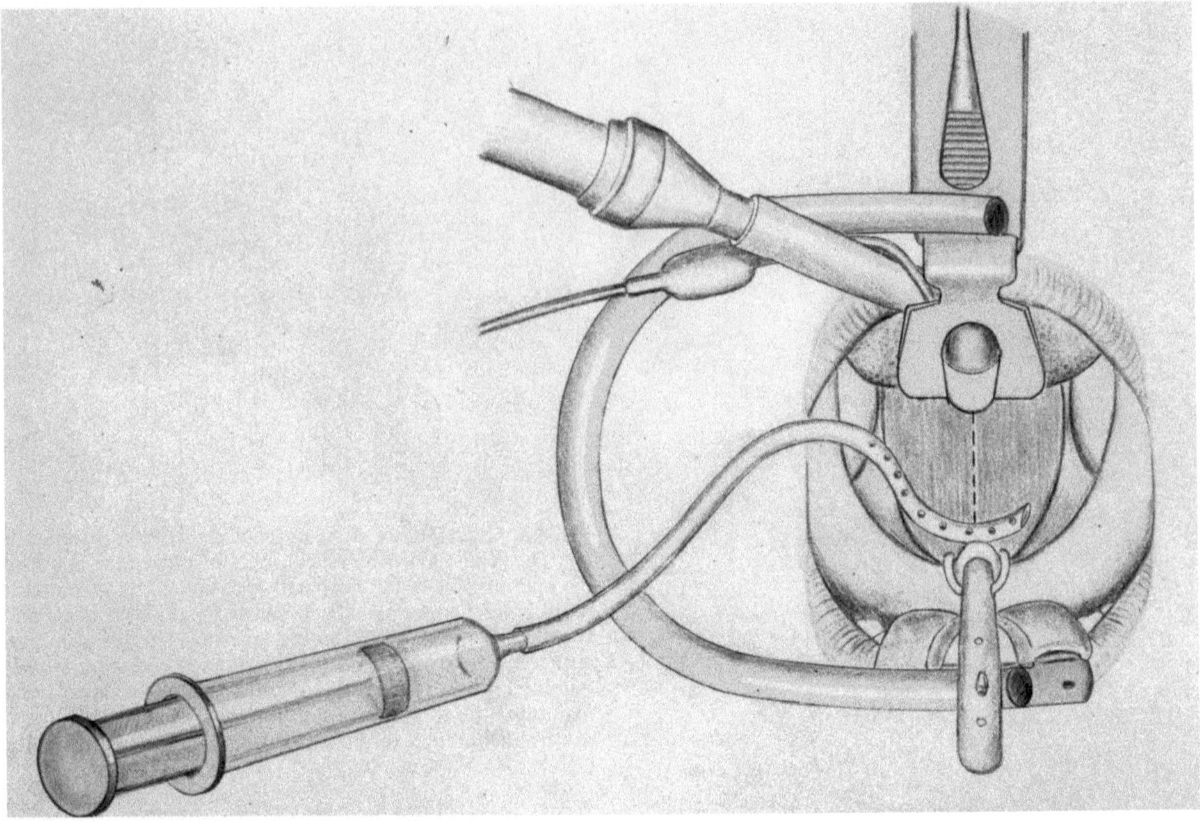

Fig. 8.5. Detail of the operative field showing a malleable tube for continuous drainage shaped in such a way as to fit into the depths of the pharynx, making continuous lavage of the area of dissection possible

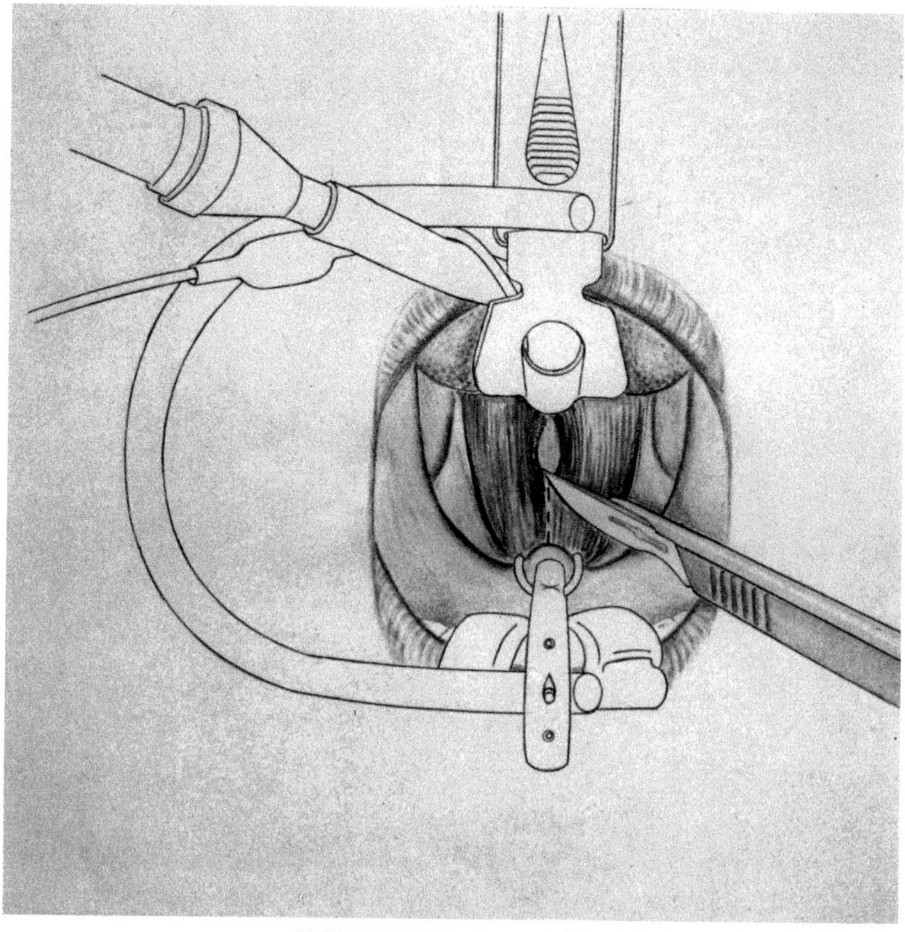

Fig. 8.6. Knife incising the full thickness of the pharyngeal wall to reach the prevertebral plane

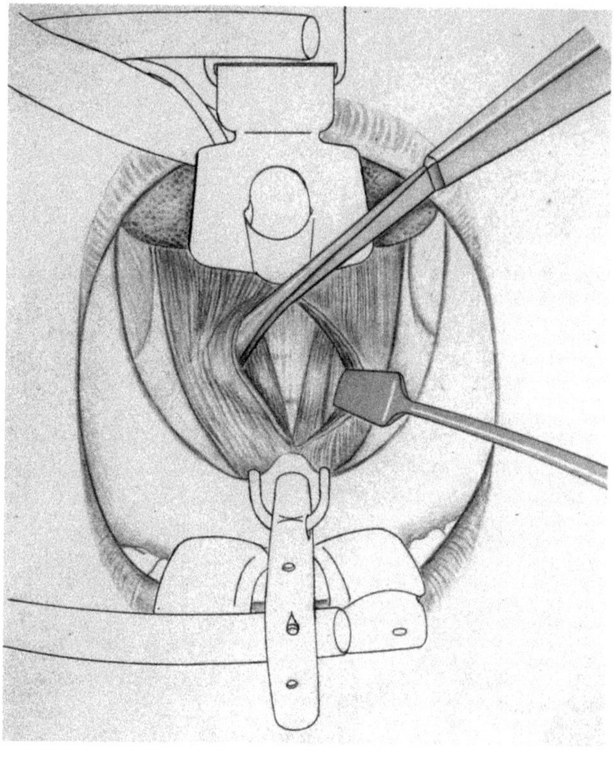

Fig. 8.7. Elevation of the pharyngeal wall and of the lateral cervical muscle

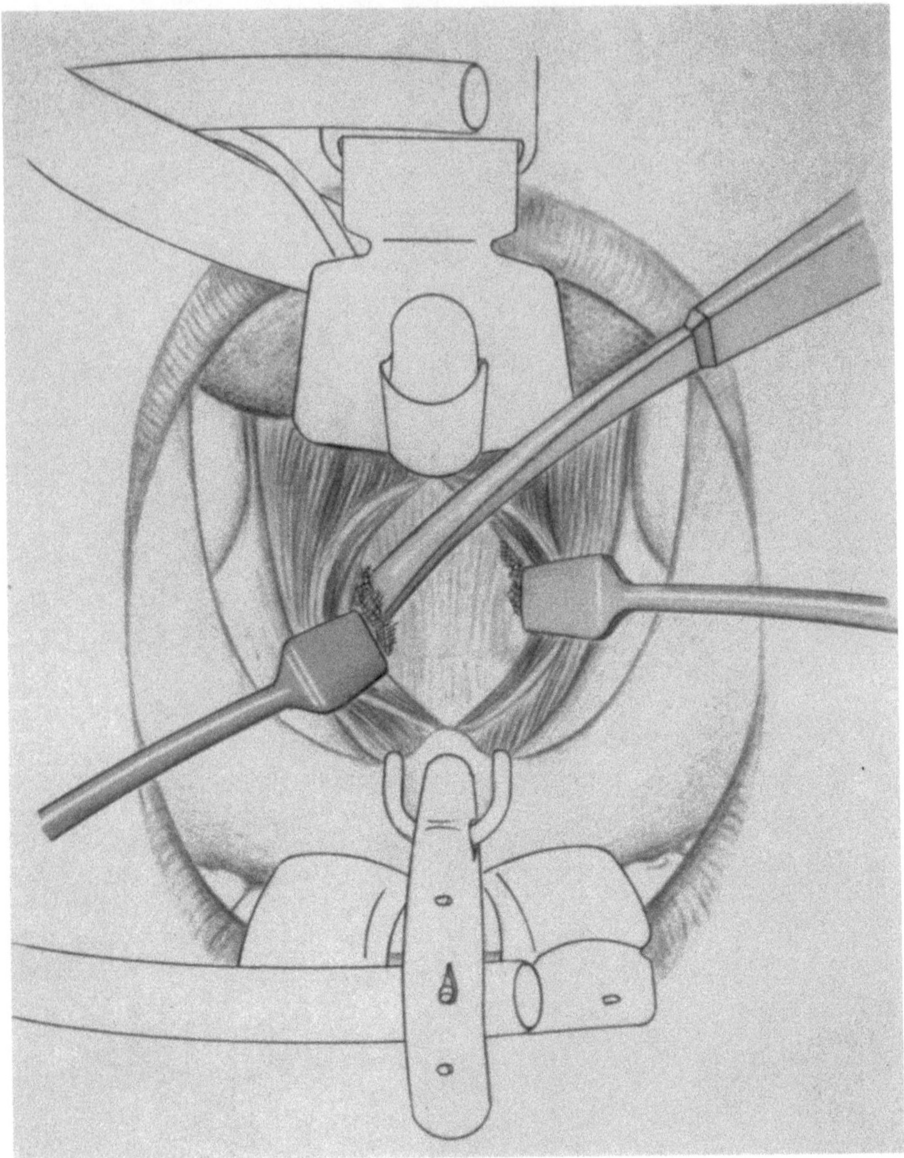

Fig. 8.8. At this point it is important to pack the lateral line of cleavage with Surgicel in order to control bleeding which will be significant as one is dissecting through the pharyngeal wall and the muscles

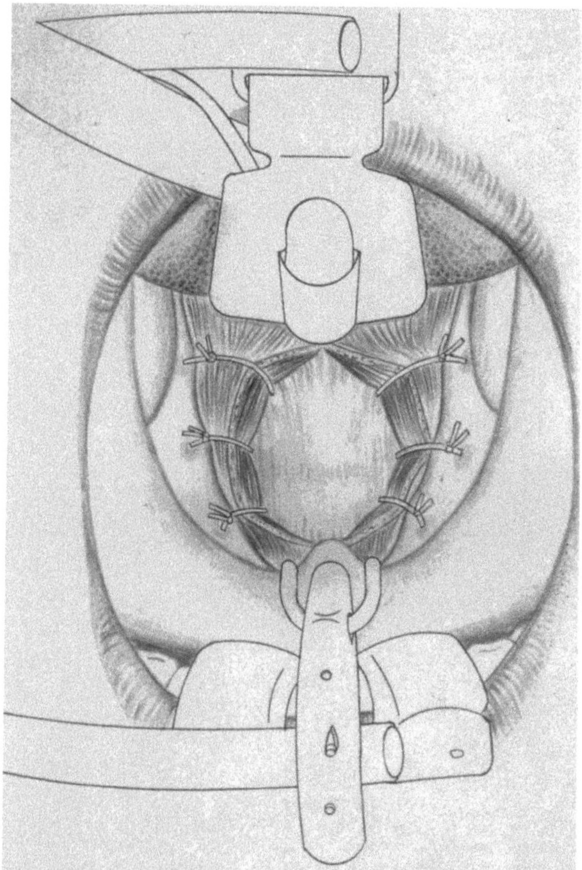

Fig. 8.9. Not only in order to achieve retraction but also to permit good illumination into the surgical site, the separated margins of the pharynx can be sutured on the lateral columns of the pharynx itself

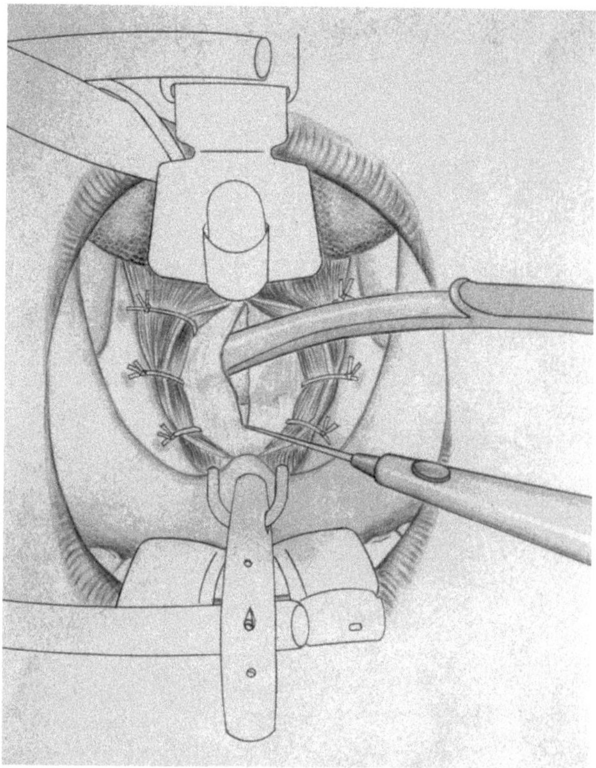

Fig. 8.10. The anterior longitudinal ligament is sectioned with electrocautery and this is followed by periosteal elevation laterally. The resulting cleavage plane will also need to be packed with Surgicel in order to control bleeding

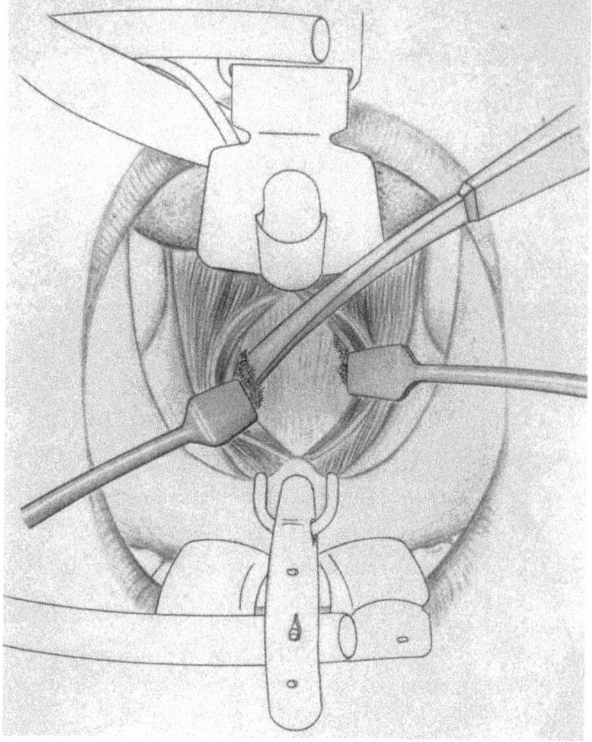

Fig. 8.11. The surface of the bone is now exposed. This exposure can extend from the arch of the atlas to both the odontoid process and the body of the axis, the C2–C3 disk, and the superior margin of the body of C3

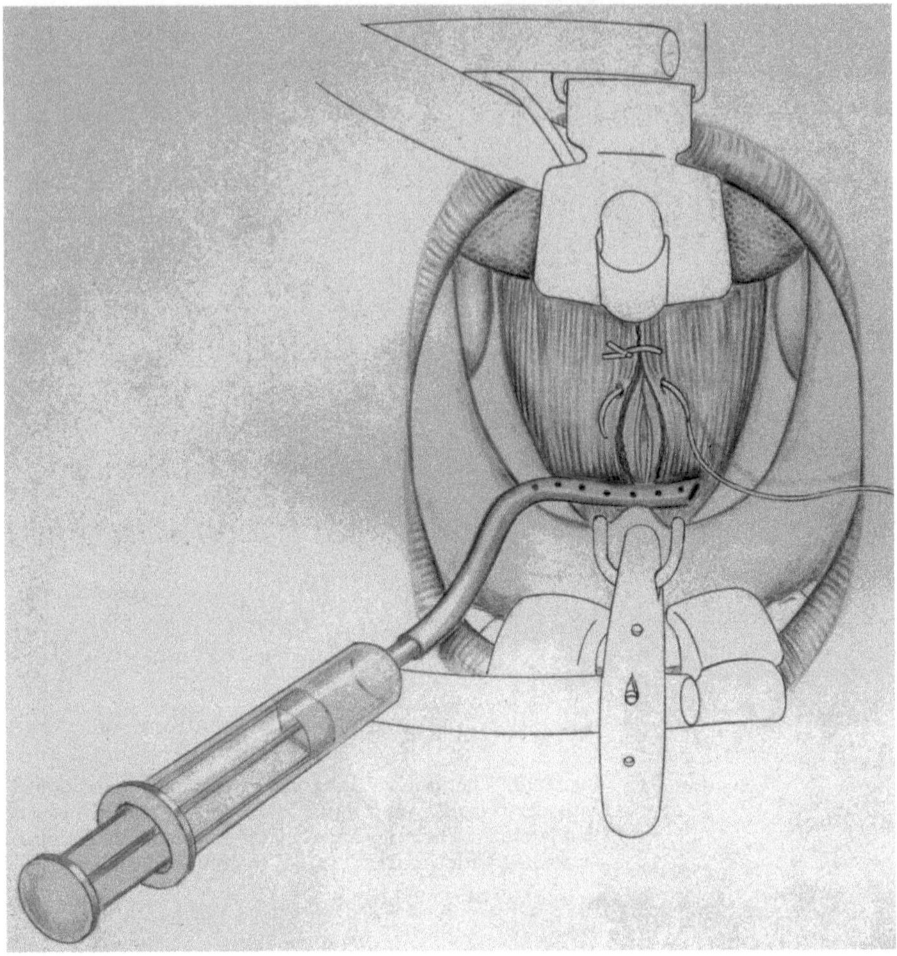

Fig. 8.12. Closure in layers is carried out with continuous suction lavage

Complications

It has alrady been mentioned that the transoral approach is known to produce significant complications and reports of this in the literature have discouraged its use. One must keep in mind that many of the complications described resulted from the inappropriate selection of this surgical approach in the treatment of severe post-traumatic instability or extensive tumor invasion, which would have been better treated with plating or massive grafts. If these are left aside, there still remain a group of complications that pertain specifically to this surgical approach. They can be divided into those that are intraoperative and those that are postoperative.

Intraoperative Complications

Soft Tissue Injury. The unskilled use of retractors or other instruments may injure the soft tissues including the tongue, the soft palate, and the lateral columns of the pharynx. These injuries range from small contusions to very extensive lacerations. When undertaking a particularly extensive resection, it is possible to reach laterally to the lateral masses of the atlas and axis. The enthusiastic use of a curet, spoon, or a clamp to remove a distant fragment may cause injury to the vertebral artery. This is an extremely serious complication since at this level the artery is inaccessible for purposes of suturing and can only be clamped. The resulting hemorrhage is often massive and hard to control. The acute ischemia produced in the basilar circulation may be lethal.

Neurological Injury. Remembering the depth of the surgical field from the surface and the difficulty in visualizing tissues, and in obtaining complete hemostasis, it is easy to imagine how it is possible to advance too far posteriorly and reach the dura mater or the spinal cord. Lesions of the dura mater may produce cerebrospinal fluid (CSF) fistulas, which may have serious consequences and must be sutured, even through this can be very difficult, the area should be covered with a fibrin paste. It is fortunate that the tentorial membrane and the posterior longitudinal ligament provide a fairly solid wall that protects the dura mater from inadvertent injury. In cases of metastic tumor with extensive invasion, involvement of this ligamentous barrier weakens it making it particularly susceptible to penetration by instruments and leading to a greater risk of injury to the subjacent dura mater and spinal cord. It is for these reasons that the operating microscope is particularly useful. As indicated above, this approach is not suitable for patients with an advanced and unstable condition, particularly one resulting from trauma and if this approach is used, it is likely that adequate reduction, fixation, or stabilization will be impossible.

Osteoarticular Injury. Severe trauma or extensive tumor destruction produce both instability and deformity. Through this approach massive grafts cannot be adequately anchored and will not be sufficiently incorporated. Internal fixation is either inadequately placed, insufficiently anchored, or protrudes into the pharynx because of the technical difficulty of operating in such a deep and difficult field.

Postoperative Complications

Soft tissues. Edema and swelling in the postoperative period may be severe enough to require tracheostomy. A hematoma, especially a large one, in this area may become secondarily infected and lead to deeper infections that extend throughout the operative site and the spine as well as produce esophageal and tracheal fistulas. The infection may spread to the mediastinum. The consequent scarring and adhesions that occur in the pharyngeal wall may produce severe dysphagia.

Neural tissues. Injury to the neural tissues, particularly when resulting in thrombosis of the medullary artery, may produce paresis, while if it involves the vertebral artery, it may produce cerebral damage. Breakdown of the surgical site may lead to CSF fistuals and eventually to meningitis.

Osteoarticular structures. If the postoperative immobilization of the patient is insufficient, disruption of the operative site may lead to instability. This is why halo traction is essential in all these cases in order to avoid movement and loosening of grafts or implants. If the surgical site becomes infected, this too may lead to a nasty osteomyelitis with subsequent loosening and displacement of the graft.

Prevention of the Complications

The most important factor that helps to avoid the disastrous complications described in the literature is the use of very strict criteria when selecting the transoral approach. One advantage today over many of the cases described in the past is the availability of antibiotics that help to minimize the risk of infection. An excellent understanding of the extent of the injury or disease may be obtained by using computed tomography (CT), computed tomographic myelography, and magnetic resonance imaging (MRI). Selective arteriography can also be helpful in defining the vascular pattern and in visualizing the characteristics of the operative site. The nature of the lesion for which a patient is about to be subjected to surgery can be ascertained with needle aspiration biopsy. All of these diagnostic methods should be used to select and plan the surgical procedure to be carried out.
Needle biopsies or even open biopsies of benign tumors or of localized malignancies and the drainage of abscesses are all correct elective indications for the transoral approach because they do not require internal immobilization. This approach is well suited for anterior decompression of the upper regions of the cervical cord, particularly in cases of congenital deformity or severe trauma such as posterior dislocation of the odontoid process.

The instrumentation is also important. The instruments used must be long and easy to grip in order to permit the full control that is essential to the delicate surgery to be carried out in the depth of the surgical field. Retractors that move aside tissues should also assure and maintain an unobstructed view of the operative site. Orotracheal tubes and drains should be kept out of the way during surgery. Frequent or continous rinsing of the operative field is important in order to maintain a clear, clean field. A very important final step at the end of the surgery is a careful inspection of the surgical wound, which should be cleansed and disinfected.

Mandible, Tongue, and Pharynx Splitting Approach

The approach described by Hall et al. in 1977 and by Stauffer in 1987 as their choice of approach to the cervical spine from the occipital region right down to C6 was the mandible, tongue, and pharynx splitting approach. In general surgery, it was recommended as the approach to the higher recesses of the pharynx by Kocher as far back as 1911. It is a direct, but rather disconcerting approach, which requires splitting of the lower lip, the mandible, the tongue, the floor of the mouth, the epiglottis, and the posterior pharynx down to, but not including, the hyoid bone. Transection of the hyoid bone can be added to achieve a greater exposure (transhyoid pharyngotomy).

Technique

The patient is placed in the supine position. A tracheotomy is essential prior to beginning this approach. The skin incision begins at the tip of the lower lip and extends down to the sublabial midline fossa (Fig. 8.13a). This incision should be accurately placed in the midline. In order to avoid visible scarring on the chin, it is advisable to make the incision across the inferior lip in the midline and then to move laterally around the chin and return to the midline just below the tip of the chin. The incision is then extended downwards, along the inferior edge of the mandible and into the neck along the midline. The upper tip of the incision in the lip can then be extended deeply through the oral mucosa. This will permit stripping of the mandible in preparation for osteotomy. The mandible should be transected accurately in midline between the two incisor teeth

(Fig. 8.13b). Reconstruction of the mandible with accurate realignment is sometimes facilitated by transection in such a way as to create an interlocking irregularity or a zig-zag pathway. A further step that we have found advantageous is to drill the holes for the reconstruction wires prior to osteotomy of the mandible, so that they are already in place at the time of reconstruction and closure.

The tongue is retracted through its apex. The incision through the tongue should be longitudinal, beginning on the dorsal surface following the median sulcus of tongue (Fig. 8.13c). The frenulum of the tongue must be divided exactly at the center in such a way as to separate the openings of the submandibular glands, which are on each side of the midline along the basal surface (Wharton's duct). The splitting of the tongue is completed by finishing the cut through its dorsal surface. Once this has been done, the floor of the mouth and the epiglottis are exposed (Fig. 8.13d). At this point, the plane of dissection is separated from the front of the vertebrae by the thickness of the posterior oropharyngeal wall. A longitudinal incision in the posterior pharynx is all that is needed to reach the vertebrae. This incision permits access as high as the clivus. Visualization may be improved either by retracting or, preferably, by dividing the uvula longitudinally. At the lower end of the incision, it is possible to reach as far as the body of C6.

Once the actual operative procedure has been completed, the layers are closed in the reverse order in which they were divided. Metal wires are used to restore the continuity of the mandible, using the holes prepared during the initial stages of the operation, as described above. Immobilization of the jaw is usually maintained for 3 weeks with dental wiring.

This approach has been described here for the sake of completeness: in fact, the dissection is quite aggressive and subject to significant postoperative difficulties. These include:

- Dental malocclusion which may result from minimal asymmetry in the realignment of the transected mandible.
- Possible loss of both motility and sensation in the tongue, partly because of scarring in the tongue itself or through the frenulum. In addition, scarring may produce occlusion of the openings of the salivary glands, which may in turn produce cystic distention of ducts (in the manner of ranulae).
- Scarring of the vestibular mucosa along the surface of the lip which may produce deformity that will interfere with lip function.

In view of the above, it is not surprising that this is not the preferred approach. It is known to be a difficult and undesirable approach that seldom provides any advantage over the direct transoral path or even the anterolateral retropharyngeal approaches, which are much more popular.

Submandibular Approach

Several extrapharyngeal transvisceral approaches have been described in the literature. These follow the cutaneous and visceral planes in the submandibular region. One of these is an approach above the hyoid bone and another the approach between the hyoid bone and the larynx.

The suprahyoid approach reaches the spine anteriorly along a pathway that begins with a horizontal skin incision. After the skin incision, the superficial veins (anterior jugular) must be tied. Splitting the superficial cervical fascia and the hyoid muscles (mylohyoid and geniohyoid) provides access to the pharyngeal wall. At this point, the hypoglottis must be protected, while the tongue and the floor of the mouth are retracted upwards to permit access to the pharyngeal space. The posterior wall of the pharynx is opened longitudinallly allowing the surgeon to reach the skeletal tissues. The subhyoid approach begins with a transverse cutaneous incision and crosses the subhyoid area which is reached after division of subhyoid muscle and the interhyroid membrane. This exposes the pharynx, which is opened at first anteriorly and then posteriorly in order to obtain access to the bone.

The submandibular approach is mentioned for the sake of completion. It is well known to have serious complications and high potential for iatrogenic injury. The consequences include speech difficulties because of laryngeal injury as well as difficulties in breathing and swallowing. The risk of infection is particularly high and even significantly higher with the transoral approach. In our experience, this approach has been totally supplanted by the extravisceral retropharyngeal approaches described. It has no advantages, but serious disadvantages.

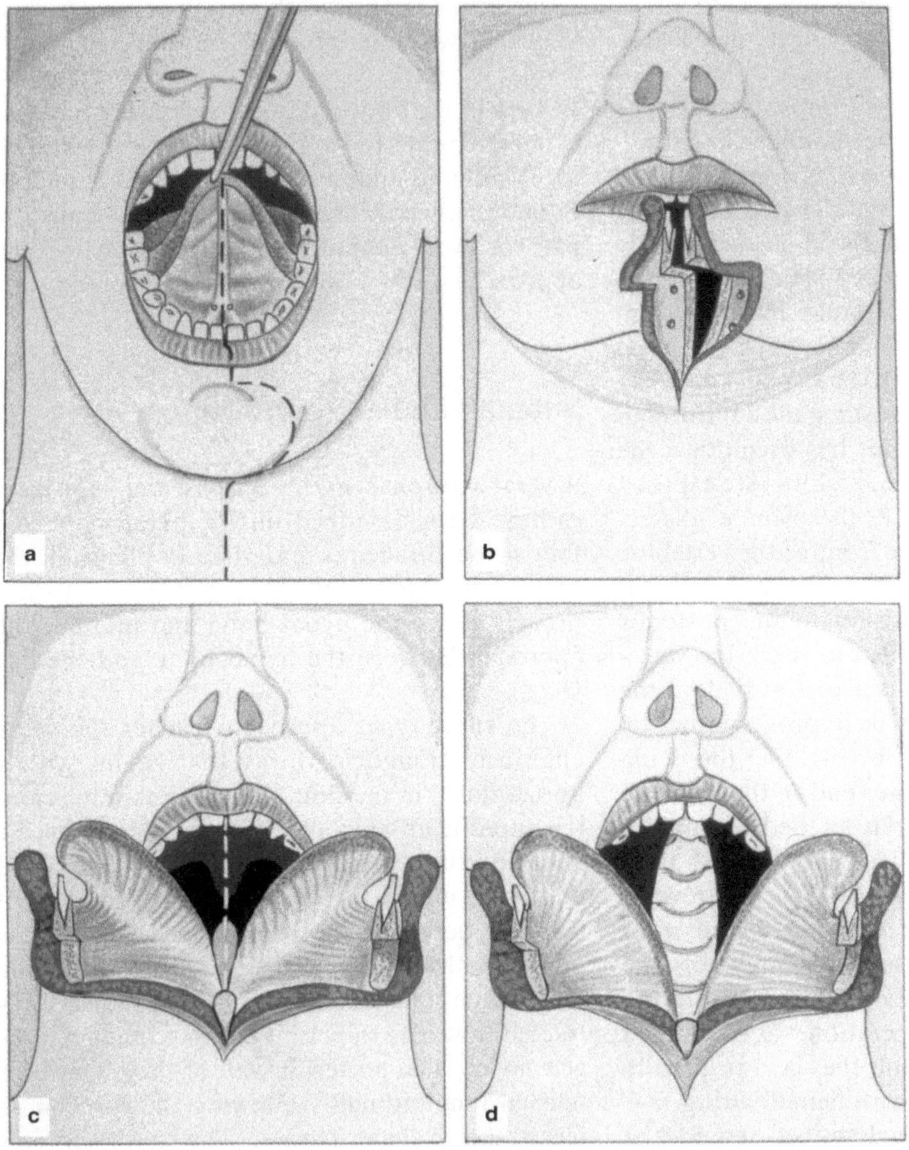

Fig. 8.13. a–d Various procedure steps of the transoral mandible and tonguesplitting approach: (*1*) incision of soft tissues (*2*) osteotomy of the mandible to ensure correct alignment of closure (*3*, *4*) access through tongue to the cervical spine

Anterolateral Approaches

High Presternocleidomastoid Approach (Retropharyngeal and Precarotid)

The high presternocleidomastoid approach gives easy access to the high cervical level of the spine all the way up to clivus. In fact, it can be regarded as a proximal or cephalad extension of the classical presternocleidomastoid approach described in cervical spine surgery. In general surgery, it is the preferred approach in the treatment of lesions of the pharynx and the proximal esophagus. In orthopedics, it has long been an established approach, described by Robinson and Smith in 1958, by De Andadre and MacNab in 1969, and by Riley in 1973. It is the author's personal preference and that expressed by many authors in the literature for the approach to the upper cervical spine and cervicooccipital level.

Technique

It is important that a halo be applied preoperatively. Not only is it useful at the conclusion of the procedure, but it is also particularly advantageous as a way of stabilizing the operative site during the procedure. With the patient awake, one applies the somatosensory evoked potential (SEP) electrodes preoperatively in order to obtain a baseline value while the patient is still alert, and a second baseline assessment is recorded once anesthesia has been induced. This is necessary because changes in the evoked potentials occur with the induction of anesthesia. During the surgical maneuvers it will be reassuring to have SEP monitoring, particularly when one is dealing with neural structures.

The patient is prepared as described and then placed in the supine position on the table. A firm support is placed under the neck in such a way as to position the head in a modest degree of hyperextension (Fig. 8.14). Once this has been done, the head can be fixed in the desired position to the head screen or the table for support, using a wide adhesive band. The chin and the upper jaw should only be free in cases where the necessity for dislocation of the mandible in order to achieve exposure is anticipated. In our experience, this precaution (as proposed by Riley in 1973) is unnecessary. We chose, as a routine, to fix the chin with an adhesive strip that extends along the horizontal arm of the mandible. The patient is now in a position where the face and head are rotated away from the side of the incision. The lobe of the ear must be retracted in order to permit the incision to be extended to the area of the mastoid. This is achieved by means of a suture through the earlobe, with the opposite ends of the sutures retracting in such a way as to pull the ear away from the site of the desired incision. Intubation must be transnasal so that the mouth is free and unobstructed. It is our practice to place a soft nasogastric tube in place preoperatively. This permits identification of the esophagus through palpation during dissection so as to avoid injury to that organ.

The skin incision starts in the submandibular region at a finger's breadth below the edge of the horizontal arm of the mandible. From the submental region, where the incision begins, the incision proceeds horizontally towards the mastoid at which point it veers downwards and somewhat medially along the anterior margin of the sternocleidomastoid muscle. The incision is extended downwards to the extent that one wants to expose the cervical spine. Ordinarily, it must only be extended to approximately the level of the cricoid cartilage, which is the level of C5 or possibly C6. In cases where greater exposure is required, it is possible to make a T-shaped incision: the first horizontally, as described above, and the second in front of the sternocleidomastoid muscle, extending the incision perpendicular to the first. As mentioned above, this is a proximal or cephalad extension of the classical approach to the lower cervical spine using a presternocleidomastoid incision; the steps of this approach are well known. The surgical dissection is performed between the visceral structures of the neck and the neurovascular bundle.

From the practical standpoint for those who are not familiar with this approach, and based on the author's experience, it is recommended that the incision be carried longitudinally downwards far distally on the cervical spine; the dissection should begin as described for the lower extension of the presternocleidomastoid approach. Once the prevertebral plane is reached, one can identify the retropharyngeal space and the neurovascular bundle. Only then should one begin the more proximal dissection. The steps in the lower longitudinal dissection should follow the usual approach of skin incision, with subsequent subcutaneous dissection and separation of the platysma. After this, incision of the superficial cervical fascia along the medial edge of the sternocleiomastoid muscle should be performed. Retraction of the sternocleidomastoid exposes the medial cervical fascia and the homohyoid muscle which can be incised between two ligatures (Fig. 8.15). The retropharyngeal region has now been reached relatively easily with separation of the visceral structures of the neck that include pharynx, esophagus, trachea, and thyroid, which are retracted medially, and the neurovascular bundle that includes carotid artery, jugular vein, and vagus nerve, which can be retracted laterally together with the sternocleidomastoid muscle. At this point, one can proceed proximally (cephalad) with dissection involving transection of the vessels which cross the operative field. Proceeding from below to above, one finds and must identify and ligate the superior thyroidal arteries and veins as well as the lingual and facial arteries (Fig. 8.16).

In practice, as one proceeds from below one must first identify the faciolingual thyroidal trunk. This is the common trunk for the thyroid, lingual, and facial veins which are tributaries of the jugular veins. On occasion, the thyroid vein may be independent and separate from the common trunk. When the origin is common, the main trunk must be ligated across the base, i.e., proximal to the origin, while the facial, lingual, and thyroid veins must be ligated more distally and individually. This step permits retraction of the venous channels exposing the hypoglossal nerve which courses immediately below these veins. Next, the superior thyroid artery is tied. If a higher level of exposure is needed, it may be necessary to identify and tie off the lingual artery and, occasionally, the facial artery. Great care must be taken in proximal dissection along the edge of the sternocleidomastoid muscle, particularly near its insertion at the mastoid, in order to avoid injury to the superficial cervical nerves and the spinal accessory nerve.

Having completed the dissection of the vertical portion of the incision, attention is turned to the horizontal portion of the incision. Here, dissection will require great care and attention. The dissections should proceed from the retromastoid area towards the front. The common facial vein and the retromandibular vein must be identified. The need to identify the retromandibular vein lies in the fact that it is a landmark in the identification of the superficial branches of the facial nerve (seventh cranial nerve), i.e., its cervicofacial terminal branch. It is easy for this nerve to be injured by retractors, as it can get pinched between the retractor and the hard mandibular bone. Once the lingual and facial vessels have been ligated, one can identify the posterior belly of the digastric muscle (Fig. 8.17). This will then provide access to the important structures of this area including the hypoglossal nerve that will be found crossing the operative field from the medial to the lateral side.

During dissection, the hypoglossal nerve can easily be identified during isolation of the lingual artery at a point where the artery passes posteriorly to the hyoglossal muscle. This suprahyoid area contains the structures that are well known in otorhinolaryngeal surgery. The hypoglossal nerve follows a path that defines two suprahyoid anatomical zones. The first is Béclard's triangle, which is denoted superiorly by the hypoglossal nerve, anteriorly by the stylohyoid muscle, and on the third side by the horn of the hyoid bone (Fig. 8.15). The second is Pirogoff's triangle, which is defined superiorly by the hypoglossal nerve, anteriorly by the myohyoid muscle, and posteriorly by the tendon of the digastric muscle. It is rarely necessary for the achievement of good exposure to divide the tendon of the digastric and of the stylohyoid muscles. Retraction of the digastric muscle will be sufficient to permit access to the prevertebral region. As part of the final exposure to the actual operative site, it is sometimes necessary to remove the submandibular gland from the field. This has been described by Riley and can be achieved by removal of the gland together with its vascular supply and salivary duct. We have seldom found this to be necessary in our experience, and, if it does interfere, it can easily be retracted rather than removed.

When identifying the hypoglossal nerve, one must also find the superior laryngeal nerve, which should be visible, once the faciolingual thyroid trunk is ligated, with the lingual artery above and the superior thyroid below. In fact this nerve should be found crossing the operative site from its origin at the vagus nerve, where it follows a path that is medial to the internal carotid and the first part of the lingual artery, it then proceeds downwards and medially on the lateral wall of the pharynx where it divides into an external and internal branch.

Once all the above structures have been identified and retracted, one has access to the surface of the spine. It is still necessary to retract the superior laryngeal nerve as it crosses from the jugulocarotid bundle. We have found it advisable not only to identify but also to free the nerve from its origin in the retrocarotid area all the way to its external portion along the pharyngeal wall. This will permit its retraction medially, if one is attempting to pass to a lower level, or laterally, if one is attempting to reach a higher level. On occasion, the nerve can be placed in such a position within the operative field that it need not be retracted. It should nevertheless be maintained under visual control at all times during the procedure. A retractor placed under the posterior belly of the digastric muscle and under the hypoglossal nerve and one placed laterally to move aside the neurovascular bundle will provide access to the vertebrae. An oblique path to the spine through the tissues described above will avoid excessive retraction of structures that can be injured if overstretched. One must therefore avoid a path that proceeds directly anteriorly.

The prevertebral space has now been reached, and transection of the deep cervical fascia will expose the prevertebral muscles. These will converge onto the anterior tubercle of the atlas. We use electrocautery to transect the anterior longitudinal ligament from below to above. Muscles are dissected away, exposing the external surface of the anterior arch of the atlas; the atlanto-occipital membrane that covers the clivus may be more difficult to visualize. Exposure will permit dissection along the body of the axis as far laterally as the joints between the lateral masses of the atlas and the axis. Inferiorly, the dissection can be extended to reach any desired operative levels.

At this point, one must use great care in dissecting laterally, for here one runs the risk of injuring the vertebral arteries. This is an all important precaution that must be kept in mind whenever one is dissecting along these upper vertebrae.

Indeed, we consider it mandatory that vertebral artery and carotid artery angiography be carried out preoperatively in cases of inflammatory or neoplastic causes of stenoses. Selective angiography in such cases is particularly useful if one is considering the possibility of preoperative embolization. It will also provide visualization of the arterial relationships with the bone which is particularly useful information that provides the surgeon with preknowledge of the vasculature in the area that he is going to enter surgically. We have found it advisable to use preoperative arteriography in a wide spectrum of diseases including cases of spondyloarthrosis, instability, and congenital narrowing. Having exposed the vertebral structures, the corrective surgery required by the pathology present can be performed, e.g., anterior decompression of the cord, removal of pathological tissue, reconstruction of a destroyed vertebral body, and stabilization with grafts or prosthetic devices. This approach is easier and safer than the transoral approach, which is known to be more difficult and to provide less exposure of the eventual operative site. The transoral approach makes it more difficult to achieve prosthetic stabilization through implants, and the approach is frought with the risk of sepsis.

Following the completion of the surgical procedure, closure is carried out in layers; the digastric muscle is closed from above, the thyroid from below, then the platysma, the subcutaneous layers, and finally, the skin. It is advisable to use suction drainage postoperatively. The patient should remain intubated for at least

24 hours postoperatively with the spine immobilized by the halo. The use of cortisone postoperatively is essential in order to avoid edema in the region, which can be massive and occasionally may be severe enough to require tracheotomy. Antibiotic coverage should be maintained for at least 5 days postoperatively.

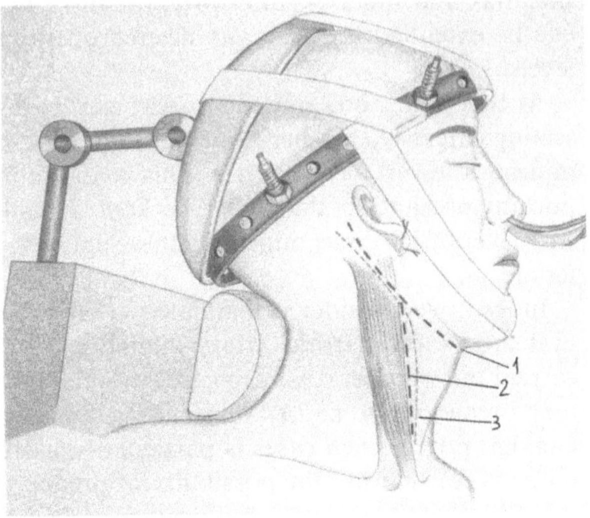

Fig. 8.14. The head is slightly turned away from the side of the incision and held in an adjustable head rest. The neck is rigidly supported. The elastic band holds only the superior part of the chin and mandible, leaving free the entire submandibular region. The nasogastric and nasotracheal tubes are put in place. A T-shaped incision is used, with the horizontal part (*1*) placed along the edge of the mandible, approximately 1 cm below it, and the vertical branch of the incision (*2*) following the edge of the sternocleidomastoid muscle. Also superimposed is the hockey stick incision (*3*). It descends from the supramandibular region to follow the anterior edge of the sternocleidomastoid muscle

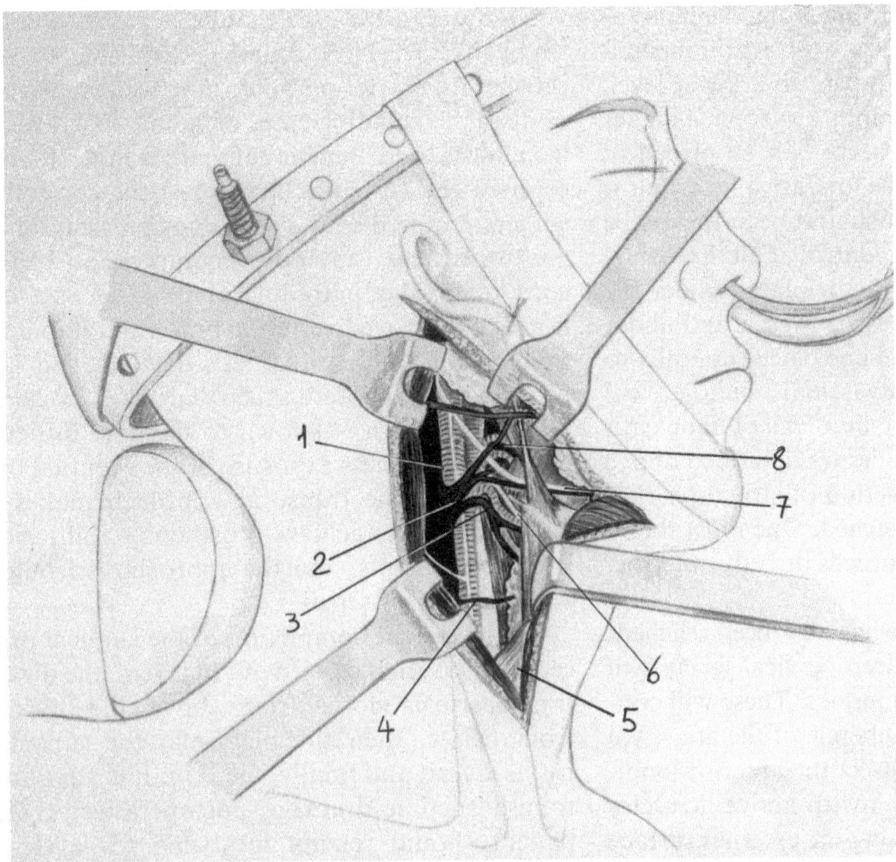

Fig. 8.15.

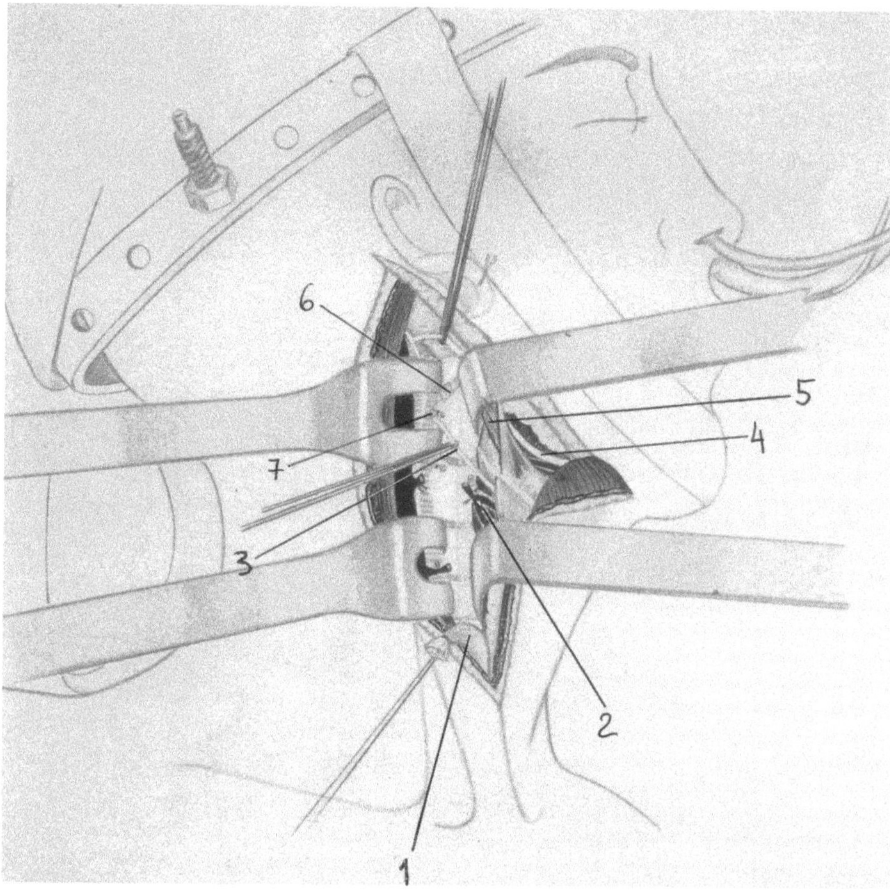

Fig. 8.16. In order to reach the prevertebral plane, the following structures must be identified and ligated (presented here in order from bottom to top). The omohyoid muscle should be cut between two ties, together with the middle cervical fascia (*1*). Above these are the superior thyroid artery and vein, and the thyrolinguofacial trunk, which here has been tied. Above these are the thyroid vein and artery, which here have been tied (*2*), then the superior laryngeal nerve (*3*), and the hypoglossal nerve (*4*). Next are the posterior belly of the digastric muscle (*5*) and the stylohyoid muscle, which are just below the external maxillary artery (or the facial artery) (*6*) and finally the lingual artery (*7*), which is here shown tied

Fig. 8.15. After the skin layers, platysma, and superficial cervical fascia have been cut, the sternocleidomastoid can be retracted laterally. Now exposed, and in order from top to bottom, we find the following structures: At the lowest level will be the carotid artery, the jugular vein, and the descending branch of the hypoglossal nerve (the vagus nerve is placed behind these two structures) (*1*), the thyrolinguofacial venous trunk (*2*) and the superior thyroid artery and vein (*3*). Continuing superiorly, one will see the medial thyroid vein (*4*), the omohyoid muscle (*5*) crossing the region overlying the middle cervical fascia, the superior laryngeal nerve (*6*), the hypoglossal nerve (*7*), and the lingual artery (*8*) that dips below the hypoglossal nerve. The next structures are the hypoglossal muscle and the submandibular gland, and finally, under the parotid gland, the external maxillary artery

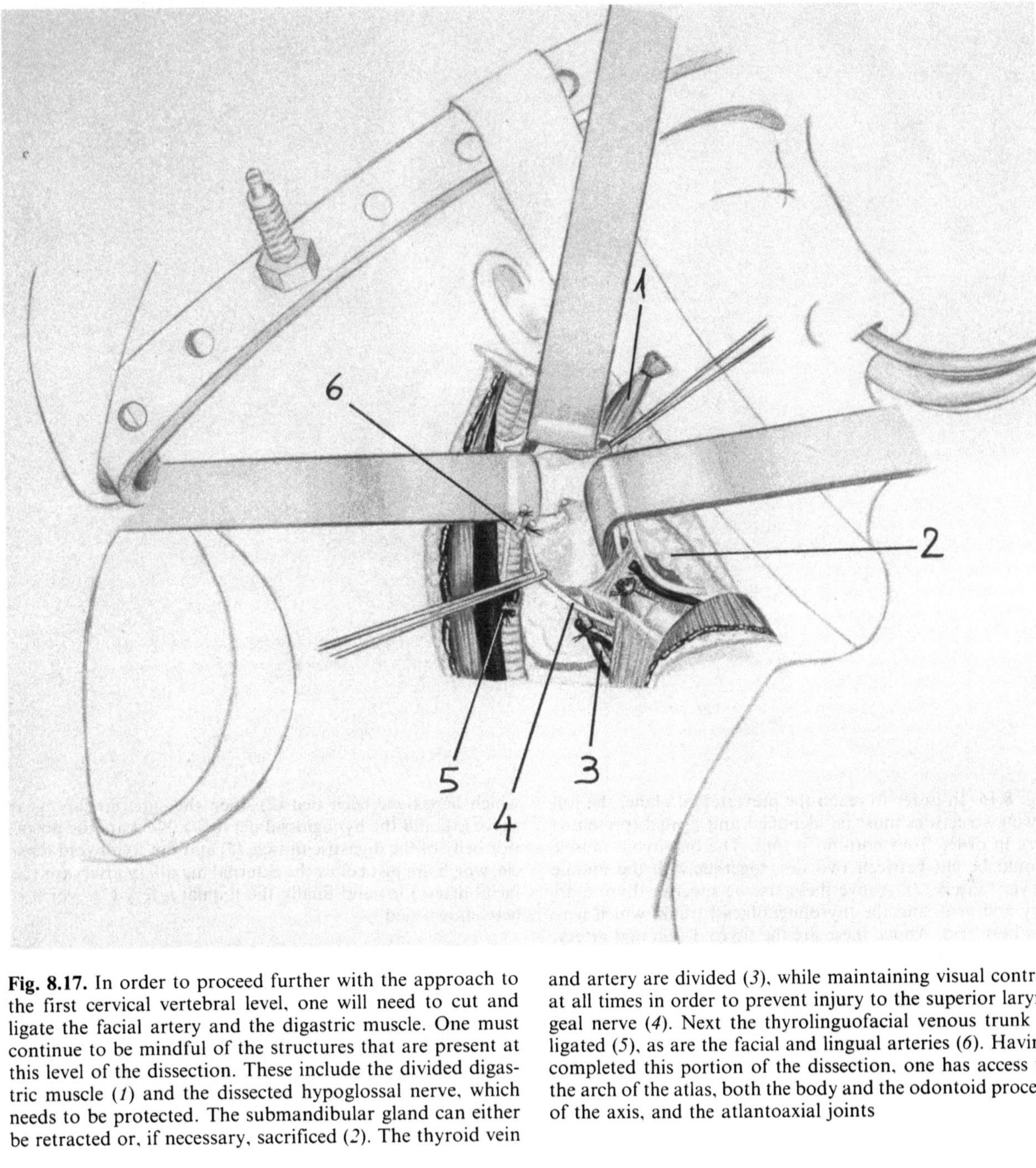

Fig. 8.17. In order to proceed further with the approach to the first cervical vertebral level, one will need to cut and ligate the facial artery and the digastric muscle. One must continue to be mindful of the structures that are present at this level of the dissection. These include the divided digastric muscle (*1*) and the dissected hypoglossal nerve, which needs to be protected. The submandibular gland can either be retracted or, if necessary, sacrificed (*2*). The thyroid vein and artery are divided (*3*), while maintaining visual control at all times in order to prevent injury to the superior laryngeal nerve (*4*). Next the thyrolinguofacial venous trunk is ligated (*5*), as are the facial and lingual arteries (*6*). Having completed this portion of the dissection, one has access to the arch of the atlas, both the body and the odontoid process of the axis, and the atlantoaxial joints

Indications

There are absolute indications for this approach which include:

1. The requirement for surgical intervention at the upper cervical spine, particularly at the cervico-occipital level when asepsis is essential and cannot be achieved through the more direct transoral approach.
2. The necessity to operate at more than one level of the cervical spine. This approach permits access from the base of the skull down through the entire cervical spine and, if necessary, to the first thoracic vertebra.

Complications

We will separate the intraoperative complications, which are the most serious, from the postoperative complications.
1. The intraoperative complications include injuries to the soft tissues and to the osteoligamentous structures. The most common are:

Soft Tissue and Visceral Injury. Perforation of the pharyngeal wall is the most commonly reported complication in the neck. The hypopharynx can be easily lacerated during dissection of the higher levels of the column, particularly if dissection is not undertaken with great care in cases with previous inflammatory disease in the area, or in cases associated with scarring and adhesions from previous surgery. The latter cases are obviously associated with the loss of the natural planes of cleavage and of the normal tissue relationships that guide the dissection. For this reason the use of a nasogastric tube is recommended that can be palpated during dissection, and which is helpful in the management of such intraoperative injuries. Should there be a laceration, the pharyngeal wall can be sutured immediately, and the tube which is already in place can then be used to feed the patient for the 3 weeks required for complete healing of the defect. Salivation may be reduced in the first postoperative days with the use of atropine. In addition, we have found it advisable to use soft bandaging of the neck. If the presence of an injury to the nasopharynx is not identified intraoperatively, then local sepsis may occur. This often leads to a fistula that will require surgical management, as it will not spontaneously close.

Resection of the submandibular gland may be associated with the formation of a fistulous tract. This follows inappropriate ligature of the salivary duct and usually results in the formation of an abscess and then a fistula because of retrograde passage of oral salivary contents into the stump of the resected duct, which can become obstructed and infected. Rarely, implantation of thyroid tissue has been reported, but this does not appear to have significant consequences.

Vascular Injury. The most frequent and most serious vascular complication is injury to the vertebral artery. It is possible for the injury to this artery to occur between the atlas and the axis, or even more proximally into the occipital foramen. As noted above, this occurs during dissection along the lateral wall of C1 and C2. While great care must be taken to avoid this, it is important that its occurrence be anticipated. The resulting hemorrhage can only be controlled by occluding the artery at an intervertebral level below that at which one is operating. This emergency repair runs the risk of injury to the nerve root and, hence, must be undertaken with great care. It is also possible for injuries to occur to the carotid artery and to the jugular vein, but these, fortunately, occur very rarely.

Neurological Injury. The most common complications of this approach are neurological. In the submandibular and perimandibular region, the operative field will be crossed by the facial nerve (seventh cranial nerve), the hypoglossal nerve (twelfth cranial nerve), and the superior laryngeal nerve. The latter is the one most often injured. The occurrence of these neurological injuries is directly related to the degree of traction and retraction used. Excessive pull on these structures will certainly result in injury. The intention of the operation is to reach the vertebral bodies. In order to achieve this, there is a tendency to emphasize medial retraction. This can be prevented by accurate mobilization before any traction is applied, by careful identification and dissection, and by using soft, manually controlled retractors rather than self-retaining or hard retractors.

Injury to the cord and to the nerve roots usually occurs as part of the specific surgical act being undertaken in the process of correcting the cause of the stenosis, and hence the risk of these is no different from that of surgery at all other levels of the spine.

2. The most frequent postoperative complications include:

- Pharyngeal or salivary fistula, as mentioned above
- Infection
- Glottic edema, which results from tissue injury and which in the most severe cases may require tracheostomy

Low Presternocleidomastoid Approach (Retropharyngeal and Precarotid)

The low presternocleidomastoid approach is the commonest direct approach to the middle and inferior cervical spine. It was first introduced as an approach to the proximal esophagus, and was then found to be an optimal approach to the cervical spine. In previous chapters, we have seen other possible approaches which, however, require great care and skill. This approach can also be used in combination with those described above to obtain access to the upper cervical spine. One may, therefore, say that this presternocleidomastoid approach between the soft tissues of the neck and the neurovascular bundle can be employed to expose any or all levels of the cervical spine from the skull all the way down to the first thoracic levels.

Technique

The patient is placed in the decubitus supine position; the head is taped to a head rest to hold it in a fixed position (Fig. 8.18). There should be slight hyperextension, but not excessive traction, since the latter will only produce tension in the soft tissues of the neck which will be detrimental to the exposure and the dissection. The combination of traction and excessive hyperextension of the head will compact tissue planes, making separation not only more difficult, but also more dangerous because structures will be difficult to identify and therefore greater traction may be required; the laryngeal nerves may be at particular risk as a result of such positioning.

Rigid support is essential for the neck. The spinal process should be well supported by a firm pillow. This will be found to be particularly helpful in preventing complications when one is applying considerable force to the vertebral body (e.g., insertion of bony grafts and the use of Cloward's drill). In such cases, a strong and rigid fixation and support of the neck assures a good counterbalance to any surgical force applied. We prefer a nasotracheal tube to an orotracheal tube, although both are possible. It is imperative that a nasogastric tube be inserted (Fig. 8.19) to act as a marker for the pharynx and esophagus during dissection. The tongue depressor and the dental protector should be such as to permit the mouth to remain slightly open. This will protect anchoring teeth in patients who have bridges or other partial and removable dental prostheses. The chin is taped to the bed and to the head rest, maintaining the slight hyperextension which should be barely sufficient to stretch the skin of the neck. The arms should be extended with a wrist band that will produce sufficient traction to lower the shoulder thereby permitting comfortable access to the patient. The gluteal region should be supported by a pillow, towel, or sheet in preparation for graft harvesting from the iliac crest. The legs should be well anchored in order to maintain stability on the surgical table. In fact, the patient should be in the anti-Trendelenburg position. This position will not only lower pressure, but favor venous drainage from the operative site in the neck.

The skin incision can be either longitudinal or transverse (Figs. 8.19, 8.20). The longitudinal incision is better for wider multilevel exposure, or when it is essential to have total intraoperative access and visual control of the entire neck. This is usually required when there are tumors, infections, or severe traumatic disruptions. The transverse incision may be preferable when one needs to operate at only one level such as in the relief of stenosis associated with arthrosis. The transverse incision is cosmetically more acceptable. We have modified the longitudinal incision in such a way that we do not follow the border of the stenocleidomastoid muscle proximally. We actually follow a line halfway between the mastoid process and the thyroid cartilage which is more central in the neck. The incision is then extended downwards until it reaches the medial border of the sternocleidomastoid muscle at the level of the cricoid cartilage. The incision then proceeds anteriorly to the sternocleidomastoid muscle, all the way down to the superior margin of the clavicle. This modification allows greater access to the front of the vertebral body than would be possible with a more lateral incision.

The approach on the right side will be described here. It must be pointed out that the operating surgeon's dominant hand will determine the position which is more comfortable with reference to the patient. Usually a right-handed surgeon will be more at home operating from the right side: all aspects of surgical operations on bone such as the use of chisels, scalpels, or curets favor a right-handed surgeon operating from the right side. In the past there has been much discussion in the literature as to whether the right or left side is preferable, particularly with reference to complications arising from the recurrent nerve. Injury to the recurrent laryngeal nerves produces vocal disturbances which not only are worrisome and cause discomfort to the patient, but which may be irreversible. It must be remembered that the path of the recurrent laryngeal nerves differs on the right and left sides. On the left it has a longer course, originating more distally in the vagus within the thorax, passing under the aortic arch, and then following the space between the esophagus and trachea in the neck. On the right side the nerve follows a much shorter course. It arises quite proximally in the upper thorax, passes under the subclavian artery, and courses between the trachea and the esophagus. It is at a much more superficial and, hence, more exposed level. In addition, it may follow a number of differing anatomical pathways. It has been reported to arise as proximal as the inferior thyroid artery, which makes it particularly vulnerable to injury if this position is not immediately identified as a variant of normal. Injury may occur because of direct traction or retraction with excessive force if the nerve is stretched between two planes that are being separated and may lead to aprosexia or axonotmesis. It is very important that these possible anatomical variations be kept in mind by the surgeon at all times during the procedure. The right-handed surgeon who uses the approach from the right side therefore has the immediate advantage that he does not have to face the problems that will be encountered if a left-sided approach is used. In our experience of over 500 patients with a variety of pathological situations, vocal complications were of the order of 6% and all were transient and of short duration. In addition to the anatomical variants, the short course of the right recurrent laryngeal nerve makes it particularly susceptible to injury if it is stretched by careless retraction; its shortness makes it less flexible and more easily injured. For this reason we use smooth, well-rounded malleable retractors which are hand held. Self-retaining retractors, designed to separate the soft tissues from the neurovascular bundle, should be categorically avoided.

The incision should cross the skin and subcutaneous tissue. Bleeding vessels, which are usually branches of the external jugular vein, should be ligated in the subcutaneous tissue (Fig. 8.21). The platysma is split and the superficial tissues can safely be retracted with a self-retaining retractor. In the exposed field, the sternocleidomastoid muscle and the superficial cervical fascia can be readily identified. The latter is split along the anterior margin of the sternocleidomastoid by sharp dissection (Fig. 8.22) and then retracted. Retraction of the sternocleidomastoid exposes the underlying neurovascular bundle (Fig. 8.23). The omohyoid muscle will next be apparent crossing the field in the middle cervical fascia. If this fascia is lifted at the proximal surface of the omohyoid muscle, it can be divided along its full length and can be separated with blunt dissection from the underlying tissue all the way down to the distal end of the incision. This entire plane can be exposed if the fascia is lifted. Sutures are passed through the belly of the omohyoid muscle in its middle portion (Fig. 8.24) and are then used to raise the muscle and the middle cervical fascia. The muscle and fascia can be transected with electrocautery, with the split extended to the limit of the exposure distally. Great care must be used not to reach the internal jugular vein at the distal end of the incision. This vein is usually quite superficial, but its course is subject to great anatomical variation. Injuries to the vein are rendered more difficult to control because of the tension in the tissues that tends to retract the vessel out of the operative field making it more difficult to reach and to ligate.

The ends of the omohyoid muscle and the cervical fascia, once retracted, expose the neurovascular bundle in the carotid sheath (Fig. 8.25). The artery is smaller and pulsating, the vein is wider and softer, and the vagus nerve, which lies posteriorly, is not in direct field of vision. Next to the neurovascular bundle, the thyroid gland is covered by the sternohyoid muscle and the sternothyroid muscle. These medial structures cover the esophagus. At the middle of the incision proximally at the level at which the omohyoid muscle was divided, if the carotid sheath is protected, one can easily slide between it and the visceral structures medially. The middle thyroid vein, which may or may not be present, is sometimes found at this point and must be ligated. Blunt dissection with the finger will find a plane of tissue separation between the neurovascular bundle laterally and the medial structures that include the thyroid gland and muscles as described above. Once this blunt dissection has been completed, the deep cervical fascia will be exposed (Figs. 8.26, 8.27). At this point blunt dissection will open up the retropharyngeal plane, exposing the vertebral surface. It may now be necessary to confirm the cervical levels exposed radiographically (Fig. 8.28).

In order to expose the higher levels of the cervical spine, the superior thyroid artery and vein, and often the thyroid, lingual, and facial trunks, may need to be sacrificed. On the other hand, if one is intending to reach the lower cervical levels, then one encounters the inferior thyroid vein and arteries. This vein can be safely sacrificed and ligated. The inferior thyroid artery however need not be sacrificed. Anatomically, it originates in the carotid and follows a circuitous path of great convexity proximally before turning towards the thyroid gland. If one frees its entire length, then one gains sufficient length for it to be retracted out of the operative field quite safely and there is no necessity to sacrifice it. However, when one is intending to reach the C7-T1 vertebral level, the artery remains in the path of the dissection and in this case one cannot avoid sacrificing it. We have not encountered functional changes in the thyroid, when the thyroid vessels were ligated as described.

Dissection has now reached the prevertebral plane. Once the deep cervical fascia has been divided by electrocautery along with the anterior longitudinal ligament (Fig. 8.12), it can be peeled off the periosteal surface of the vertebral bodies. The dissection can be carried laterally as required, but it is usually not necessary to dissect as far as the transverse apophyses. The only instances when this is necessary is when one needs to reach the vertebral arteries, but even in such cases one should not extend beyond the lateral margins of the bodies in order to avoid the cervical sympathetic chain. Once the longitudinal ligament has been lifted from the vertebral body, there may be extensive bleeding from the bone which often requires sealing with bone wax. The bleeding from the surface of the vertebral body becomes even greater as one moves laterally. We have found it advantageous to use Surgicel smeared onto the bony surfaces with a spatula as soon as the bone surface is exposed, even before the tissues are retracted (Fig. 8.30). This should be done on all surfaces exposed by dissection, bilaterally. Not only will this control bleeding, but it will help raise the edges of the anterior longitudinal ligament which has been split, making the use of a self-retaining retractor easier (Fig. 8.31). As noted above, in order to avoid injuries to the soft tissues of the neck, the self-retaining retractor should be applied only to the anterior longitudinal ligament and its arms

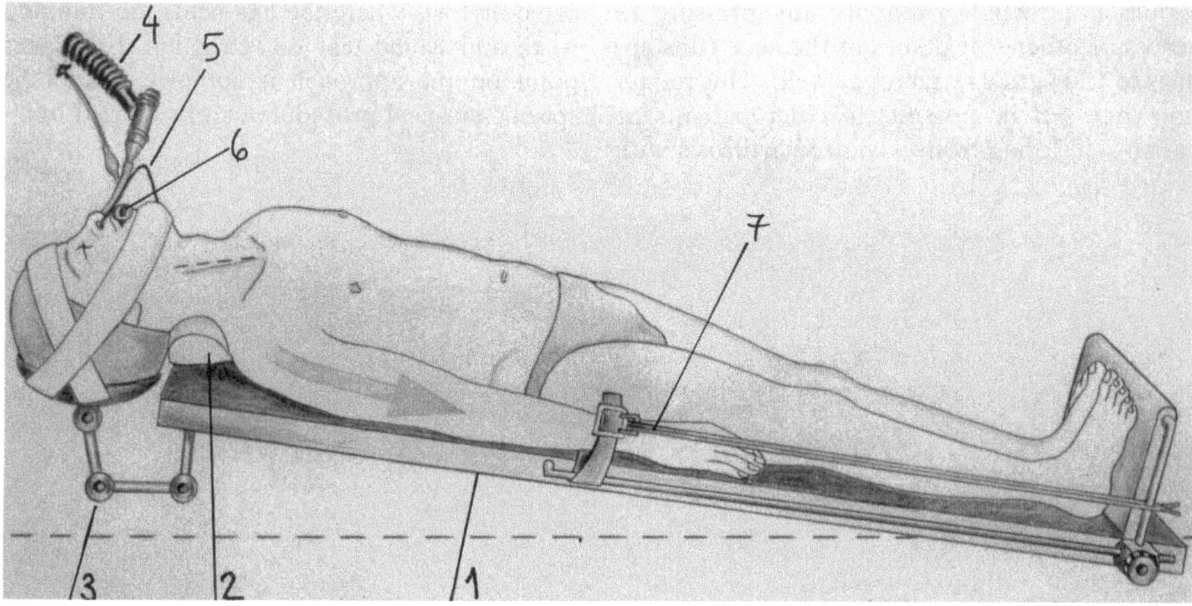

Fig. 8.18. The patient is placed in the anti-Trendelenburg position (*1*) with a rigid support under the neck (*2*). The head is supported by a mobile and adjustable rest (*3*). Elastic bandages hold the head in position with slight hyperextension of the chin. Nasotracheal (*4*) and nasogastric (*5*) intubation is shown in place along with a tube-type tongue depressor (*6*). The arm is subjected to traction (*7*) in order to lower the shoulder. In the neck, one can see the placement of the typical presternocleidomastoid incision

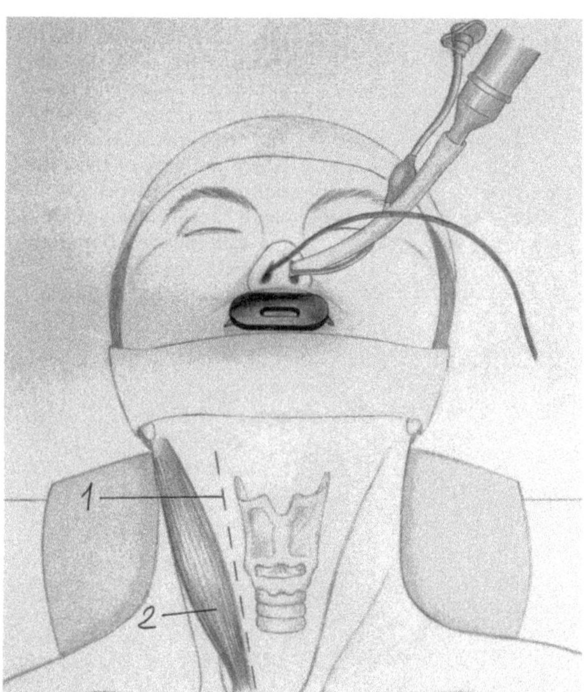

Fig. 8.19. A detail of Fig. 8.18 showing the incision (*1*) which superiorly is quite medial, but at the lower end of which approximates the anterior edge of the spernocleidomastoid muscle (*2*). This placement of the incision is essential in order to reach the higher levels of the cervical spine; a more lateral skin incision in the more typical presternocleidomastoid area would require a greater degree of retraction. The incision illustrated provides a more direct approach to the vertebral surface and particularly its medial or central region

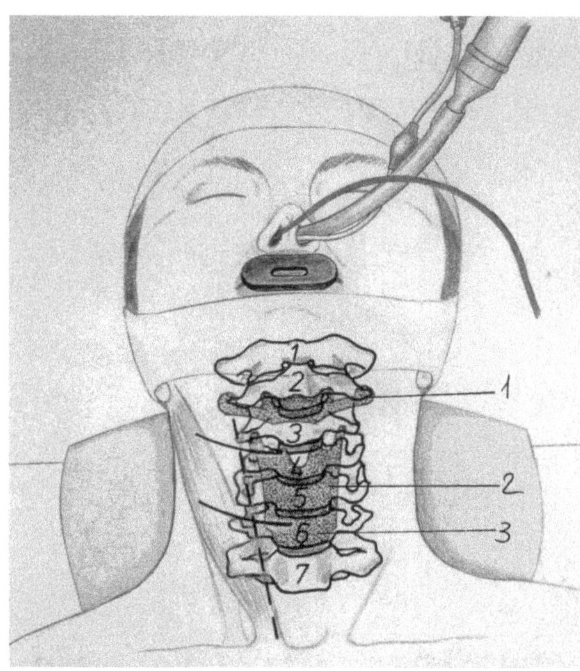

Fig. 8.20. Anatomical relationships that are used in determining the more esthetically acceptable placement of incision for access to one or two vertebral levels. The hyoid bone (*1*), the thyroid cartilage (*2*), and the cricoid cartilage (*3*) serve as reference points for the level of access for C3–C4, C4–C5, and C5–C6, respectively

should not include or apply any pressure to nerves or other soft tissues of the neck (this applies to Cloward's retractor as well). This retraction may not be possible in older patients or patients suffering from advanced arthrosis with osteophytosis where the ligaments are thin and weak and would tear on retraction. From this point on the approach is completed, and the specific surgical procedure can be carried out.

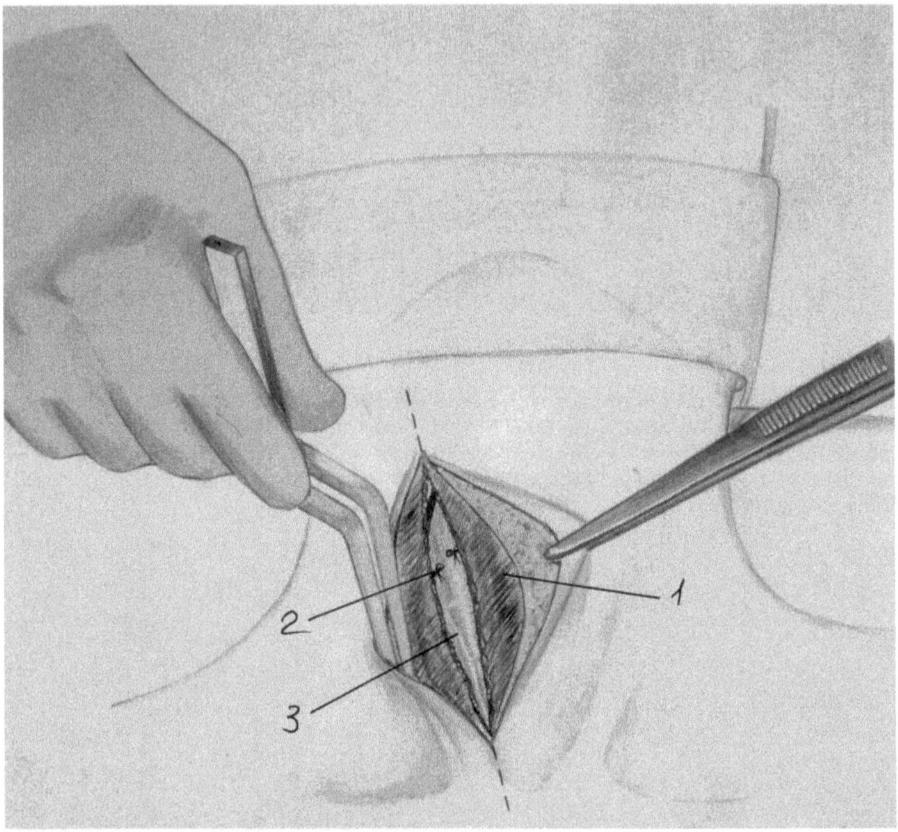

Fig. 8.21. Following the incision of the skin, the subcutaneous tissue and the platysma (*1*) are exposed and the superficial veins which are part of the external jugular network are tied (*2*). The sternocleidomastoid muscle (*3*) is now exposed and covered by the middle cervical fascia

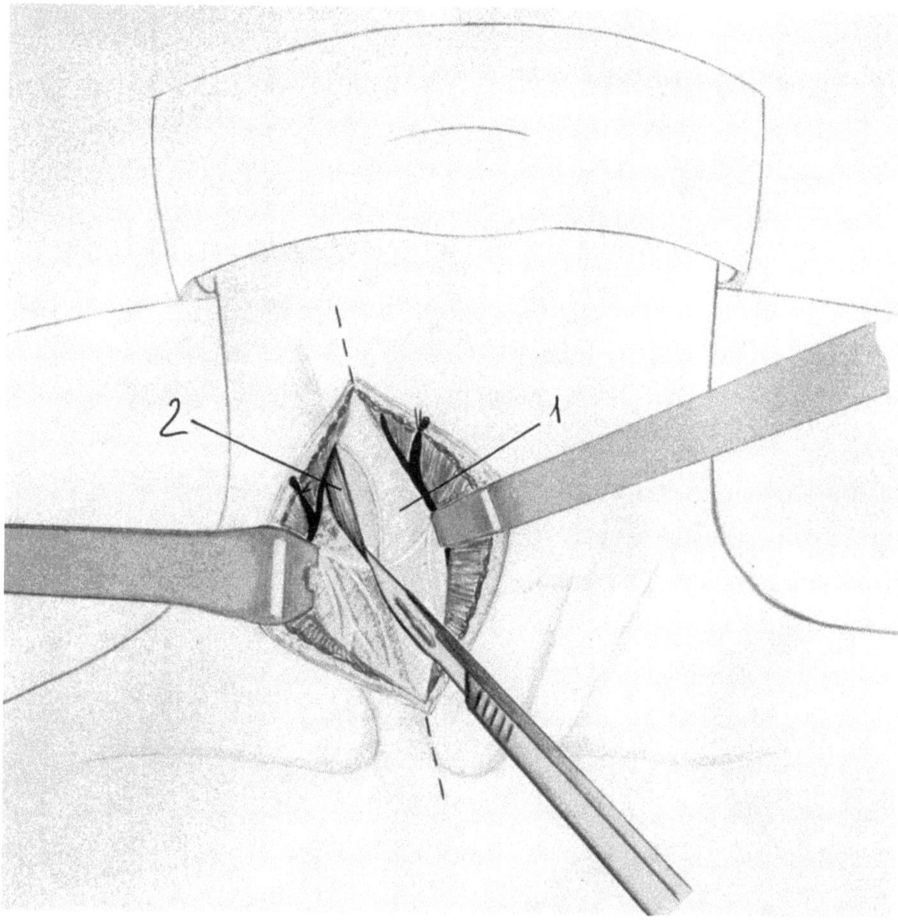

Fig. 8.22. The scalpel cuts the superficial cervical fascia (*1*) exactly at the edge of the sternocleidomastoid muscle (*2*). Following the edge of the muscle allows the muscle to act as a delineating margin facilitating the alignment of the incision

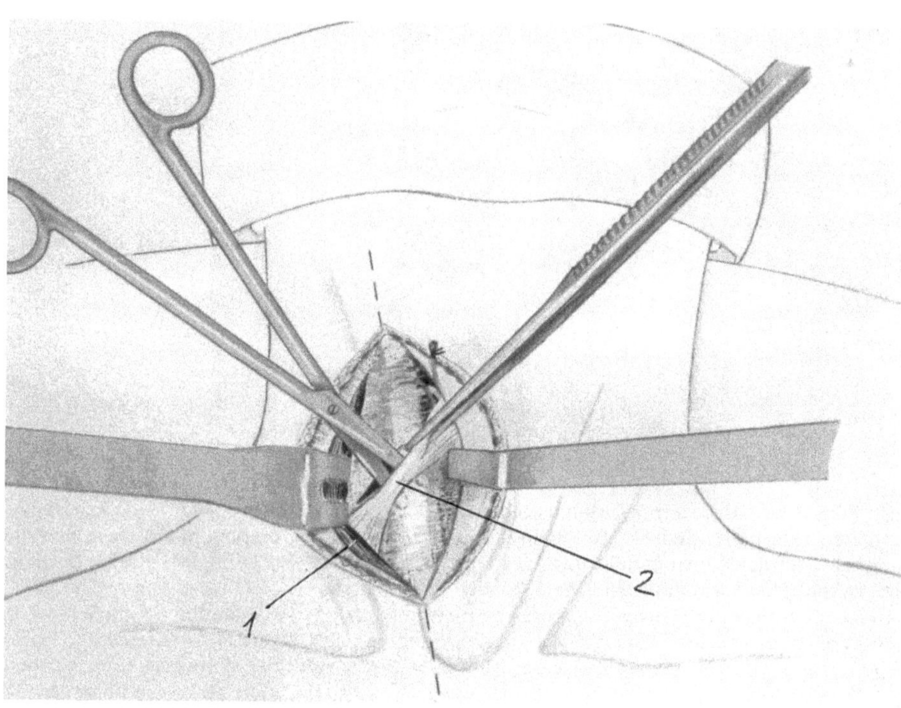

Fig. 8.23. Once the sternocleidomastoid muscle has been retracted exteriorly (*1*), one can identify the middle cervical fascia in the underlying plane of the section that envelops the omohyoid muscle (*2*). The omohyoid muscle is raised with the tips of the scissors, permitting a blunt instrument to be used to raise it along with the distal portion of the middle cervical fascia

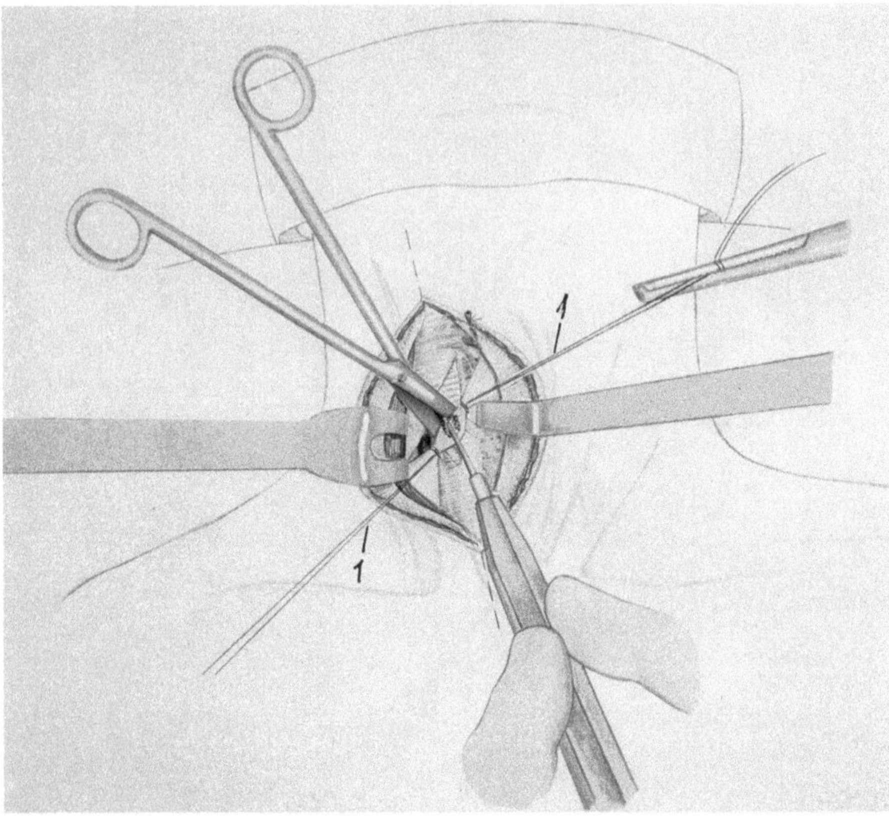

Fig. 8.24. Two sutures (*1*) are placed proximally and distally in the omohyoid muscle (these will be used for resuturing the muscle at the end of the surgical procedure). The muscle is raised with blunt scissors which protect the fascia and the muscular plane. The muscle is incised along with the fascia using electrocautery

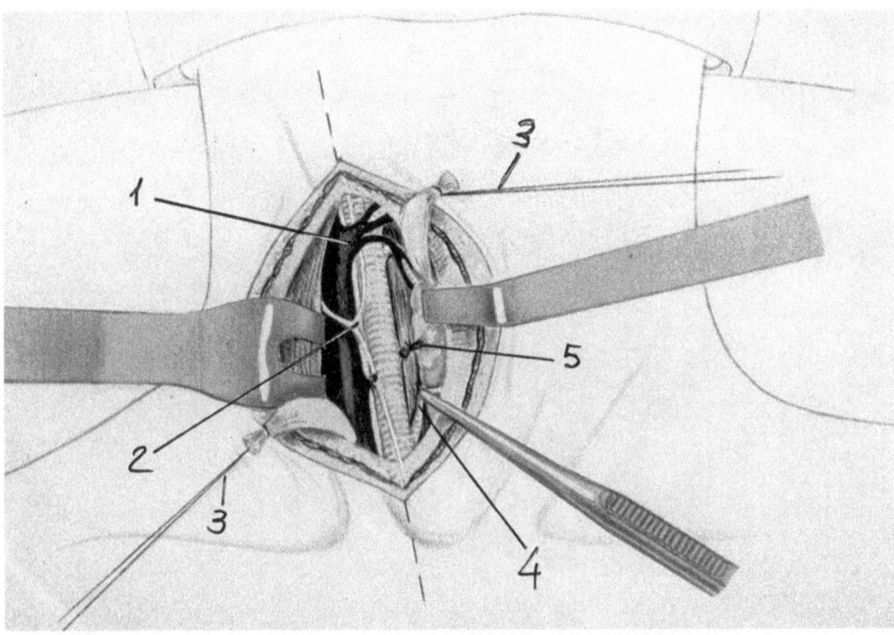

Fig. 8.25. Once the sternocleidomastoid muscle has been retracted externally, and the two bellies of the omohyoid have been retracted, using the sutures described in Fig. 8.24, the thyroid gland will appear in the operative field and can be retracted medially. This will expose the most important structures of this region. This includes the thyrolinguofacial venous trunk (*1*) and the neurovascular bundle of the neck (the common carotid, the internal jugular vein, the vagus nerve, and the descending branch of the hypoglossal, *2*). The omohyoid muscle is identified by its ligature (*3*). The inferior thyroid artery must be identified and dissected free, so as to enable one to move it freely. It need not be ligated unless one is intending to reach levels below C6 (*4*). The middle thyroid vein is shown tied off (*5*); it is found crossing the level of the hyoid muscles to reach the thyroid. Immediately below it is the wall of the pharynx

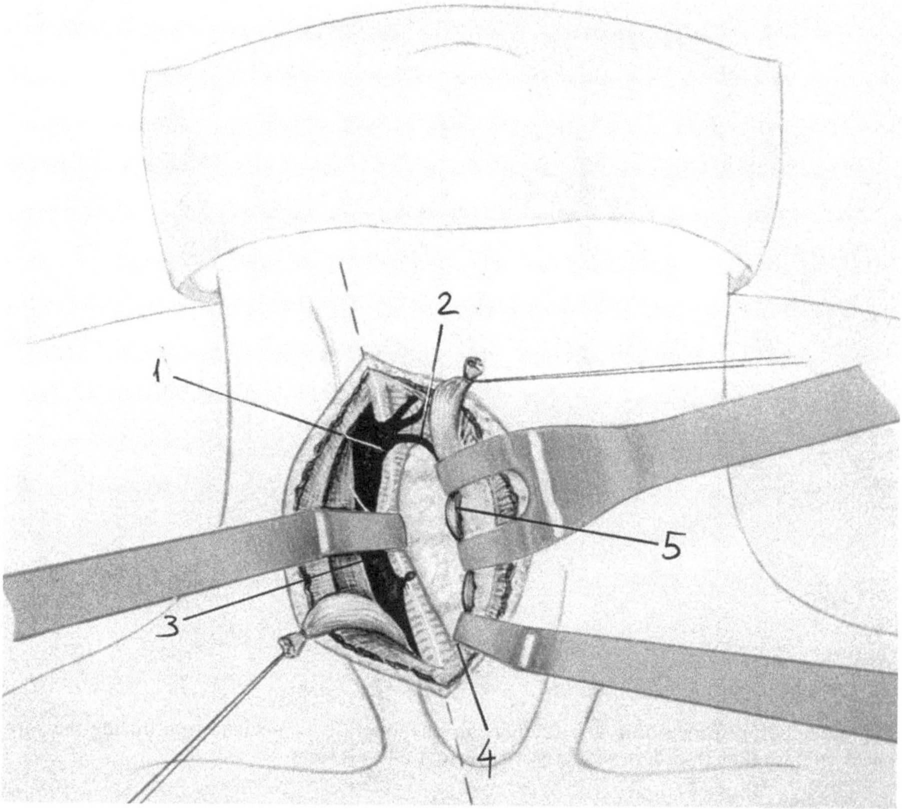

Fig. 8.26. By retracting the neurovascular bundle of the neck laterally and the larynx and wall of the pharynx medially, one reaches the prevertebral plane which is covered by the deep cervical fascia. The structures identifiable in the drawing include: the thyrolinguofacial venous trunk (*1*), the artery and superior thyroid vein remaining in their bed (*2*), the neurovascular bundle of the neck, retracted laterally (*3*), the inferior thyroid artery, which is dissected out and retracted (*4*), the thyroid and the wall of the pharynx, which are medially retracted (*5*)

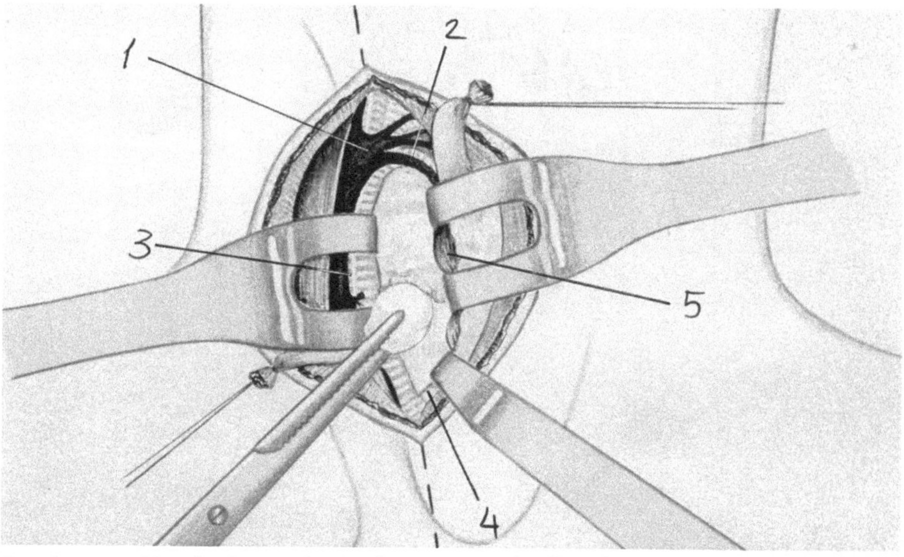

Fig. 8.27. Deeply, the vertebral plane is covered by the deep cervical fascia which is seen being wiped with a sponge held by a Cocker forceps. This is used to free the deep cervical fascia in the prevertebral space, and also to dissect out the posterior wall of the pharynx superiorly and medially. Seen in the diagram are: the thyrolinguofacial venous trunk (*1*), the superior thyroid vein and artery (*2*), the neurovascular bundle of the neck (*3*), the inferior thyroid artery, lying free but being retracted (*4*), the wall of the pharynx and the thyroid being retracted medially (*5*)

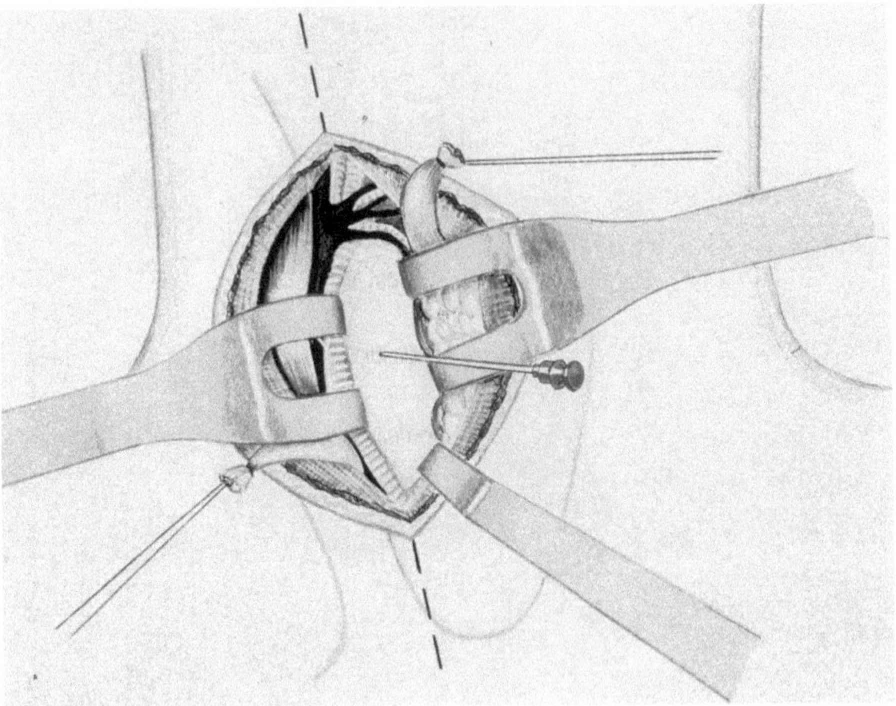

Fig. 8.28. Before proceeding any further, an intraoperative check film is taken in order to identify the vertebral levels for orientation during the surgical procedure

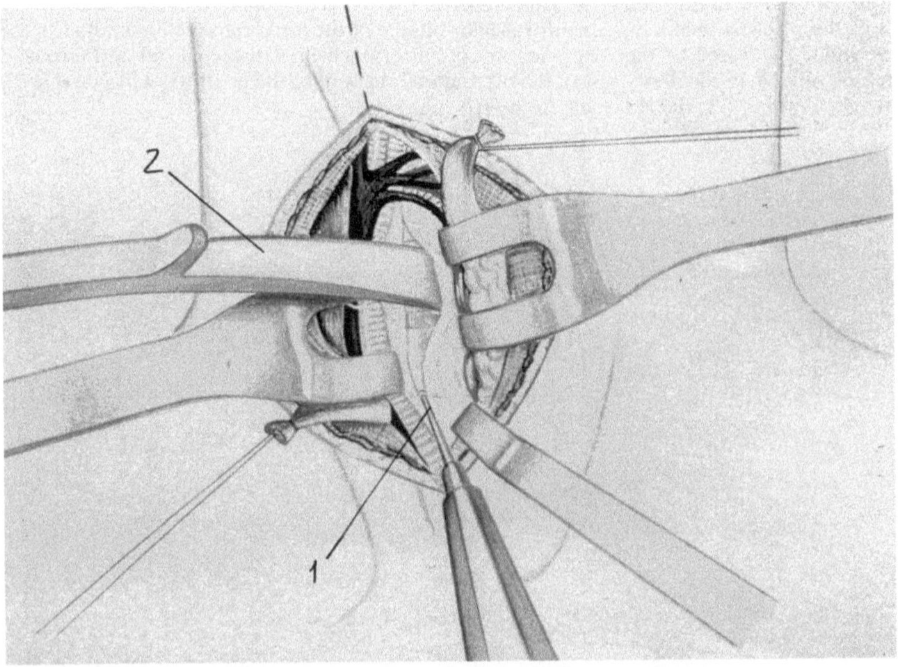

Fig. 8.29. Electrocautery is used (*1*) in order to cut the anterior longitudinal ligament. This provides access to the actual vertebral surface. Periosteal elevation (*2*) is extended along the surface of the vertebral body as far as the lateral edge. The anatomical relationships are identical to those described in the previous figures

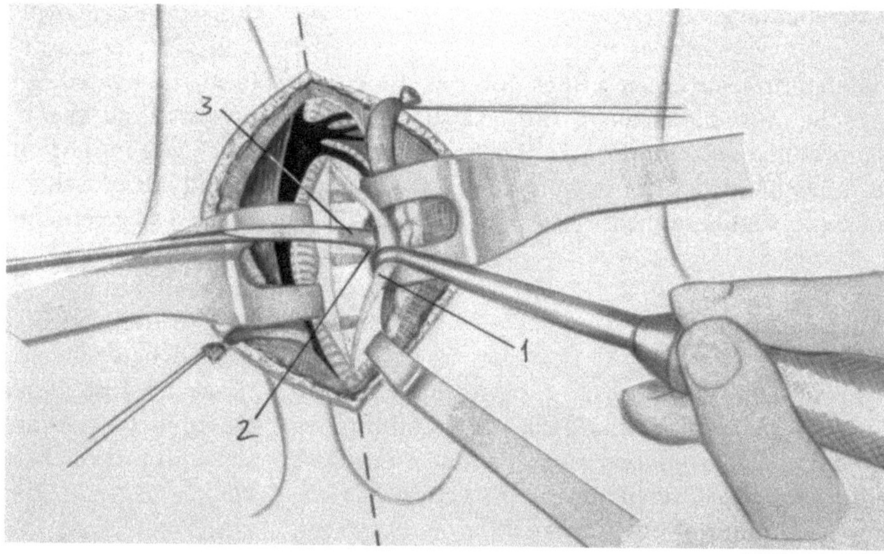

Fig. 8.30. The anterior longitudinal ligament (*1*) ist detached as far as the most lateral portion of the body, keeping in mind that this is a step that will create extensive bleeding. Surgicel (*2*) is packed with a rounded spatula into the cleavage between the periosteum and the subjacent bone (*3*). Bilateral packing with Surgicel is important in controlling bleeding in the operative field

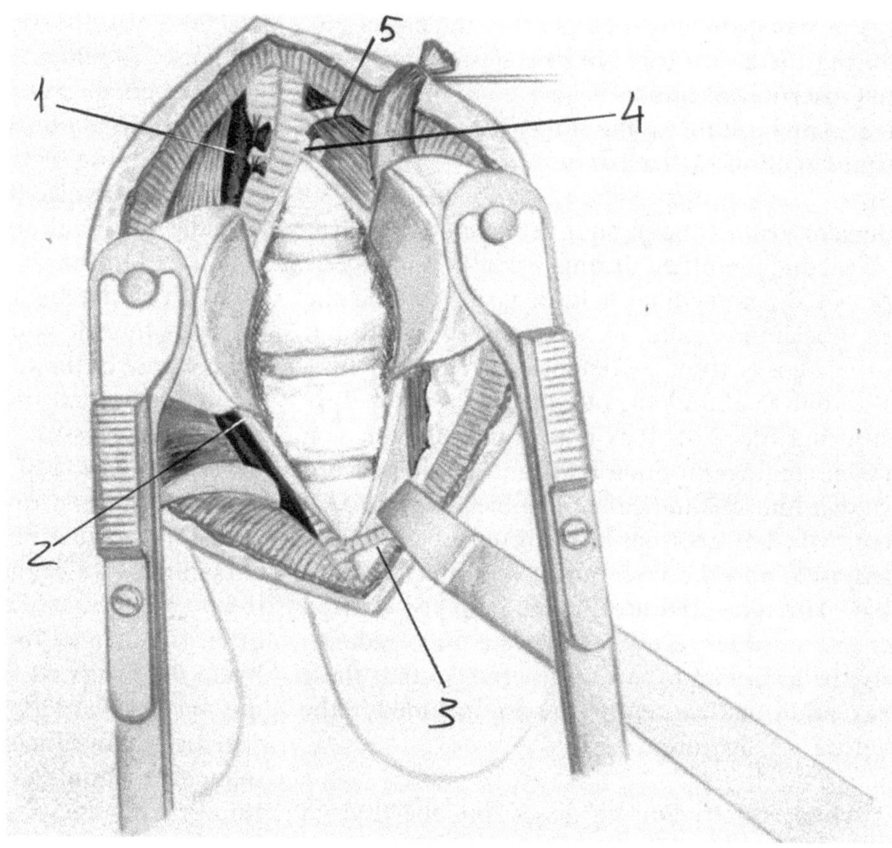

Fig. 8.31. Having reached the prevertebral plane, a self-retaining retractor can be used, but it is best anchored along the edges of the elevated anterior longitudinal ligament. Should the ligament not be capable of providing a base for the retractor, then one must be extremely careful with its use, since one of its arms will be in a position to injure the wall of the pharynx. It may be better in such cases to use a hand-held retractor. The position of the structures at this point is as follows: The thyrolinguofacial venous trunk has been sacrificed and ligated (*1*), The neurovascular bundle of the neck has been retracted laterally (*2*), The inferior thyroid artery has been pulled laterally with a hand-held retractor (*3*), The superior thyroid artery has been sacrificed and tied (*4*), The lingual artery lies just visible at the upper edge of the dissection (*5*)

Complications

The complications described for this approach are the most numerous because this is the most commonly used approach. The complications can be divided into vascular, soft tissue, and neurological complications.

Vascular Injury

Carotid Artery. Injuries to the carotid artery are usually the result of the use of self-retaining retractors that apply pressure to the artery, but injury can also occur during dissection. This is most common when draining inflammatory foci, sometimes with fistulae, and in cases of advanced and widely disseminated tumors in the region. If the artery is not adequately protected from the instrumentation being used, particularly sharp instruments such as drills and chisels, or during the use of force in distracting tissues for the insertion of grafts, it may be injured. Small tears can be sutured, but larger tears may necessitate ligation of the artery.

Jugular vein. It the jugular vein is not well visualized and identified during dissection, it may be out of the immediate field of vision behind the sternocleidomastoid muscle. Its wall is soft and can be easily torn, particularly in older patients. Bleeding is abundant, but can be controlled by suturing the wall. It is important that the surgeon remains emotionally is control and proceed calmly and methodically. The bleeding must be controlled by pressure, the tear must be carefully assessed, and the vessel must be totally accessible. This may require opening up the carotid sheath in order to expose the vein and to identifiy the artery and the vagus nerve, so that these two additional structures are not included in the sutures or ligatures.

Thyroid vessels. During dissection, the thyroid vessels may be injured. The superior thyroid artery can be ligated, and sometimes is, when it cannot be retracted from the operative field. The same applies to the vein. The thyrolinguofacial trunk, as noted above, may block the progress of dissection and exposure, and does not tolerate well any degree of traction. It must be sacrificed and ligated. The middle thyroid vein, when present, and the inferior thyroid vein should be ligated. The inferior thyroid artery, as already discussed above, must be carefully freed if it is to be retracted. If it is not going to be in the direct field of dissection, it must be maintained under visual control at all times. Injury to the inferior thyroid artery is a frequent event when self-retaining retractors of the soft tissue are used, particularly in older patients where the vessels are hardened by arteriosclerosis, with loss of elasticity and calcification of the wall.

The Vertebral Arteries. Injuries to the vertebral arteries occur when one is operating in the lateral portion of the vertebral body towards the transverse processes, and when osseous dissection involves the vertebral artery foramen. It obviously should not occur when one is operating only on the vertebral bodies. On occasion, extensive dissection within the body may produce a collapse of the lateral wall of the body and, hence, involve the transverse apophysis, so that the vertebral artery is caught in a sudden collapse of the hard, surrounding, osseous structures. Fortunately, in the majority of cases, the artery is flexible enough to bend and adapt to the collapse of the surrounding bone. If, however, injury occurs, the bleeding will be massive. Immediate pressure with Surgicel must be followed by ligation of the artery once it has been dissected out and freed from its bony shell. On occasion, because of the fragmentation that occurs in the wall of the vertebral artery foramen, it may be necessary to descend to a lower level, often right down to C6, in order to be able to ligate the artery. It is not unusual for injury to the vertebral artery to occur as a result of a specific technical maneuver. The most common maneuver leading to injury is the use of retraction that involves the passage of portions of the retractor, often with a sharp or hooked end, laterally under the vertebral body in order to obtain exposure (e.g., when using a Homann retractor). While the exposure obtained by such retraction may appear to be advantageous, its consequences can be disastrous and it is best to avoid them altogether.

The Thoracic Duct. When operating near the cervico-thoracic junction, particularly on the left side of the neck, one may inadvertently encounter the thoracic duct or other major lymphatic channels. It is at the level of the first thoracic vertebra that the thoracic duct passes on its way to the subclavian. If one is operating at this level, then one must remember the presence of this structure. Right-handed surgeons who operate from the right side will obviously not encounter this difficulty.

Neurological Injury

As noted above, the most common neurological injuries are those involving the recurrent laryngeal nerves. They usually result from excessive traction or from dissection that does not follow the established pathways. The superior laryngeal nerve is present in dissections aimed at reaching the upper levels of the neck from C3. At this level, the nerve will be found to cross the field in its approach to the pharyngeal wall. The inferior laryngeal nerve is subject to a greater number of anomalous paths, arising from the vagus nerve anywhere from the middle to the inferior cervical region and often in association with the inferior thyroid vessels.

These nerves are injured whenever one misses the retroesophageal prevertebral space and inadvertently enters the space between esophagus and trachea where this nerve is found. The branch of the hypoglossal nerve that crosses the middle cervical region can be sacrificed with few consequences. The cervical sympathetic chain can be injured in its superior region near the stellate ganglion when one is dissecting in the lateral cervical muscular plane (the long muscles of the neck). It is usually injured when one fails to remain subperiosteal in dissecting the lateral aspect of the vertebral body in the approach to the transverse apophyses. This injury leads to both esthetic and functional complications in that it produces a full Horner's syndrome. This will include the full homolateral complex of anophthalmia, myosis, and palpebral ptosis.

Soft Tissue Injury

Often soft tissue injuries are the most serious. Of these the most frequent are injuries to the esophagus and the pharynx, which require immediate surgical repair and thus are of particular importance to the surgeon, who must identify them intraoperatively and immediately deal with them. When the middle cervical fascia and the omohyoid muscle have been split, the esophagus and the pharynx are immediately exposed. The walls of these structures at this levels are not only thin, but also soft and easily injured by aggressive dissection. Small tears to the structures can and have been missed intraoperatively. If any doubt arises, the presence of the nasogastric and nasotracheal intubation will permit orientation during intraoperative examination, and hence confirmation of whether any injury has occurred. The careless application of self-retaining retractors may produce tears at the time of their application and during any application of force later in the progress of the dissection. If these complications are identified intraoperatively and repaired immediately, one needs only maintain the patient on a nasogastric tube for 2–3 weeks postoperatively, with a compressive bandage on the neck. Parenteral nutrition and feeding through the nasogastric tube will be sufficient, particularly when augmented by the use of atropine to decrease salivation. It is important to remember that if such complications arise, one may have to avoid the use of massive osseous grafts or the application of foreign bodies such as orthopedic plates or other implants.

If the tear is not identified intraoperatively, then one must be on the alert for this possibility when drainage persists for several days postoperatively. We have found that an easy way to definitely confirm the presence of a tear is to give the patients 5–10 cc methylene blue to drink; after a few minutes, the dye will appear in the drainage from the wound. At this point, the surgical incision must be reopened and the tear must be repaired. If this is not done as soon as it is detected or if it is missed, with the passage of time abscess cavities and sinuses will be formed deep in the tissues of the neck. These can track extensively and reach into the mediastinum, making management more and more difficult as time passes.

The thyroid gland is protected by the muscles of the neck and can only be injured by retractors or by sharp instruments used in dissection. Injuries are associated with hemorrhage, which is immediately obvious at the time and which can be controlled by a full thickness suturing of the tear.

Presternocleidomastoid Approach (Retropharyngeal and Retrocarotid)

In the past the retrocarotid retropharyngeal presternocleidomastoid approach was used to obtain surgical access to the vertebral artery (Henry 1957). In addition to providing good exposure of both the intra- and extraosseous portion of the vertebral artery, it also gives access to the lateral side of the cervico-occipital region including the transverse apophyses, the intertransverse foramina, and the nerve roots of the first cervical vertebrae. If necessary, the incision may be extended distally to permit exposure of the lower cervical vertebrae. This approach to the high cervical spine was also described by Whiteside and Kelly (1966).

Technique

The patient is placed in the supine position with all the precautions and preparation described in the previous section, including placement of the halo and the head screen. The head is turned to the side opposite to the operative side (incision) (Fig. 8.32). The patient should have nasotracheal and nasogastric intubation with the earlobe retracted by suturing in order to expose fully the mastoid region, and there should be SEP monitoring. A hockeystick incision is begun in the retromastoid region, 2 cm behind the apex of the mastoid, and is curved inferiorly; it is extended horizontally around the mastoid, and then down the anterior border of the sternocleidomastoid muscle. The initial dissection should be directed to the identification of both the external jugular vein crossing in front of the sternocleidomastoid and the greater auricular nerve (Fig. 8.33). The nerve must be freed and anchored superiorly in order to safeguard it from injury (which would produce a retroauricular area of hypoesthesia). The next step is to separate the sternocleidomastoid muscle from the mastoid process, leaving only a few fibers that will be useful in reinserting the muscle during closure. Removal of this muscle is only necessary if extensive exposure is required, and may not be necessary for limited surgical procedures such as biopsy, drainage of abscesses, or the removal of small lesions. Next, one must identify the spinal accessory nerve, which can be located by following the belly of the sternocleidomastoid muscle distally; the nerve will be found approximately 3 cm from the insertion of the muscle and may be partly embedded in the muscle itself (Figs. 8.32–8.36). The nerve should be freed and retracted, either anteriorly or medially, together with the blood vessels that comprise the neurovascular bundle. If exposure is required below the level of C2 and even towards the distal end of the cervical spine, the nerve will remain in the way (Fig. 8.36). In order to avoid having to sacrifice the spinal accessory nerve, it must be dissected free proximally all the way up to its exit from the skull near the jugular vein, so that it can then be retracted together with the sternocleidomastoid muscle. At this point, the transverse process of the atlas, which protrudes slightly laterally, is palpable halfway between the angle of the jaw and the mastoid process. The posterior belly of the digastric muscle must be identified and retracted either superiorly or medially in order to obtain adequate exposure, as required by the procedure to be carried out.

During this dissection, great care must be taken in dissecting posteriorly and superiorly from this zone. This is the area through which the extraskeletal portion of the vertebral artery passes cephalad from the transverse foramen of the atlas. Having reached the transverse process of C1, then the access needed to continue the dissection for exposure medially and inferiorly is provided. At this point, the transverse processes in the prevertebral plane are exposed behind the carotid sheath, which can be mobilized and retracted anteriorly. Further dissection will permit access to the retropharyngeal space separating the previsceral areolar tissue (Sharpey's fibers). Immediately visible, and covering the first cervical vertebrae with fibers that extend as far as the anterior tubercle of the atlas on its medial side, is the prevertebral muscular plane (long muscles of the neck). In order to expose the anterior arch of the atlas, the body of the axis, or the base of the odontoid process, one must dissect this prevertebral muscular plane; the lateral joints between the masses of the atlas and the axis and the base of the odontoid process, at the point in which it articulates with the atlas, can be then approached.

The prevertebral muscular tissues can be dissected subperiosteally and retracted anteriorly, but one must be careful not to injure the cervical sympathetic chain (Fig. 8.36). This dissection, however, will be essential if access to the transverse apophyses is required. In order to reach the vertebral body, the long muscles of the neck must only be separated from the central region of the vertebral body and retracted towards the transverse processes. Detachment of the muscles may be limited only to the area required by the specific procedure to be carried out, i.e., the procedure may require exposure of the entire vertebral surface or just of the lateral aspect including the transverse process.

When the specific procedure has been carried out, closure will include the establishment of suction drainage with suturing of the sternocleidomastoid muscle at its mastoid insertion and closure of the platysma, the subcutaneous tissue, and the skin incision. Halo immobilization is continued postoperatively.

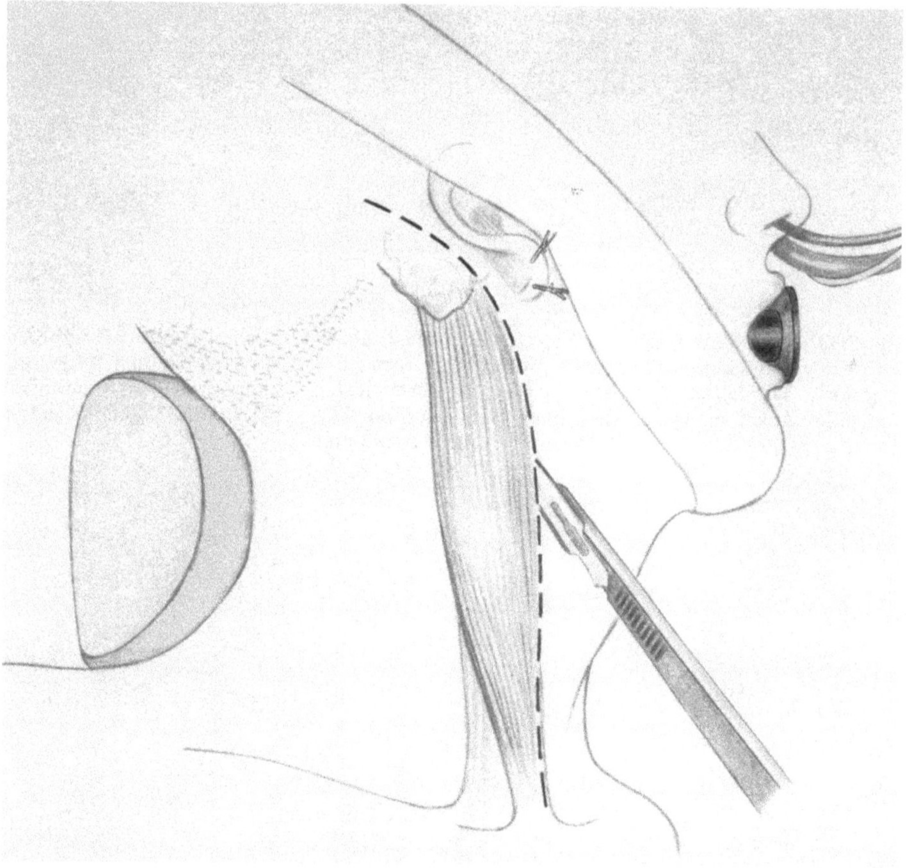

Fig. 8.32. The patient is placed on the table with the head rotated towards the side opposite the incision. Nasotracheal intubation is in place. The chin and mandible are fixed with an elastic bandage. The earlobe is retracted and sutured away from the operative area. A hockey stick incision is illustrated, beginning approximately 2 cm behind the mastoid, and turning distally to follow along the edge of the sternocleidomastoid muscle (its anterior margin)

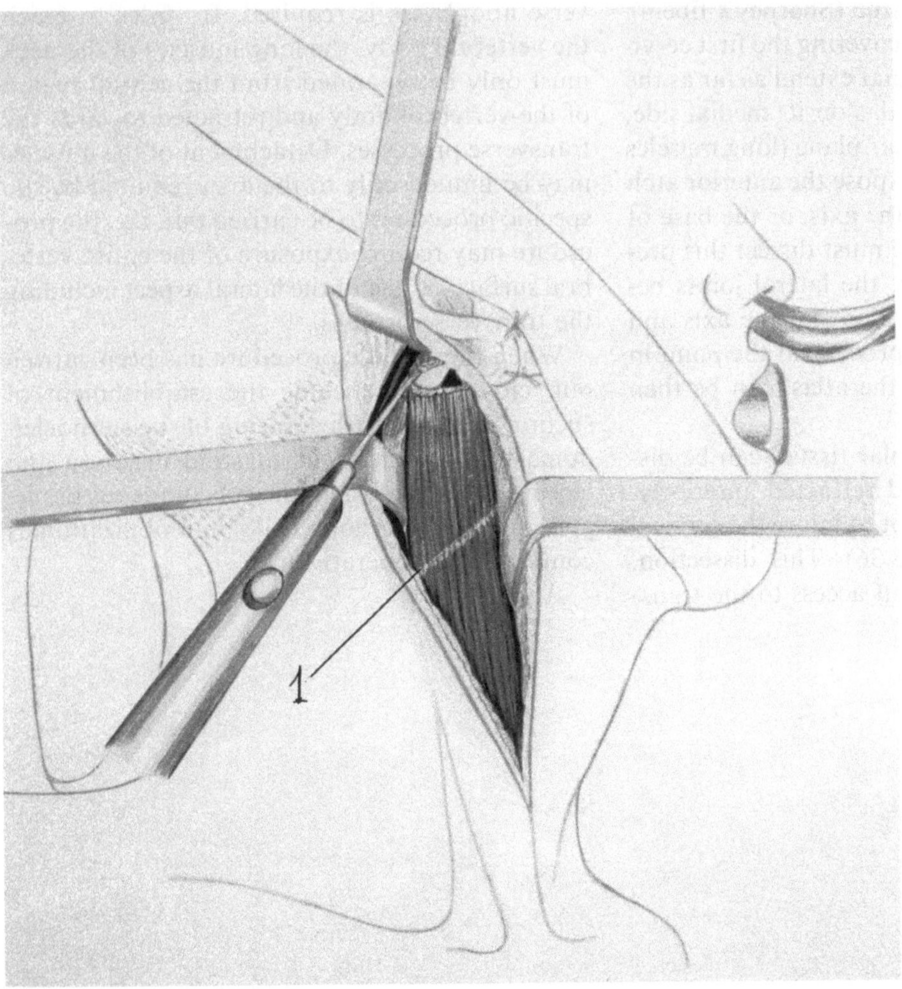

Fig. 8.33. The external jugular vein, once identified, along with the greater auricular nerve is protected by retraction superiorly. The cautery is used to separate the sternocleidomastoid muscle from the mastoid bone at its insertion. The spinal accessory nerve (*1*) lies inferiorly to the mastoid and remains protected. Approaches to the higher cervical levels may require that the nerve be dissected out and retracted anteriorly, while for more distal approaches, it can remain in place with the sternocleidomastoid muscle

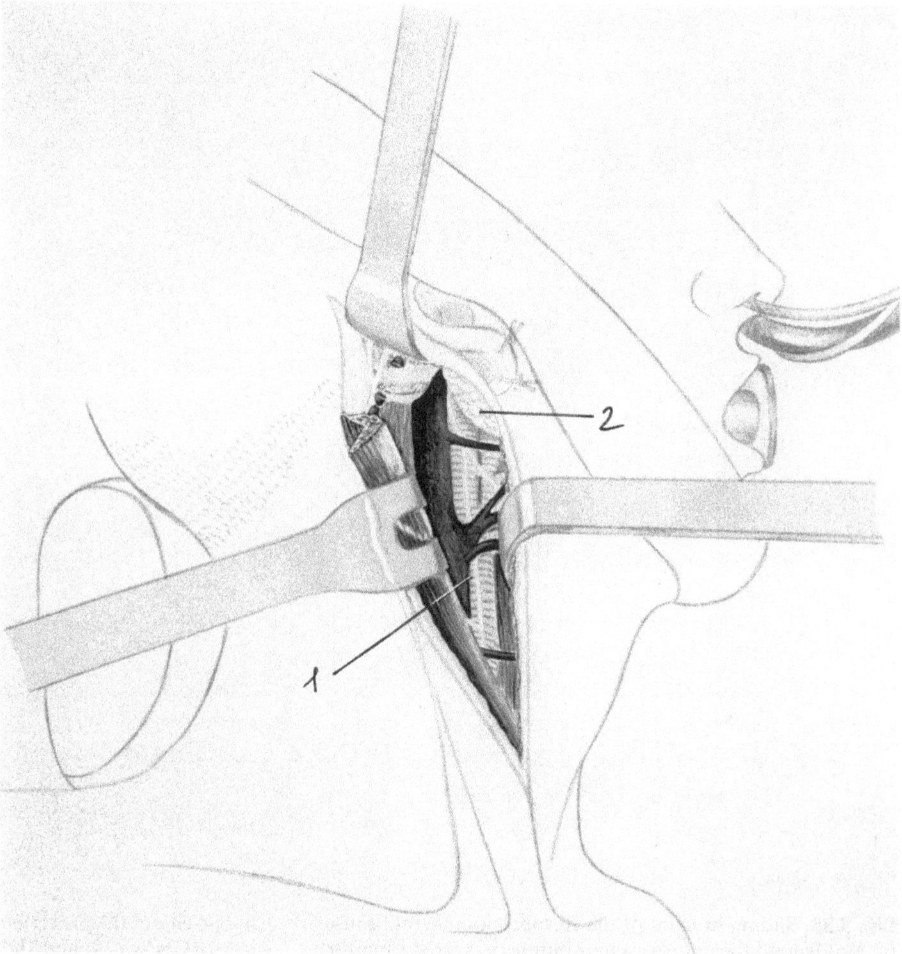

Fig. 8.34. The neurovascular bundle of the neck (*1*) lies below the sternocleidomastoid muscle and the inferior margin of the parotid gland (*2*)

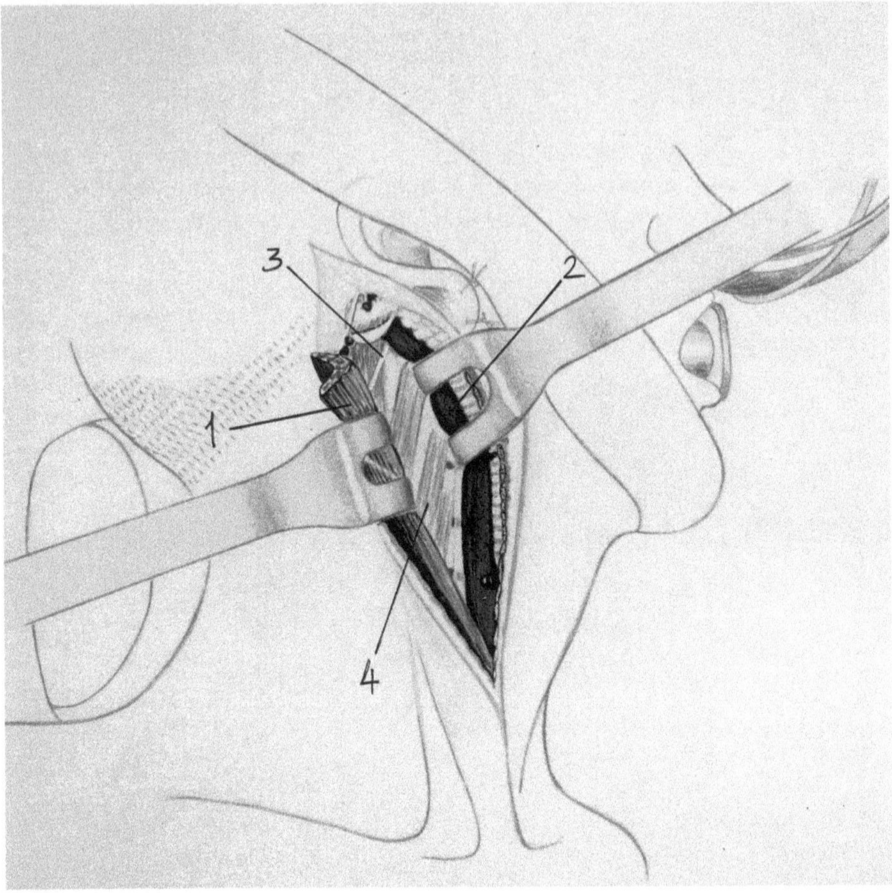

Fig. 8.35. Sliding in front of the sternocleidomastoid muscle (*1*) and behind the neurovascular bundle retracted superiorly (*2*), one enters the prevertebral space. Here one will find the accessory nerve (*3*) and the prevertebral muscles (*4*)

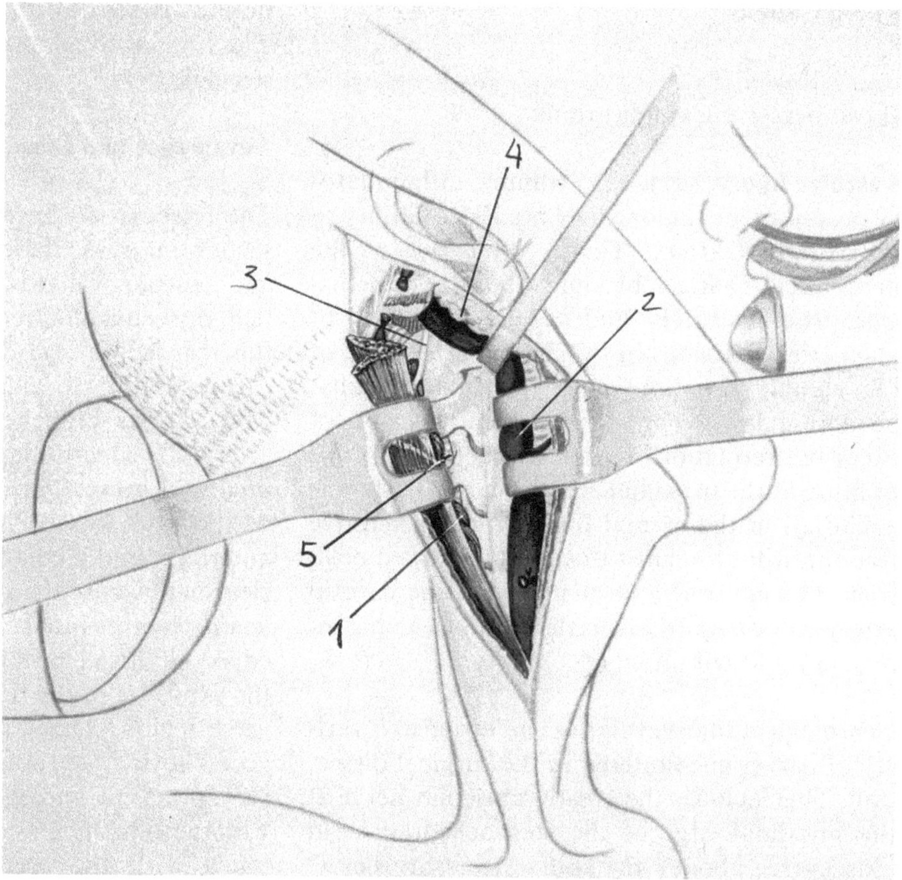

Fig. 8.36. The prevertebral muscles (*1*) are detached and retracted. The neurovascular bundle (*2*) is raised forward by retraction. Only for access to the medial aspects of the body of C2 and the arch of C1 is it necessary to apply retraction of the neurovascular bundle superiorly. It is difficult to retract the jugular vein and the carotid artery, because they are fixed at their point of entry at the base of the skull in such a way as not to permit any motility at this point. In order to avoid injury to the blood vessels, or anoxia in their distribution, a hand-held retractor is used, and the tension is released periodically in order to permit free circulation through the vessels. Also visible are the spinal accessory nerve (*3*), the parotid gland (*4*), and the intertransverse canal with the vertebral artery (*5*)

Complications

Intraoperative Complications

Vascular Injury. In cases of trauma, inflammatory processes, or tumor, there is a risk of injury to the vertebral artery. This is often due to the anatomical changes brought about by the disease process. Rarely, and usually as a result of inexperience, lesions of the carotid artery and of the jugular vein have been reported. Usually, intracranial vascular injuries occur because of excessive retraction. It is easy to explain this, because at the proximal end the carotid artery is anchored in the cranial foramen and excessive traction will be against this rigid and fixed position. The consquences of injury to the carotid artery will obviously be reflected in ischemic injury in its distribution.

Neurological Injury. Injuries can occur to a variety of nerves encountered in the surgical dissection. This includes the greater auricular nerve at the proximal edge of the sternocleidomastoid muscle (see above), the spinal accessory nerve, the facial nerve, and the cervical sympathetic chain. The spinal accessory nerve can be injured either by careless dissection or unnecessary and excessive traction. The facial nerve may not only be overstretched by retraction, but may also be compressed between the retractors and the mandible. The cervical sympathetic chain can be injured in the dissection of muscle in the lateral cervical plane in the approach to the transverse apophyses.

Postoperative Complications

Glottic edema is the most common postoperative complication in view of the extensive tissue trauma induced by the surgical dissection. In our experience, the need for preoperative tracheotomy is not always mandatory; we feel it essential only in cases of severe trauma or extensive tumor in which the dissection is expected to produce severe and extensive tissue injury. In all other cases we maintain postoperative intubation, as described above, for at least 24 hours and attempt to minimize or control edema with steroids.

Advantages and Disadvantages

The retrocarotid approach avoids surgical dissection in areas where there are major vascular and neurological structures that must be identified, dissected, and retracted from the field. For this reason, we regard it as superior to the precarotid approach, which would force one to deal with various branches of the external carotid artery, the superior laryngeal nerve, and the hypoglossal nerve. Once the neurovascular bundle of the neck has been identified and retracted anteriorly and medially, one has a more or less clear pathway to the spine, devoid of any significant structures that must be dissected, retracted, or sacrificed. Secondly, this approach allows the exposure of the full length of the intertransverse region from C1 down to C7, with good access to the lateral aspect of the spine. It is a very practical and useful approach in dealing with tumor compression of the cord. When combined with the precarotid approach, it can provide a particularly extensive exposure that will permit cord decompression and removal of extensive tumor deposits.

This method, however, in spite of its great advantages throughout the cervical spine, does not give good access above C1. It cannot be used to reach the atlanto-occipital region that will be obstructed by the neurovascular structures which cannot be adequately retracted out of the field of vision. The carotid artery, the jugular vein, and the vagus and hypoglossal nerves have a fixed position as they exit the skull, and it is very difficult and dangerous to attempt to retract them. Serious problems include both neurological injury and vascular insufficiency involving the distribution of the internal carotid artery. A technical difficulty is that the dissection is angulated in such a way as to make good illumination of the operative site difficult, so that visualization of structures may be less than optimal.

Retrosternocleidomastoid Approach

The retrosternocleidomastoid approach allows access to the whole cervical spine, from C1 to C7, and it is utilized mostly to get the cervical sympathetic chain, the anterior lateral surface of vertebral bodies, the transverse processes, the intertransverse spaces, and the vertebral artery.

Technique

The patient is placed on the operating table in a supine and anti-Trendelenburg position (Fig. 8.37). A rigid support is placed under the neck, while the head is lying in a mobile support, fastened with bandages passing around the forehead and under the mandible. The earlobe is sutured to the skin to make access easier. Incision of skin starts from the upper portion of mastoid process and extends downwards, following the posterior edge of stenocleidomastoid muscle (Fig. 8.38).

After the subcutaneous tissue and platysma have been cut, the sternocleidomastoid muscle is exposed (Fig. 8.39). One must be particularly careful, when performing the proximal part of the incision, to avoid injury to the superficial occipital vein and mastoid branches of the superficial cervical plexus. A good access to underlying planes is obtained by cutting the superficial cervical fascia along the posterior edge of the sternocleidomastoid muscle, thus reaching the carotid artery. The retrostyloid space is located in the upper part of incision: it is possible here to palpate the transverse process of the atlas 1 cm below the mastoid apex. Distally, it is easier to retract the sternocleidomastoid muscle, the neurovascular bundle, and the visceral structures of the neck. Prevertebral muscles are detached from the skeletal plane and then retracted (Fig. 8.40).

It is necessary first to locate the cervical sympathetic chain: After this has been done, it is easy to reach the anterolateral portion of the vertebral bodies, the transverse processes, the intertransverse spaces, and the vertebral artery.

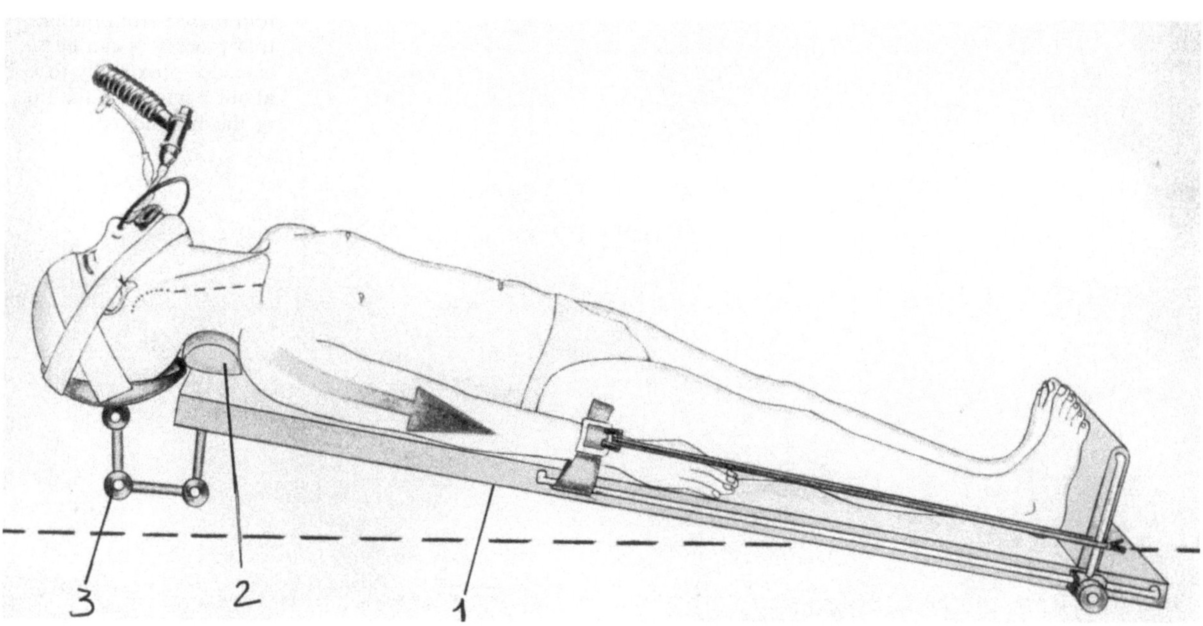

Fig. 8.37. The patient lies on the operating table in the anti-Trendelenburg position (*1*). There is a rigid support under the neck (*2*). The adjustable head support (*3*) is shown with the head rotated to the side opposite the surgical approach. Nasotracheal and nasogastric tubes are in place

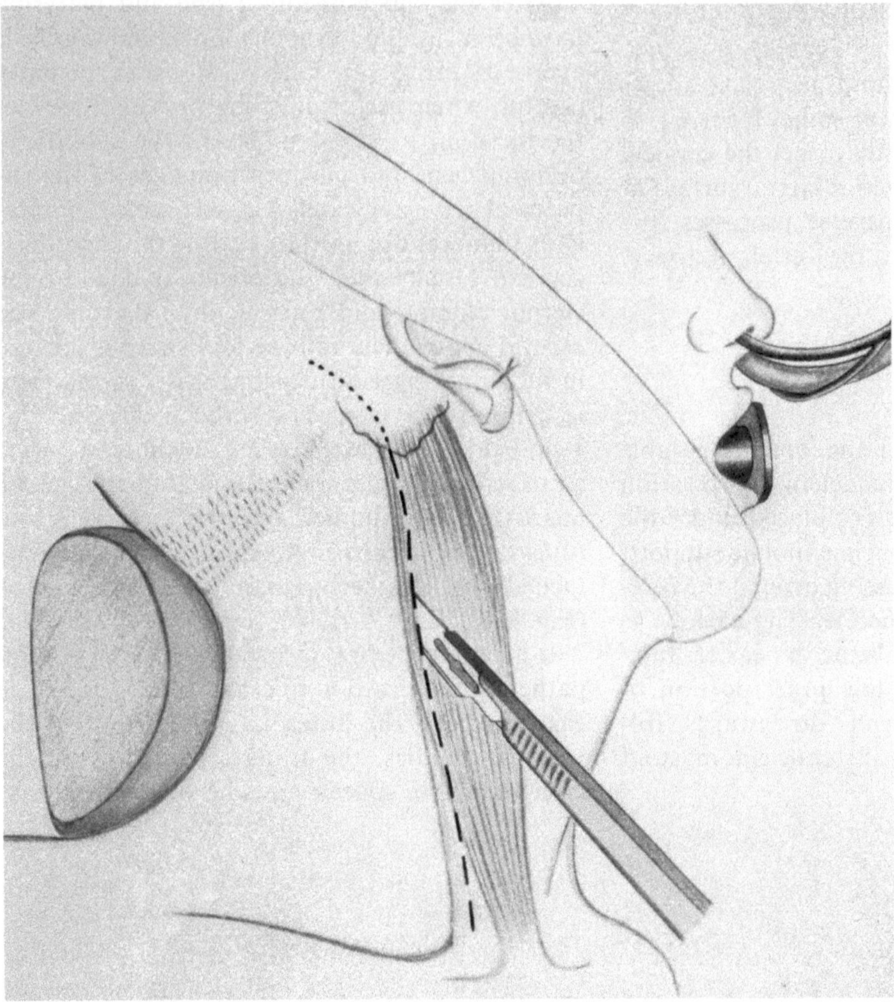

Fig. 8.38. The incision follows the sternocleidomastoid muscle from the mastoid process. It can be extended proximally to about 2 cm above the tip of the mastoid

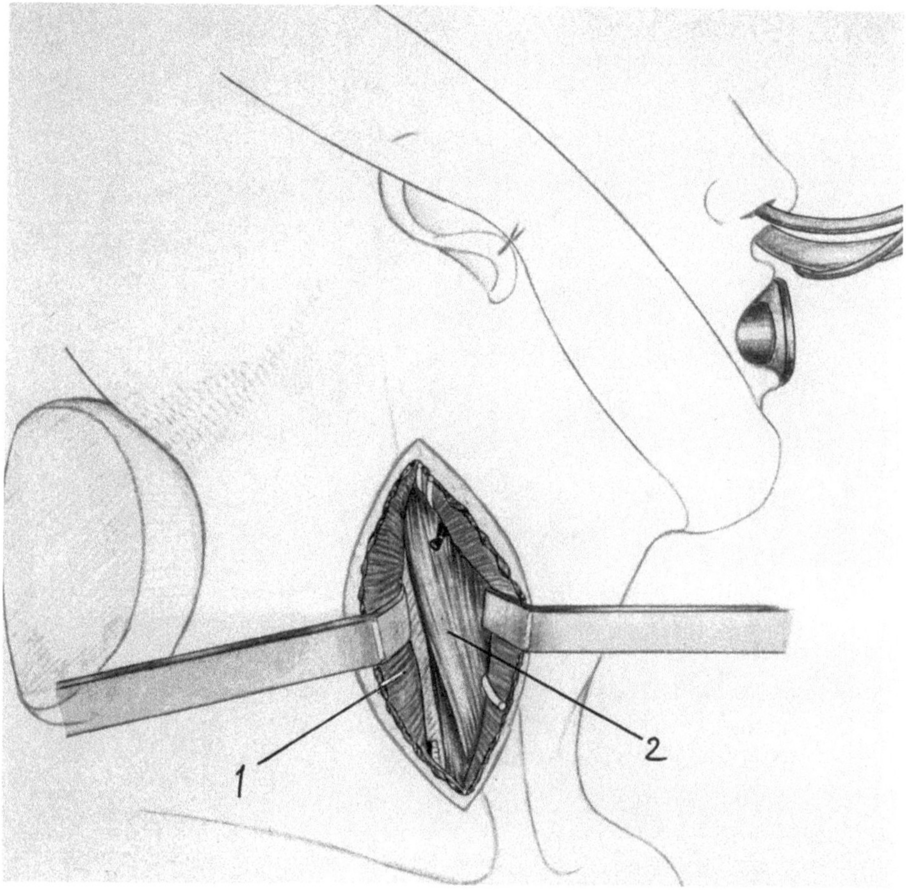

Fig. 8.39. Following incision of the skin, subcutaneous tissue, and platysma (*1*) the sternocleidomastoid muscle (*2*) is exposed. The posterior margin of the muscle is enveloped by the superficial cervical fascia, which is cut along the posterior edge of the muscle to obtain access to the subjacent planes

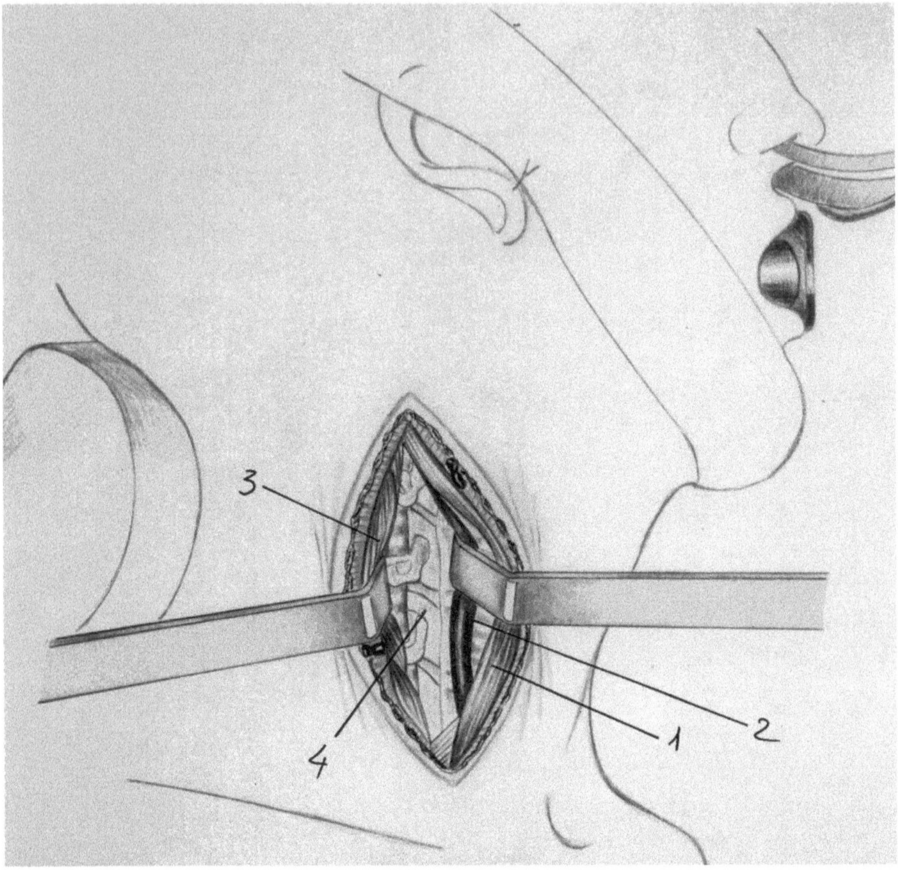

Fig. 8.40. Medial retraction of the sternocleidomastoid muscle (*1*), the neurovascular bundle (*2*), and the visceral structure of the neck allows one to enter the prevertebral plane. The prevertebral muscles are detached and retracted (*3*). One can then reach the lateral zones of the intertransverse spaces of the vertebral bodies (*4*) if one needs to undertake any procedure in this area

Posterior Approach

The posterior approach obviously provides the best access to the posterior elements of the cervical column. In the upper cervical spine (C1 and C2) and at the occipitocervical junction, the following structures may be reached:

- The posterior aspect of the occiput and foramen magnum
- The greater occipital nerve
- The occipitocervical membrane
- The higher extension of the posterior extracranial portion of the vertebral artery
- The posterior arch of the atlas
- The atlantoaxial membrane
- The laminae and apophyseal regions of C2
- The posterior interapophyseal joints of C1–C2 and C2–C3

This approach also permits access to the following structures in the lower cervical spine (C3 to C7):

- The interspinous ligaments and apophyses
- The laminae
- The ligamentum flavum
- The posterior apophyseal joints

Through this posterior approach, the posterior elements may be removed (apophyses, laminae, ligamentum flavum) and access obtained to the posterior aspect of the cord and roots. In some cases, if necessary, with careful retraction and protection of the neural structures, it is possible to reach the anterior side of the vertebral canal (actually the lateral side of the posterior wall of the vertebral body and the intervertebral disk spaces), the pedicles, and the root canals (primarily the posterior portion). With this approach, however, one should not expect to be able to reach or to undertake any surgery in the central region of the vertebral bodies. This would involve particularly difficult if not impossible retraction or displacement of neural structures, which might well produce severe neurological damage.

Technique

The patient should be placed in the ventral decubitus (prone) position on the operating table. The sitting position with the head supported by a head rest has also been described, but the prone position is preferred except in cases of cervical osteotomy, in which the patient must be awake, and the procedure for dealing with ankylosing spondylopathy, which is carried out under local anesthetic. The patient must be placed on an orthopedic table using specifically placed rigid supports. These should be placed across the thorax and the sternum and longitudinally across both the iliac crests to maintain freedom of movement of the abdomen with compression and thus to permit unobstructed diaphragmatic movement in respiration throughout the duration of the procedure. Pressure on the abdomen will increase intra-abdominal pressure and, particularly, venous pressure in the spleen, and this may well increase venous pressure in the operative site leading to excessive bleeding. If this is combined with a limitation of diaphragmatic movement in respiration, the patient's oxygenation may also be affected. The legs and thighs are well fixed to the table by straps, while the feet are supported by a pillow on a fixed base (Fig. 8.41). The hands should be held to the side of the body by wrist bands attached to an elastic band. This places the arms in tension to a degree that the shoulder tips will be lowered. A Tensioplast type of adhesive band passed over the shoulder is anchored in such a way as to further lower the shoulder tips.

The head is placed in a horseshoe-shaped headrest that is mobile and adjustable and which follows the outline of the forehead, leaving only the eyes, the nose, and the mouth accessible. This will also provide access for nasogastric and endotracheal tubes for anesthesia. The following are important precautions. It is important that the eyes remain free of the padded head support. Serious injury to the cornea and to the eye itself can result from pressure of a badly positioned support. To avoid this, very careful attention must be paid to the placement of the head. Furthermore, the eyes should be also protected by an antiseptic cream, held slightly open with a small tape, and should be completely protected with gauze packing.

The endotracheal anesthetic tube should be carefully anchored in the mouth. Carelessness in doing this will have repercussions in that tubes may be displaced when the patient, who was intubated while lying on his back, is rotated and placed in the required operative position. Great care must be taken, therefore, to avoid these eventualities that will unnecessarily delay or complicate the surgery. Criss-crossing tapes should be used to position the head firmly in the head rest. In addition, the tapes will provide tension on the skin.

In cases where the patient has a severe instability, because of tumor or other reasons, and has been in a halo traction preoperatively, then it will be the halo that will be anchored to the head rest rather than the head itself. The position of the head is also important. There should be flexion of the head only and not of the neck with respect to the trunk. The head should be pulled forward and not flexed anteriorly. Whenever possible, traction should be applied to the head in order to cancel the normal physiological lordosis and the head should be slightly turned forward. This positioning has several advantages. Superficially, the skin folds that cross under the occiput will be stretched out. The interspinal and interlaminal spaces between C1 and the occiput and C1 and C2 will be opened out, facilitating any surgical activity in these areas once dissection reaches these deeper regions. The neck should not be pulled too far forward with respect to the shoulders, since this anterior placement of the neck with respect to the trunk may be associated with hyperextension, and the increased lordosis will interfere with the surgical approach and dissection. Great care should be taken to avoid the following:

- *Rotation of the head with respect to the neck.* This is of particular importance in the occipito-cervical region where it can create significant difficulties.

- *Lateral displacement of the neck with respect to the trunk* which would create problems during surgery in the lower cervical spine.

The operative table should be in the anti-Trendelenburg position in order to decrease pressure and hence the risk of bleeding at the operative site. Having prepared for the skin incision, the surgeon must orientate himself by identifying specific landmarks that will help to outline the approach. It is important that the incision be midline in order to avoid poor or unacceptable repair and scarring. From above, the external occipital protuberance, which can be felt through the skin, and the spinous processes of C2 and C7 (the most prominent) may be identified. A line is drawn uniting these landmarks which have been marked once identified. Bleeding during the approach can be minimized by using local anesthetic with epinephrine. The infiltration with local anesthetic should begin at the spinous processes and proceed laterally from these into the paravertebral tissues (Fig. 8.42).

The choice of the side of the incision is the personal choice of the surgeon. It depends on the side from which the surgeon is most comfortable. Usually, a right-handed surgeon prefers the right side and vice versa. The skin is thick and the skin incision longitudinal. The subcutaneous tissue is also dense, particularly along the spinal apophyseal line. The length of the incision is determined by the level at which the surgery is to be carried out. The incision usually begins 2 or 3 cm above the external occipital protuberance if one is intending to reach the occipitocervical region. If one is intending to operate on lower levels, then the incision need not extend beyond the level of the external occipital protuberance.

Following the initial skin incision, the subcutaneous fat layer is cut. A self-retaining retractor is used to open the wound and allow the achievement of hemostasis with electrocautery. Next, the midline should be identified to permit delineation of the lateral paravertebral regions. The superficial aponeurosis is then incised at the midline, the nuchal ligament is identified; this is a membranous fibrous layer adherent on its anterior aspect to the spinous processes which represents the medial insertion of the trapezius muscles of the neck. It is an important structure that plays a crucial part in the maintenance of stability in the cervical spine. It extends from the occiput to the posterior tubercles of the atlas and along the spinous processes from C2 to C7. Once it has been divided, preferably by electrocautery and perfectly in midline, separating its attachment from the subjacent osseous elements of the spinous processes, dissection must remain outside the muscle bulk on either side, which now appears more superficial.

At the upper end, over the occipitocervical junction, the incision now reaches easily to the occipital bone at the external occipital protuberance. Having reached this level, the periosteum can be elevated from the occiput, using an appropriate periosteal elevator over the entire posterior surface of the occiput. The periosteal elevation is not difficult. Beginning at the midline it is extended for 15–20 mm laterally. The only precaution to be taken is to preserve the greater occipital nerve of Arnold, which passes under the greater inferior oblique muscle of the head, and crosses the semispinal muscle of the head as well as the splenius and trapezius. Superiorly, as it nears the occiput, it becomes more and more superficial, travelling together with the terminal branches of the occipital artery on either side of the occiput. This greater occipital nerve is usually located 15 mm lateral to the midline, and is easily avoided if the surgeon scrupulously stays within the subperiosteal region during the dissection and within the medial region of the dissection. Having cleared the occipital surface and the external occipital protuberance, then one must carefully identify the spinous apophysis of C2. This will be a specific landmark in identifying the posterior arch of the atlas. Having removed the muscles with electrocautery from C2 and remaining absolutely medial, one can then identify by palpation the posterior arch of the atlas and its tubercle (Fig. 8.43).

With a midline incision the muscles are separated and then the elevation of the ligamentous muscle insertion from the tubercle of C1 is continued. The periosteum is then stripped from the arch of the atlas laterally (Fig. 8.44). One must be aware of the presence of the vertebral artery in this part of the dissection. This artery passes in the area by circumventing the lateral mass of the atlas at the same level as the posterior arch. As the surgeon follows the posterior arch of the atlas away from the central region (the tubercle) it is important that he remain meticulously in the subperiosteal plane. This elevation must be done carefully and need not extend beyond 15 mm from the midline. A suggestion in technique is to use blunt dissection in stripping the arch; a sponge can be placed on the periosteal elevator and the periosteal space created is packed with strips of Surgicel (Fig. 8.45).

In dissection directed to the lower cervical spine, that is the more distal regions, electrocautery may be used for stripping. Again, one must stay meticulously close to the periosteum of the spinous processes and the laminae of C2–C7. This will permit elevation of the lateral cervical muscles (these include the semispinal muscle of the head, the long muscles of the head and neck, and, situated in the deeper planes and higher, the oblique and rectus muscles along with the interspinal and transversospinal muscles). The detachment and stripping of the paravertebral surface can be done easily with electrocautery. Periosteal elevators are difficult to control and, in cases where the stenosis is due to tumors or in cases where there is an element of instability, their use can result in neurological injuries. Instead it is easier to use electrocautery particularly to reach the more lateral portions of the dissection and electrocautery can alway be fully controlled. Whenever periosteal elevators are used, the tip should be covered with gauze, making it suitable only for blunt dissection. At this point, muscle elevation and exposure of the apophyseal joints of the spine have been completed. The self-retaining retractors can now be positioned and the surgeon has full access to the entire posterior region of the neck.

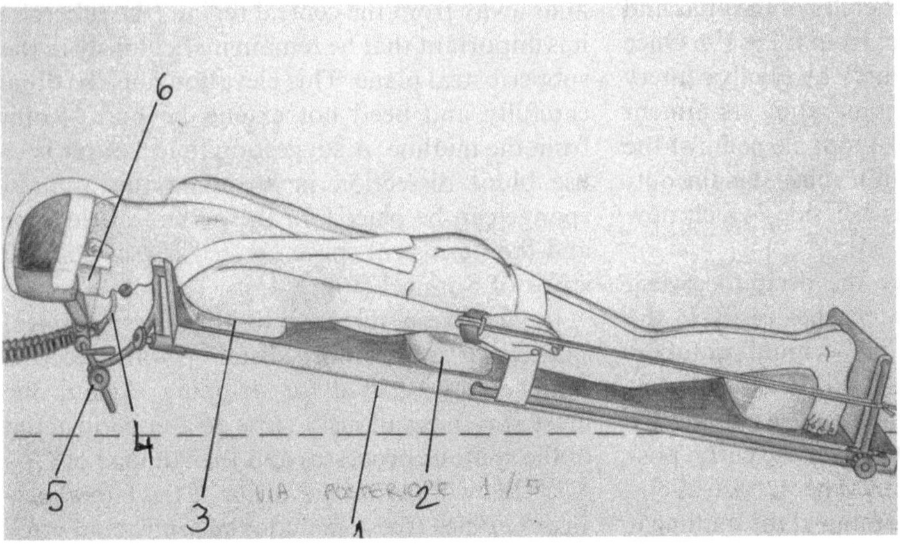

Fig. 8.41. The patient is placed on the operating table in the anti-Trendelenburg position (*1*). Supports are placed on the iliac crests (*2*) and on the sternal region (*3*) in order to permit free movement of the abdomen. Nasotracheal intubation is demonstrated (*4*). The forehead is placed on a mobile adjustable rest (*5*). The eyes are free of obstruction outside the support of the forehead (*6*). The head is held in position with tapes. Adhesive tapes apply caudad traction on the shoulders, and the arm is also under longitudinal traction

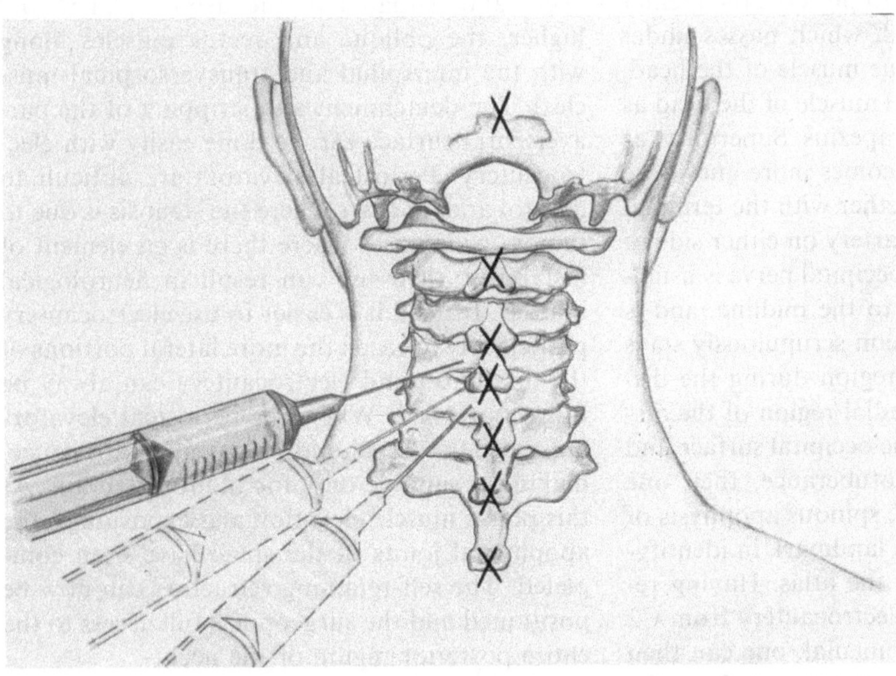

Fig. 8.42. Anatomical landmarks are marked on the skin to identify the external occipital protuberance in the spinous processes. Local anesthetic with epinephrine is injected in order to minimize bleeding at the level of the spinous processes and laminae

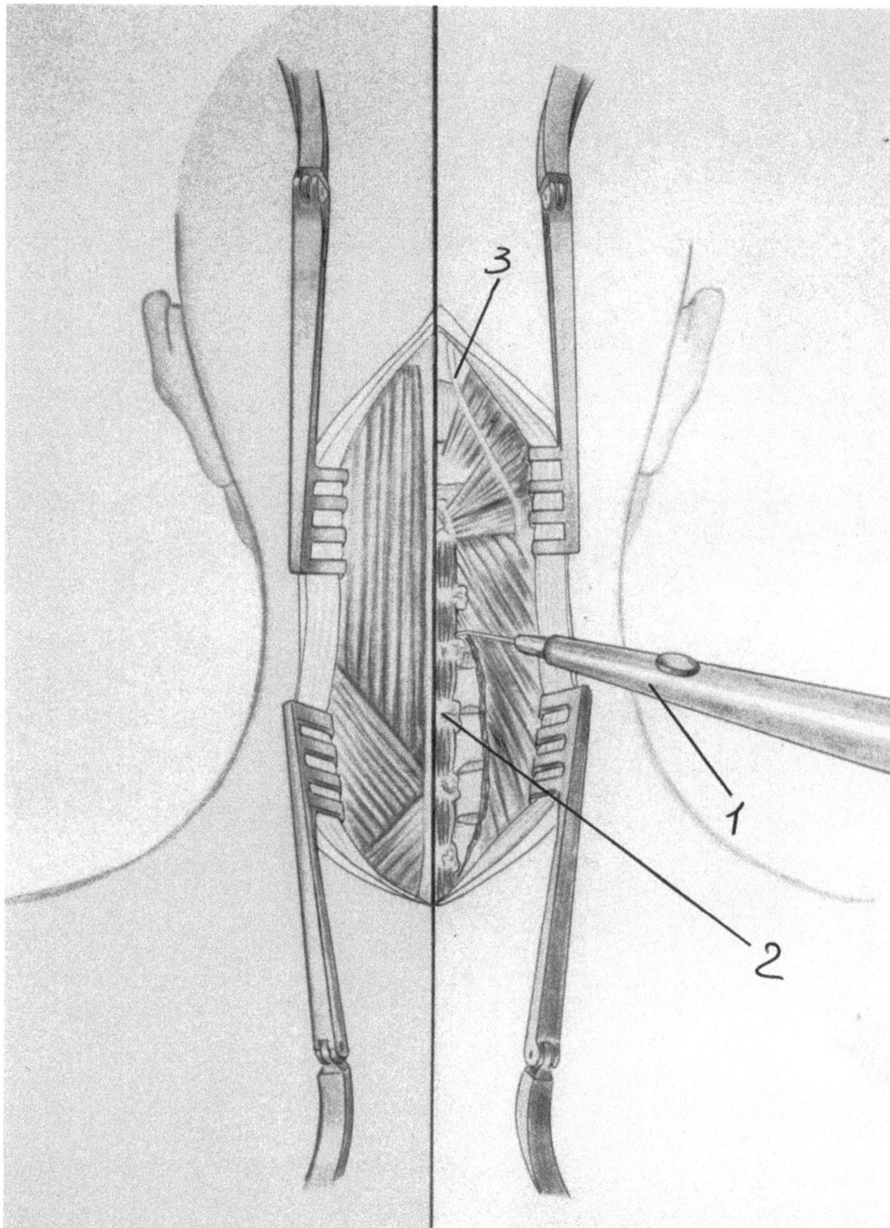

Fig. 8.43. Using electrocautery, the paravertebral muscles are severed (*1*) first on one side and then on the other. Electrocautery is preferable in cases of tumors and cases of post-traumatic instability. As one proceeds proximally, great care must be used in the separation of the small occipital muscles from the spinous process of C2 (*2*). This is in order to avoid extending the dissection too far externally where one runs the risk of injuring the greater occipital nerve (*3*)

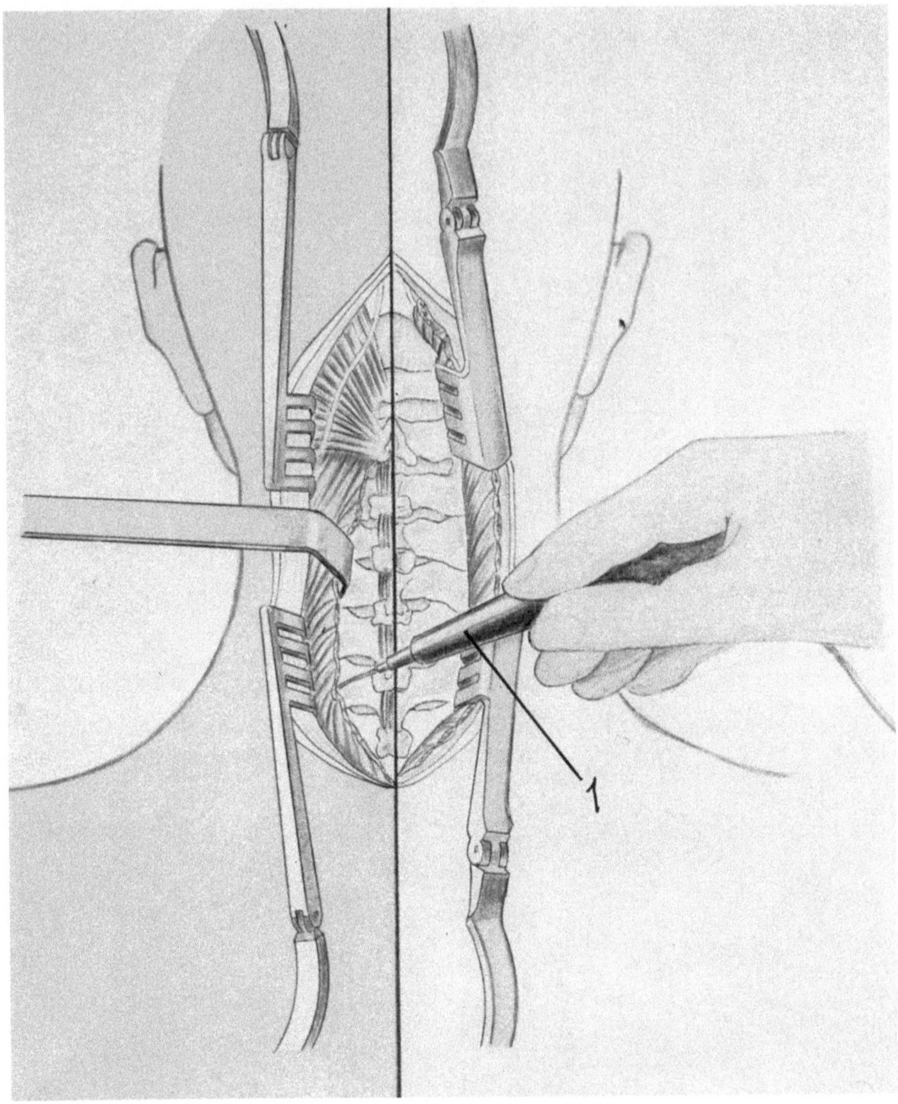

Fig. 8.44. Separation of the muscles is undertaken with the electric scalpel (*1*)

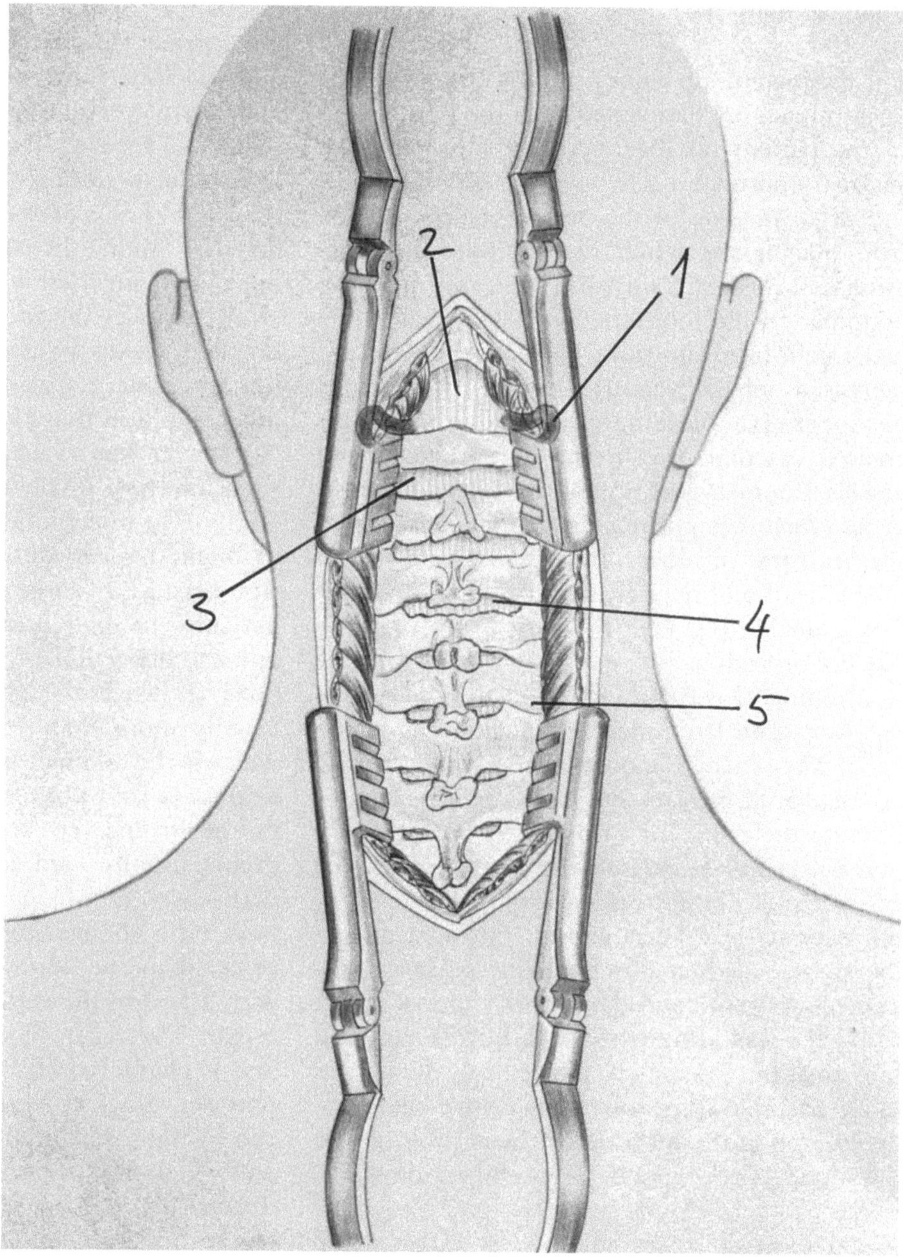

Fig. 8.45. This is the final stage of the dissection at the skeletal level showing the vertebral artery (*1*) still covered by muscles. Also visible are the occipitoatlantoid membrane (*2*), the atlantoaxial membrane (*3*), the ligamentum flavum (*4*), and the posterior interapophyseal joints (*5*)

Complications

The most common complications of the posterior approach are associated with the positioning of the patient on the operating table and the surgical approach itself.

Bad positioning of the patient usually results from placing the patient directly onto the operating table in such a way that compression of the abdomen will interfere with diaphragmatic movement in respiration. The consequences are increased splenic venous pressure and greater intraoperative bleeding from the ensuing increased vascular pressure in the parameningeal vessels. Poor oxygenation of the patient can also occur. *Incorrect positioning of the head* and of the head rest produces an unfavorable position of the head and neck with respect to the trunk. This can disadvantage the surgeon in carrying out his procedure because of the inappropriate positioning of vertebral components. *Injuries to the eyes* result from incorrect positioning of the head. They include lesions of the cornea, either because of direct pressure from the head rest or because the eye is inappropriately protected.

Loose endotracheal tubes for anesthesia will be easily displaced, not only during positioning of the patient once anesthetized, but also during the surgery. When this happens, surgery must immediately stop and the patient must be rotated on the operating table back into the intubation position. This can be particularly dangerous in an unstable spine which may have been rendered even more unstable by the early stages of the surgical procedure before stabilization is carried out.

Neurological injury may result either from movement of the patient while he is being positioned on the table, or from direct injury, particularly from periosteal elevators in cases of tumors or in patients with instability. The more common of these complications are dural tears that can lead to CSF fistulae. These can occur when one is working near the dura mater, such as happens during the opening or widening of the external margin of the foramen magnum or in the detachment of atlantoaxial and atlantooccipital membranes. In addition, injuries may occur to the greater occipital nerve of Arnold. This can happen during a too lateral dissection that is not carried out completely outside the muscles and which extends between the lateral occipital and lateral cervical muscle masses in the high regions of the neck. Nerve roots may be injured during the dissection when it is extended beyond the lateral limits of the apophyseal joints. When dissecting along the lateral surface of the joints, one may inadvertently injure the superficial cervical plexus or the roots that give origin to the brachial plexus (which is more serious). This usually occurs in patients with severe traumatic injuries and in those with tumors.

Vascular injuries may also occur. The most serious are those involving the vertebral artery. In addition to direct injury to the vertebral artery, as might happen during posterior decompression because of large tumor masses, the artery may also be injured during periosteal elevation and the dissection of the posterior arch of the atlas. If the elevation is carried too far laterally, usually more than 15 mm from the tubercle, which is the midline, and if it is carried out in an aggressive and poorly controlled manner, then injuries to the vertebral artery do occur. These events usually tend to occur more frequently with cases in which the normal relationships have been changed, either by extensive trauma or by advanced tumor. Injury of the arterial wall with a tear in the vertebral artery is difficult to repair. The region does not permit easy access and is characterized by the presence of important neurological structures, such as the lower end of the medulla, all of which may be at risk and which limit the surgeon's ability to address the vascular damage. Clips may be used to control hemorrhage only if the field is extended laterally. Other vascular complications may be associated with the deep cervical artery that passes along the posterior cervical region quite laterally near the apophyseal joints. Also injuries to the posterior venous plexus can occur, but these do not create severe consequences and can be easily controlled.

Combined Approaches

Multiple approaches become necessary when the stenosis is due to involvement of the entire circumference of the canal such as might occur in cases of tumor. The various approaches can be combined as part of a plan intended to achieve the necessary surgical intervention in order to definitively deal with the cause of the stenosis. Combined approaches can be used simultaneously at one sitting or can be staged at different times several days apart. When the surgery is staged, the problems encountered are those that have been previously described for the individual surgical approaches. The problems however can be quite different when multiple approaches are used at one operation. The specific requirements and problems related to the combined approaches such as position of the patient and specific surgical procedures will be discussed from personal experience.

Combined Unilateral Anterior Approaches

In some patients suffering from anterior causes of stenosis, it is possible to combine anterior approaches through the same skin incision. The typical example is that of invasive lesions involving the vertebral body in both its central and lateral regions and extending to the transverse apophyses. The basic pre- and poststernocleidomastoid approaches to both the high and low cervical spine have been previously described. It must be pointed out that the length of the incision depends not only on the level at which the surgery is to be carried out, but also on the number of levels that will need to be operated on. Proximally, the hockey stick incision or the T-shaped incision is used (the latter has a horizontal portion parallel to the arch of the mandible and a vertical portion that runs along the sternocleidomastoid muscle). Following skin incision and during dissection to identify the important structures, one uses landmarks such as the superficial cervical fascia along the anterior margin of the sternocleidomastoid muscle to enter the area of the homhyoid with the middle cervical fascia. Here, one must clearly identify the neurovascular bundle of the neck, often an easy task. After this has been done, and still at the presternocleidomastoid level, one may slide in front of the neurovascular bundle or behind depending on the patient's specific surgical requirements. Using this approach, one can simultaneously operate centrally on the vertebral bodies and more laterally as far as the transverse apophyses.

It is relatively easy to reach the middle of the inferior cervical spine by passing in front or behind the neurovascular bundle of the neck. In fact, from C4 to C7 the bundle can be easily retracted anteriorly or posteriorly, permitting easy access to the desired level. However, when one needs to reach the upper cervical spine, or at least C1 and C2, then the constituents of the bundle are encountered as they approach their foramina at the base of the skull. At this point, retraction is difficult and not without significant risk of injury and complications. In such cases, the sternocleidomastoid muscle can be separated from its insertion and flipped downwards to allow better access and visualization both behind and in front of the neurovascular bundle. This pathway may be neither direct nor provide a very wide exposure, but it certainly provides sufficient access to the body of C2 and C3, with acceptable but less comfortable access to the body of C1. Furthermore, when dealing with advanced neoplasms that are associated with metastases to the lymph nodes in the lateral cervical regions through this approach, one can resect the sternocleidomastoid muscle together with the jugular vein and the lymph node chain as part of the definitive management of the neoplasm.

Combined Bilateral Anterior Approaches

Bilateral approaches may be used simultaneously at one surgical sitting. This combined approach is useful in dealing with invasive types of pathology or in cases of functional stenoses. The commonest example of such cases is tumor involvement of the entire vertebral body. Nevertheless, it is important to remember that the surgical trauma produced by this contemporaneous right and left anterior approach may be significant. Therefore, unless it is absolutely necessary to undertake this at one sitting, a staged procedure separating the right- and left-sided surgery by several days is preferable. In fact, in cases of massive tumors that require extensive resection, an initial resection should be performed on one side, with appropriate stabilization and reconstruction of the segment or segments involved. At a second sitting, removal of the tumor may be completed from the contralateral side. Often this sequential management is utilized when one needs to reach the transverse apophyses of the vertebral bodies, particularly when the involvement requires surgery on both sides that may reach the vertebral arteries bilaterally.

A bilateral simultaneous anterior approach is, however, indicated when the stenosis is high at the level of C1 and C2. In these cases, the purpose is to achieve fusion of the upper cervical vertebral bodies through the lateral approach. Such a bilateral arthrodesis between the atlas and the axis was described by Barbour in 1971. This was realized through fusion of the lateral masses of the atlas to the axis at the level of the lateral joints with two screws.

Obviously the indications for these procedures are very specific and limited. Primarily these are the cases in which one cannot undertake a posterior arthrodesis of C1–C2, usually because of the absence of the posterior arch of the atlas (either through fracture or previous laminectomy). The same also applies when it is not possible to undertake a cervico-occipital fusion. In the technique described, screws are used to immobilize the two atlantoaxial joints.

Technique

For the simultaneous bilateral approach, the patient should be placed on the table with the head resting on a head rest (Fig. 8.46). The head cannot be fixed. The skin is prepared bilaterally. The earlobe is retracted out of the field of surgery on both sides, and fixed in place by sutures. The head should be rotated towards the same side as the skin incision. The landmarks to be identified by palpation are the mastoid, the angle of the jaw, and the transverse apophysis of the atlas. The incision begins behind the mastoid process, passes over it, and curves along the first portion of the edge of the sternocleidomastoid muscle for a distance of 5 cm. As indicated previously one must identify the greater auricular muscle and the external jugular vein, both of which cross the sternocleidomastoid muscle. The insertion of the sternocleidomastoid muscle is separated at the mastoid process. It is retracted downwards and externally. The spinal accessory nerve should be distal to the incision and out of the field of view. Having retracted the sternocleidomastoid muscle, one must identify the posterior belly of the digastric muscle, which can then be retracted anteriorly. This exposes the tip of the transverse process of the atlas. Next, the hypoglossal nerve, the posterior belly of the digastric muscle, and the neurovascular bundle are retracted. The transverse apophysis of C1, which is covered by the deep cervical fascia and which is a landmark guiding us to the anterior surface of the atlas must be identified (the surgeon must strictly follow the bony surface). The lateral mass of the atlas should be easily identified, along with the atlantoaxial joints. The prevertebral muscles are then detached and retracted. One should not enter any dangerous areas, in spite of the abundance of neural and vascular structures in these areas, if one is careful to remain on the surface of the transverse apophysis of the atlas, right along the bony surface. Great care should be taken with retraction. No undue stretching or pressure should be used to avoid any injury to the carotid artery, the jugular vein, the hypoglossal and vagus nerves, and the digastric muscle. The same precaution should be taken with the vertebral artery, which at all times should be located above the plane of dissection.

Simultaneous Combined Anterior and Posterior Approaches

The simultaneous combined use of anterior and posterior approaches should be undertaken in patients with tumors that require total or subtotal removal of a lesion and in cases of severe trauma, where both the anterior and posterior elements are involved. In cases of tumor, one can begin either from an anterior or a posterior approach. The intention of this initial approach is to begin the removal of the tumor and achieve stabilization. Once this has been accomplished, the wound is completely closed. The patient's condition permitting, the patient is moved into the appropriate position for the second part of the combined approach to begin. The second stage may also be deferred by several days if necessary. This strategy can be frequently applied in posttraumatic stenosis. In the presence of a recognized posterior lesion such as subluxation of the apophyseal joints, one may elect to begin from the back and surgically reduce the dislocation with fusion of the apophyseal joints.

The mechanism of pathogenesis in this type of subluxation is the result of excessive and abnormal movement of the apophyseal joints and hence involves the disk, which may be disrupted and impinge on the anterior aspect of the canal.

In the stages of reduction, the surgeon attempts to realign the osseous components, bearing in mind that fragments of the disk may remain within the canal. Experience indicates that the best way to identify this eventuality is to perform an intraoperative myelogram. The surgeon gives the injection in his operative field, while the radiologist takes care of the radiographs and the exposure from outside the operative field. If fragments of disk are identified anteriorly, there are two possible ways of dealing with the problem. If the fragment is laterally placed, with a hemilaminectomy and retraction of the nerve root and cord, the fragments can be identified and removed from the back. However, if the fragment of disk is large and centrally placed, it is preferable to close the superficial muscular layers posteriorly, flip the patient over on the table, and undertake formal anterior decompression immediately to remove these fragments.

There are no specific complications associated with the described methods using combined anterior and posterior approaches. Nevertheless, difficulties do arise in cases where it becomes necessary to undertake a simultaneous anterior and posterior approach. These occur with patients in whom the required surgery demands the simultaneous exposure of the anterior and posterior vertebral structures. A typical example of this is post-traumatic nonunion or malunion, particularly in patients who have displaced vertebral bodies following a fracture subluxation, i.e., cases of subluxation of the apophyseal joints, especially neglected fracture subluxations, both of which have been consolidated in their position of displacement. Bony spurs and bony bridges have been formed in these cases, along with calcification of the anterior longitudinal ligament. The bones are in a fixed position of malalignment of the apophyseal joints. Only after taking down the osseous buttresses and bridges of the anterior longitudinal ligament can one reduce the fixed subluxation and restore the apophyseal joints to congruity (Fig. 8.47). Obviously, neither the anterior nor the posterior approach alone will be sufficient to permit the surgeon to reduce such fixed dislocations. In these patients the double approach must be used. The vertebral bodies must be freed and reduced with realignment of the walls of the bodies. This restores the continuity and diameter of the vertebral canal. Obviously, one can only achieve this through a simultaneous combined approach (Fig. 8.48).

The patient is in the lateral decubitus position. The trunk rests on the operating table right up to the axilla. The shoulder and the arm extend beyond the table and are supported at a level lower than that of the trunk. the head rests on its side on a head rest to which it is firmly fixed with tapes. In our experience, it is preferable to apply halo traction preoperatively. This provides postoperative immobilization and also helps in intraoperatively placing the head and neck. This position of the patient requires that the surgon be seated in front of the patient for both the anterior and posterior approaches. The steps required for reduction must be taken simultaneously by the surgeon and an able and skilled assistant. At all times there must be fluoroscopic control. Surgery should be carried out carefully and methodically. For monitoring cord function, particularly in order to be warned if cord compression is produced by the maneuvering, we use SEP throughout the operation.

During this procedure, the neck is entirely free and is basically held in suspension between the trunk and the head by the pull of the halo traction. Therefore, the surgeon must remember that he is maneuvering structures that are not being supported, and since they are devoid of any counterforce to the instrumentation, all activity must be carried out with the greatest of care. This implies avoiding the use of chisels and the preferential use of air drills to remove osseous fragments and bone buttresses that obstruct reduction.

References

Barbour JR (1971) Screw fixation and fractures of the odontoid process. S Aust Clin 5:20–24

De Andrade JR, MacNab I (1969) Anterior occipitocervical fusion using an extra-pharyngeal exposure. J Bone Joint Surg [Am] 51:1621–1626

Fang Hsy, Ong GB (1962) Direct anterior approach to the upper cervical spine. J Bone Joint Surg [Am] 44:1588–1604

Hall JE, Dennis F, Murray J (1977) Exposure of the upper cervical spine for spinal decompression by a mandible and tongue splitting approach. J Bone Joint Surg [Am] 59:121

Henry AK (1957) Extensile exposure, 2nd edn. Livingstone, Edingurgh, pp 53–80

Hodgson AR, Francis E (1960) Anterior spine fusion for the treatment of tubercolosis of the spine. The operative findings and results of treatment in the first one hundred cases. J Bone Joint Surg [Am] 42:295–310

Kocher T (1911) Surgery of the pharynx. In: Kocher T (ed) Operative surgery. Black, London

Riley L (1963) Surgical Approach to anterior cervical spine. Clin Orthop 91:16

Simmons EH, Du Toit JR, Guillaume (1978) Lateral atlanto-axial arthrodesis. Orthop Clin North Am 9:1101

Smith GW, Robinson RA (1958) The treatment of certain cervical spine disorders by anterior removal of the intervertebral disc and interbody fusion. J Bone Joint Surg [Am] 40:607–624

Southwick WO, Robinson RA (1957) Surgical approaches to the vertebral bodies in the cervical and lumbar regions. J Bone Joint Surg [Am] 39:631–644

Stauffer ES (1987) Mandibular splitting approach to the upper anterior vertebral canal. In: Kehr P, Weidner A (eds) Cervical spine I. Springer, Berlin Heidelberg New York, p 330

Verbiest H (1963) From anterior to lateral operations on the cervical spine. Neurosurg Rev 1–1:47

Whiteside TE (1978) Lateral retropharyngeal approach to the upper cervical spine. Orthop Clin North Am 9(4):1115

Whiteside TE, Kelly RP (1966) Lateral approach to the upper cervical spine for anterior fusion. South Med J 59:879–883

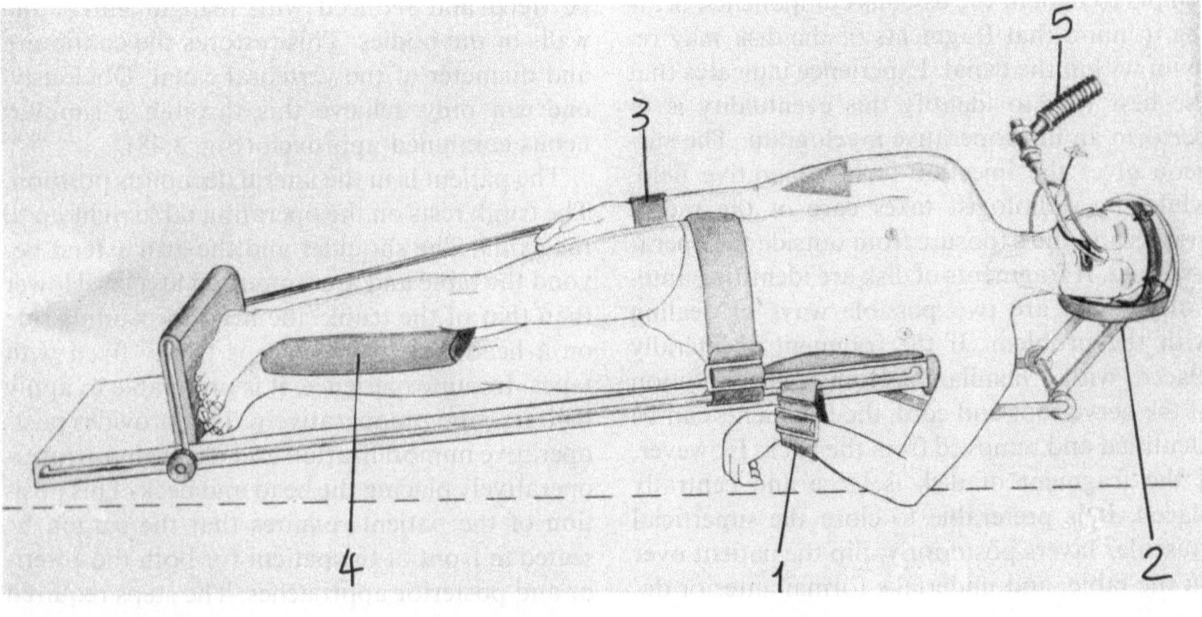

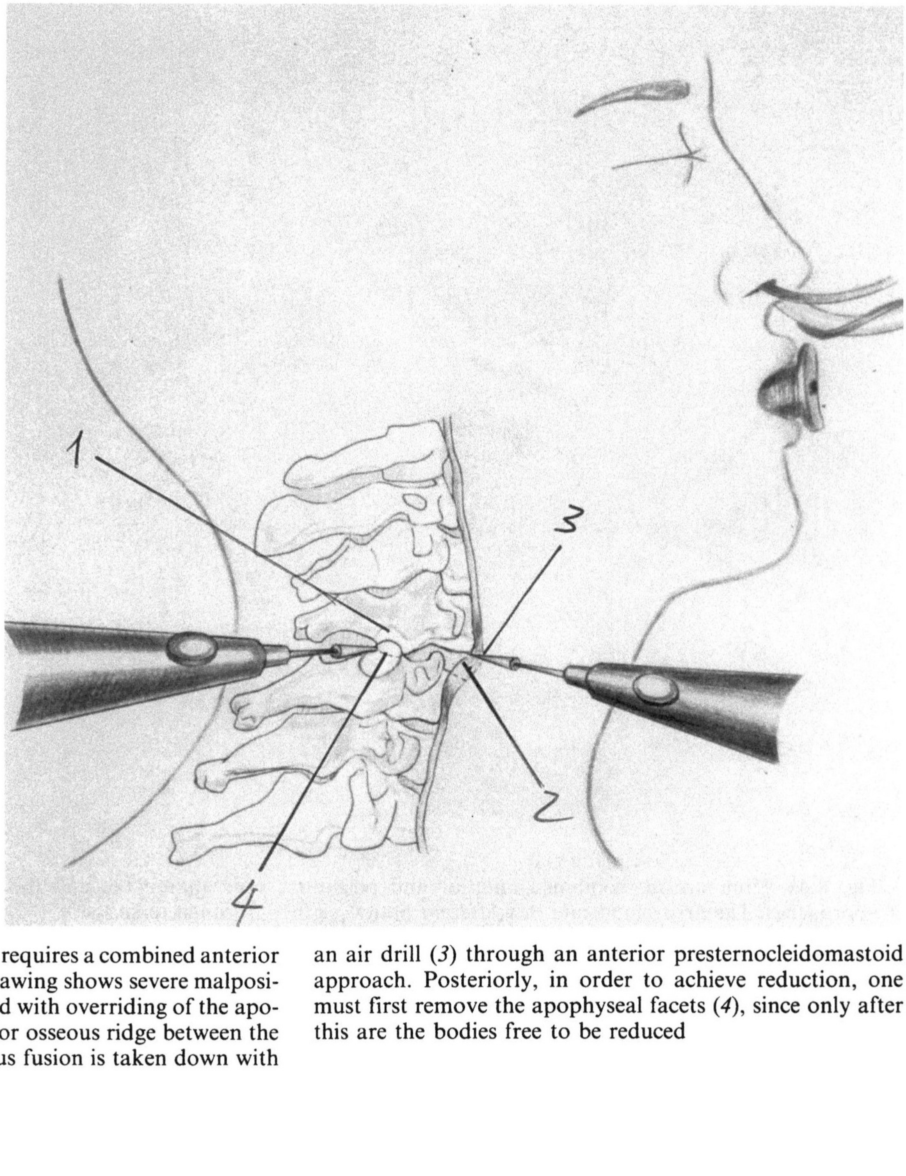

Fig. 8.47. A classical case which requires a combined anterior and posterior approach. The drawing shows severe malposition following trauma associated with overriding of the apophyseal facets (*1*) and an anterior osseous ridge between the vertebral bodies (*2*). The osseous fusion is taken down with an air drill (*3*) through an anterior presternocleidomastoid approach. Posteriorly, in order to achieve reduction, one must first remove the apophyseal facets (*4*), since only after this are the bodies free to be reduced

◀ **Fig. 8.46.** When one is undertaking a simultaneous anterior and posterior approach, the patient should be placed on his side on the table. The entire body lies on its side, completely on the table right up to the axilla. The shoulder and the arm extend beyond the bed. A wrist support supports the arm (*1*). An adjustable support holds the head in the lateral position (with or without halo traction) with the head adjusted to the same level as the shoulder (*2*). The upper arm is pulled towards the feet (*3*) in order to lower the shoulder. The bed is in a slight anti-Trendelenburg position. The legs are well supported with a pillow between them (*4*). This position allows for a simultaneous anterior presternocleidomastoid approach and a posterior longitudinal approach along the spinal processes. Nasotracheal and nasogastric tubes are in place (*5*)

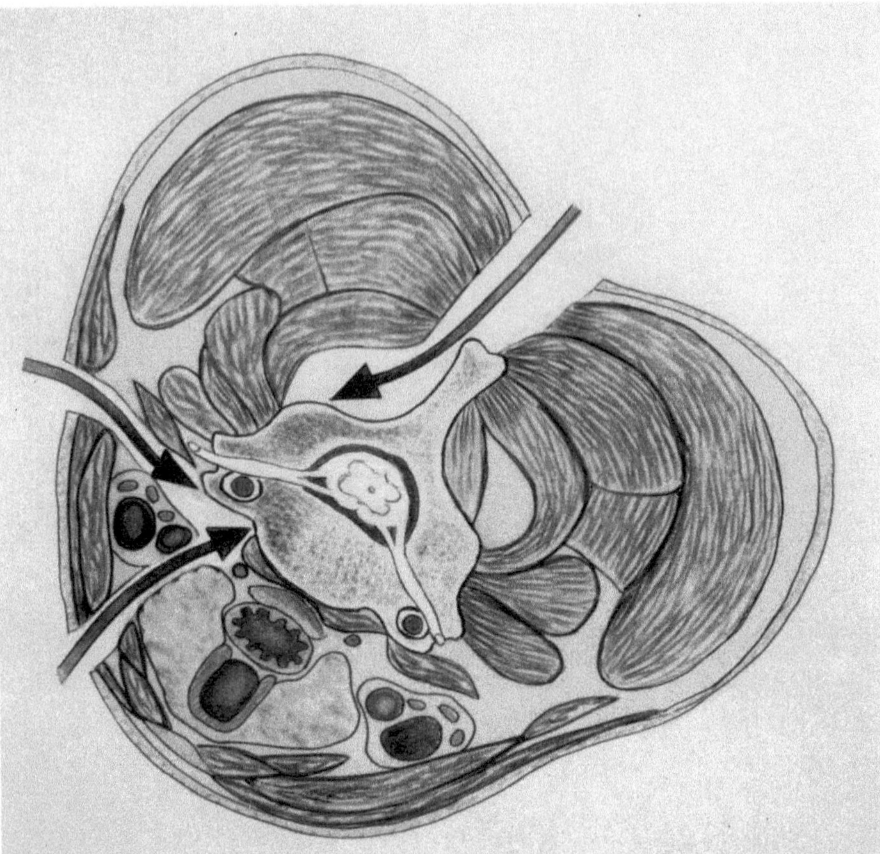

Fig. 8.48. Simultaneous combined anterior and posterior approaches. The arrows indicate the different pathways of the approaches and the structures which can be reached through them

CHAPTER 9

Surgical Techniques

Anterior Decompression

The surgical approaches that can be employed in order to obtain access to the cervical spine have been described in Chap. 8. Obviously, the choice of the approach will depend to a greater or lesser degree on the surgical procedure to be carried out once the exposure is completed. *The purpose of any procedure must be the complete removal of the cause of the stenosis.* When stenosis is the result of anterior compression, use of the anterior approach is preferred; the release of the compressed structure through the anterior approach, however, may be carried out in a variety of ways, depending on the actual pathology present. The best approach that will permit the best exposure in each case will be determined by whether the pathology is neoplastic, arthritic, or traumatic. On occasion, identical pathology can be approached by different methods, depending not only on the surgical procedure to be carried out, but also on the skill and experience of the surgeon in using a specific procedure (e.g., Cloward vs Smith-Robinson vs multilevel surgery). The more common surgical procedures and their practical aspects will be discussed in the following.

Anterior Decompression. Using Modified Cloward Instrumentation

The approaches described in the previous chapter guided dissection to the point at which the ventral aspect of the vertebral bodies is reached and the anterior longitudinal ligament is about to be stripped. The procedure described by Cloward for anterior decompression begins with a diskectomy (Fig. 9.1). A long scalpel is used to incise the edges of the vertebral bodies both in the horizontal and in the longitudinal planes of the spine. When large osteophytes are present, these protrude from the vertebral bodies and may overlap the entire intervertebral space. A curved chisel should be used to osteotomize these, so that flat vertebral surfaces can be obtained (Fig. 9.2). This will then permit a more complete diskectomy. The main purpose of removing the osteophyte and of evening out the vertebral end plate surfaces is to make sure that the bodies are perfectly even and no eccentricity results. This is particularly important when attempting to penetrate deep into the intervertebral disk space. If the anchoring surface of the drill is not even, then asymmetry may result. In order to assure that all disk tissue is removed, we have found the use of a Cloward spoon, either straight or curved, to be very useful in gaining greater accessibility to the disk material, which makes possible a more complete removal (Fig. 9.3). To achieve this the dissection must be extended as deeply as possible, right up to the posterior edges of the contiguous vertebral bodies. A depth gauge or sound should be used to determine the depth for purposes of instrumentation (Fig. 9.4).

As the next step it is most important to insert the guide exactly at the center of the vertebral bodies to be drilled (Figs. 9.5, 9.6). The lateral edges of the vertebral bodies to be drilled must be clearly visible so that the surgeon will have complete orientation during this procedure. If the drilling is eccentric or angled, serious complications may result. Extreme examples of such complications are injuries to the vertebral artery and to the nerve roots at the inferoposterior end of the root canal (Fig. 9.7). The sleeve is tapped along the guide with a hammer until it is perfectly anchored in the vertebral bodies, with its four tips pushed well into the bodies themselves. This is critical, since the sleeve is not perfectly anchored, the depth of drilling may be incorrectly measured and may permit entry into the spinal canal with injury to the cord. With each drilling, the sleeve must be advanced with a tap of the hammer. For this reason, a rigid support for the patient's neck is essential in preparing the patient and in positioning him on the operating table (Figs. 9.8, 9.9). It is the only way in which the spinous processes can be fixed and well supported enough to withstand the force of insertion of the guide and its sleeve and for drilling accurately into the vertebral bodies. The sleeve must be firmly held in place before one begins to drill into the vertebral body. A calibrated guide must be used in order to ensure that the depth of the drilling is controlled and does not exceed that which was measured at the time of diskectomy (Fig. 9.5). Once the drilling is completed, the drill and the sleeve are removed and the hole formed must be quickly examined while suctioning. There will be significant bleeding which usually originates in the deepest portions of the cavity in the region of the posterior margin of the vertebral bodies where the nutrient vessels are located. To control this bone wax may be pressed into the deep region and then smeared along the walls of the cavity. To reach into the depths of the cavity with bone way, an applicator loaded with bone wax is most useful (Fig. 9.10).

Hemostasis is most important in order to permit the surgeon to visualize his operative site without any interference from excessive bleeding. Any remaining disk fragments can now be removed and, once this is complete, the surgeon can visualize the extent of penetration, and hence have a visual measure of what remains to be drilled. Guided by repeated visual inspection, the surgeon should slowly advance penetration. It is important that this be done carefully and slowly in graduated steps in order to avoid unnecessary complications. The processes of gradual and controlled drilling, repeated inspection of the wall and of the depth of the penetration, and achieving hemostasis with bone wax are time consuming, but are the only sure way to progress carefully up to and not beyond the necessary level. During these repeated steps, the surgeon will appreciate the necessity for rigid support of the patient's head and neck that provides a counterforce to his efforts. Soft support would only lead to movement of the vertebral body posteriorly with each attempt at penetration, and would allow the osseous edges to be pushed into the cord and its related neurological structures. Having advanced to within a few millimeters of the posterior walls of the vertebral bodies, curved curets (either 45° or 90°), which are extremely valuable to the surgeon at this time, are used (Fig. 9.11). They can be carefully slid behind the remaining vertebral cortex through the disk space, lifting the posterior longitudinal ligament away from any osteophytes that are present. Large osteophytic spurs must be removed slowly, piecemeal, and stepwise. One must always look for a line of cleavage along the surface of osteophytic spurs, particularly in the most severe cases; these can usually be found if one is dissecting from the disk space, particularly towards the lateral sides where insertion of the spoon in this plane of cleavage will allow the exophytic spur to be lifted away. Cloward drills do not penetrate well into hard bone. This is to be expected in cases of advanced spondyloarthritis with significant sclerosis of the posterior cortex and the margins of the vertebral bodies. However, the curet may also not be able to break through this rather thick and sclerotic bone. In these cases, an air drill is useful in thinning out these sclerotic walls from inside so that they become weak enough for the curet to break through and eventually complete the removal (Figs. 9.12, 9.13a).

When the removal of the osseous tissue is completed, the posterior longitudinal ligament is seen as a soft structure at the deep end of the operative field. The posterolateral tissue at the unci can now be removed. At this point, the exposure should provide ample space, enabling the surgeon to identify the inner end of the root canal. Under direct visual control, the curet can be guided towards the canal in order to grab and remove first the posterior portion and then the posterolateral portion of the unci (Fig. 9.13b). This procedure is relatively safe if it is carried out under direct visual control, unlike the transdiskal approach described in other procedures for removing the unci.

At this point, assuming that decompression has been achieved and no other levels are to be operated upon, harvesting of the iliac graft can begin. From the wing of the ilium, which should initially have been prepared and draped, one must remove a cylinder of bone that includes both cortices. It is best to obtain the graft from just below the iliac crest posteriorly where the bone is thickest (Fig. 9.115).

A 3-cm longitudinal incision makes it possible to dissect away the muscles and the fascia from the bone. The graft should be taken using an instrument with a diameter of at least 3 mm greater than the hole drilled into the vertebra. All periosteal tissue and all soft tissue components must be removed from the harvested graft.

It is suggested that a hole be drilled in the center of the graft. Once the graft is in place, any bleeding that might occur behind it will be able to escape and no pooling or build up of tissue pressure will result. The graft can be shaped with a bone file in order to give it two opposing flat sides (Fig. 9.14a). The graft will be placed in a hole that was drilled with a round contour, but which under the conditions of insertion will be stretched and elliptical with flattened sides.

At this point, the surgeon is attempting to produce an arthrodesis in distraction in such a way that the arthrodesis seals the disk space, which is cleared of its contents and which, by producing distraction, enlarges the root canal bilaterally. For this reason, the graft should be 3 mm in diameter greater than the hole drilled, since once it has been inserted into the trough within the bone, it assists in maintaining distraction. Professor Boni designed a distractor that helps in achieving this separation (Fig. 9.14). As seen in Fig. 9.14, it has two points on each side that are designed to fit precisely into the grooves produced by the drill guide. These can be tapped into place with a hammer in order to ensure that they are solidly fixed. The use of a combination of traction and distraction permits the insertion of the bony graft, which will then be firmly anchored once the distraction is released (Figs. 9.14–9.16). An important technical point is to ensure that the graft is pushed completely into the vertebral body with its surface even with the surface of the surrounding vertebral body. This facilitates soft tissue closure without any undue stress on the tissues (Figs. 9.14, 9.17).

Should the stenosis involve more than one level, it is possible to repeat the Cloward procedure at each of the involved levels (Figs. 9.18, 9.19). It must be remembered that if one body is to be drilled twice, the remaining bone will be weakened and will easily collapse. In such cases one may need to drill off center in order to retain a good osseous bridge. Certain precautions must be taken in drilling vertebral bodies off center. To ensure that the drill guide is fixed onto the guide wire, it may be necessary to produce a shelf on the side of the vertebral body below and above the level of operation, either with a straight curet or with a ball drill. Once this drilling is completed, then all the steps described above can be followed and repeated at each level as required (Fig. 9.5). Obviously more than one graft must then be harvested and prepared.

Technical Errors and Complications

The following errors should be avoided in anterior decompression using Cloward instrumentation:

Incorrect positioning of the guide and drill. The correct positioning of the guide and drill on the vertebral bodies on either side of the disk space to be drilled must be emphasized. If this is not accurately done, the direction of drilling will be eccentric and angled. Posterior osteophytes tend to be central and, therefore, their eventual excision may be rendered unnecessarily more difficult. Whenever anterior osteophytes are encountered, it is important to remove them with chisels to create a smooth and uniform base, thereby restoring the anterior surface of the vertebral bodies. Only when this has been accomplished should the guide and drill be definitively positioned.

All too frequently the guide and hence the drill are positioned laterally and off center. This is a technical mistake with potentially serious consequences. The vertebral body must be exposed to such an extent as to permit visualization of the entire anterior aspect and both lateral aspects so that their orientation is clearly identifiable. If drilling is off center, the drill may penetrate the lateral regions of the body and reach its uncal (posterolateral) portion towards the base of the pedicle, or even laterally enough to reach the intertransversal space and injure the vertebral artery.

If the guide is not perfectly seated in a plane parallel to that of the vertebral body because of the anterior osteophyte, it advances obliquely through the vertebra. In such cases, one side of the drill may be still in the bone, giving the surgeon the impression that one is still drilling bone, while the other part of the tip extends right into the canal, with a high risk of injury to the meninges and cord (Figs. 9.7, 9.9).

Obviously, this is an extremely dangerous situation. The incorrect use of the drill, in our experience, is the cause of the most severe complications reported during this procedure.

Incorrect assessment of the depths of drilling. It is important to proceed in small, repeated steps when deepening the drilling. This may take longer, but it provides a greater degree of safety to the procedure. When approaching the posterior wall, the advancement of the drill must be carefully assessed and gradual and the depth reached by the drill must be routinely confirmed after each graduated advance. This will assure that the safe depth is not exceeded. As described, an error in the depth reached by the drill may have serious consequences with injury to the cord.

Failure to reach the posterior wall of the vertebral body. If the surgeon has not drilled as far as the cortical surface, particularly large osteophytes that bulge posteriorly may be extremely difficult to remove with a curet. By being cautious, advancing the drill slowly in predictable steps, and using curved curets to assess the depth reached by the drill, it is possible to identify the line of cleavage between the original cortex and the osteophyte. Only at this point should one proceed to the formal removal of the osteophyte. If the posterior wall is not accurately reached, the tissues will not be freed and the result will not be satisfactory.

Injury to the cord or the nerve roots may occur when posterior and posterolateral bulges are being removed. This is apt to occur when the surgeon proceeds without visual control and if he has failed to identify the planes of cleavage accurately.

Injury to the vertebral artery. During the removal of the posterolateral wall of the vertebral body at the uncus, it is possible to injure the vertebral artery. As the dissection proceeds laterally during removal of the tissue from the uncus, one must always bear in mind the possibility that the tip of curet may extend too far laterally and reach the intertransverse canal.

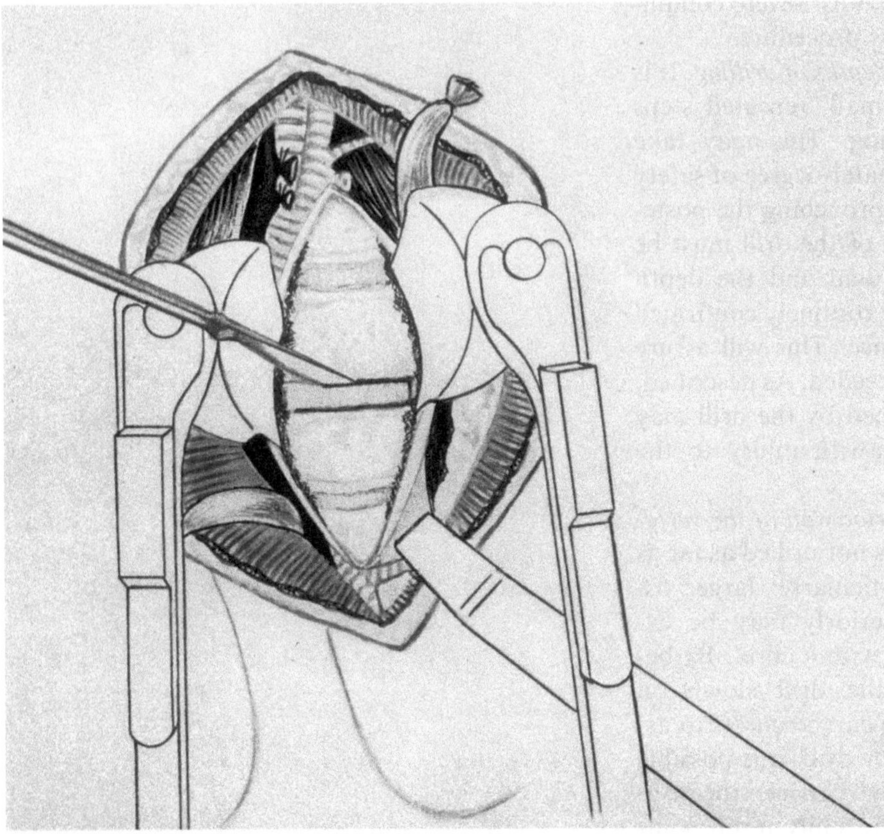

Fig. 9.1. To begin the diskectomy, a scalpel is used to enter the intervertebral disk space

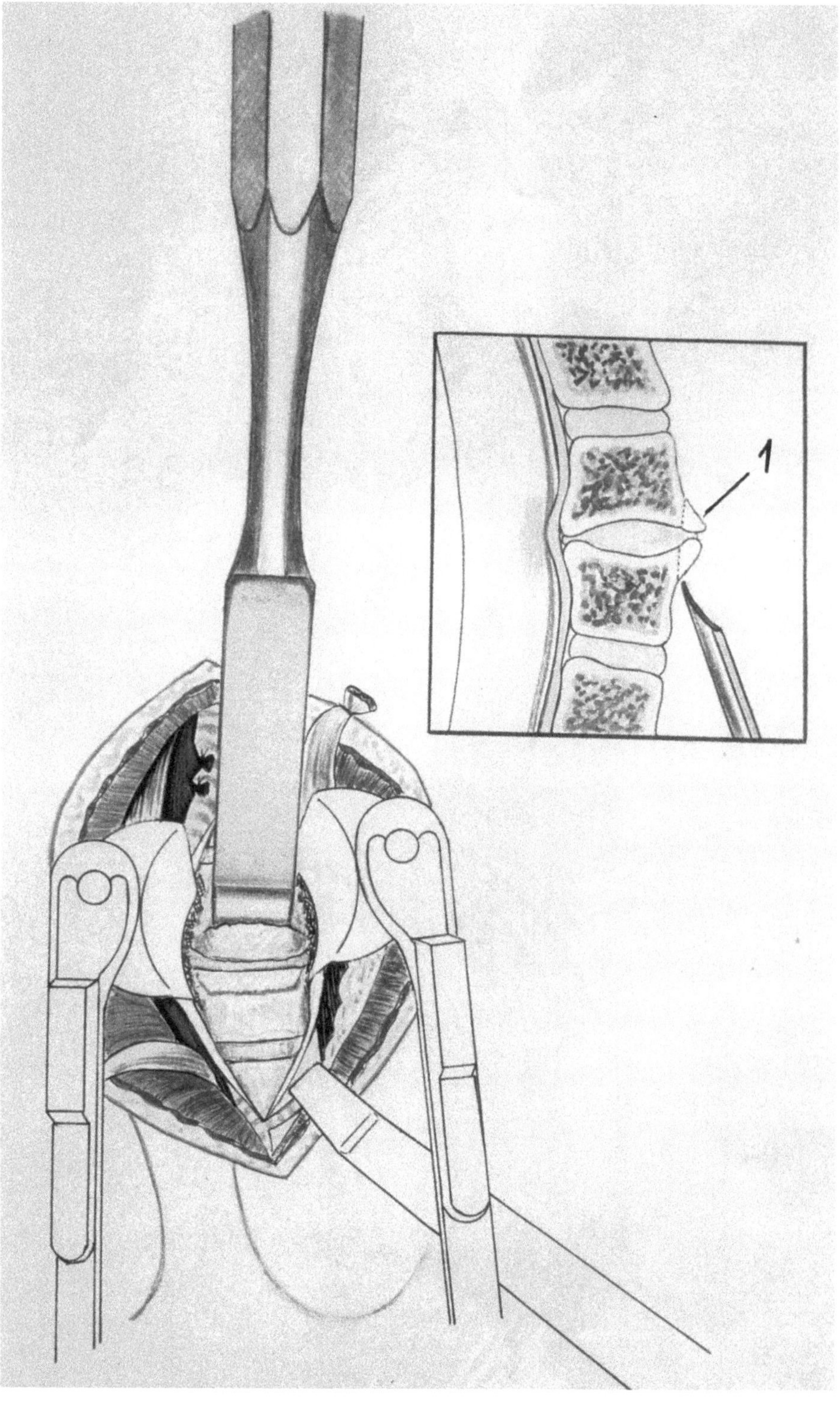

Fig. 9.2. If osteophytes protrude anteriorly (*1*), it becomes necessary to remove them with a chisel in order to provide a smooth and uniform base for the drill guide and hence the Cloward drill

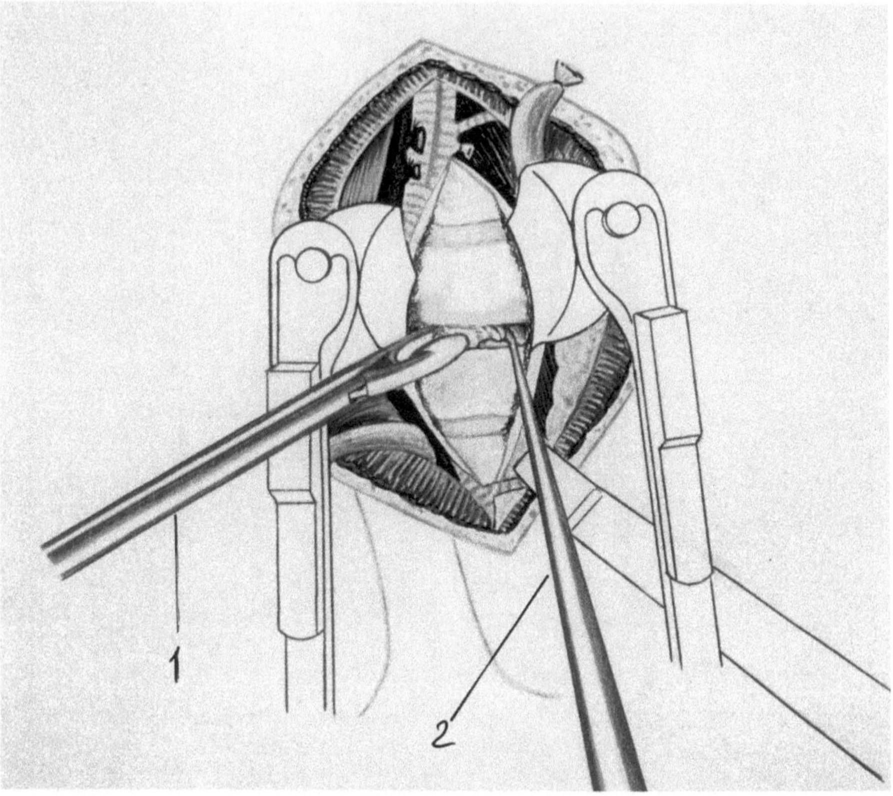

Fig. 9.3. The disk can be removed with disk forceps (*1*), assisted by curved curets (*2*). The curets permit removal of the deeper fragments of disk

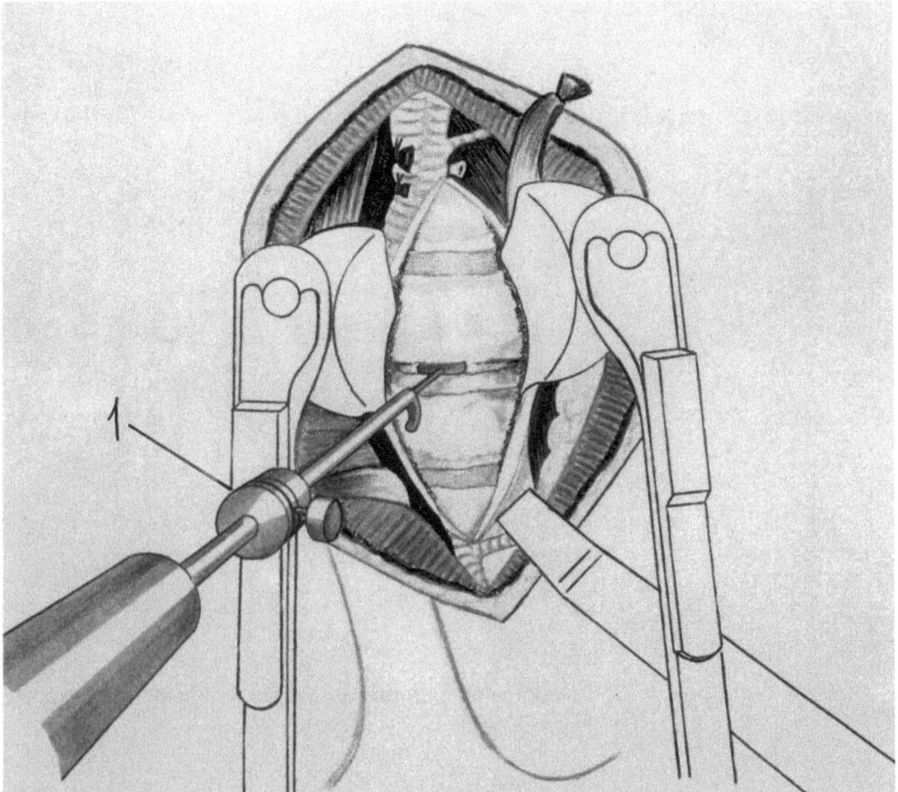

Fig. 9.4. The gauge (*1*) measures the required depth of drilling, allowing the drill to advanced in measured steps

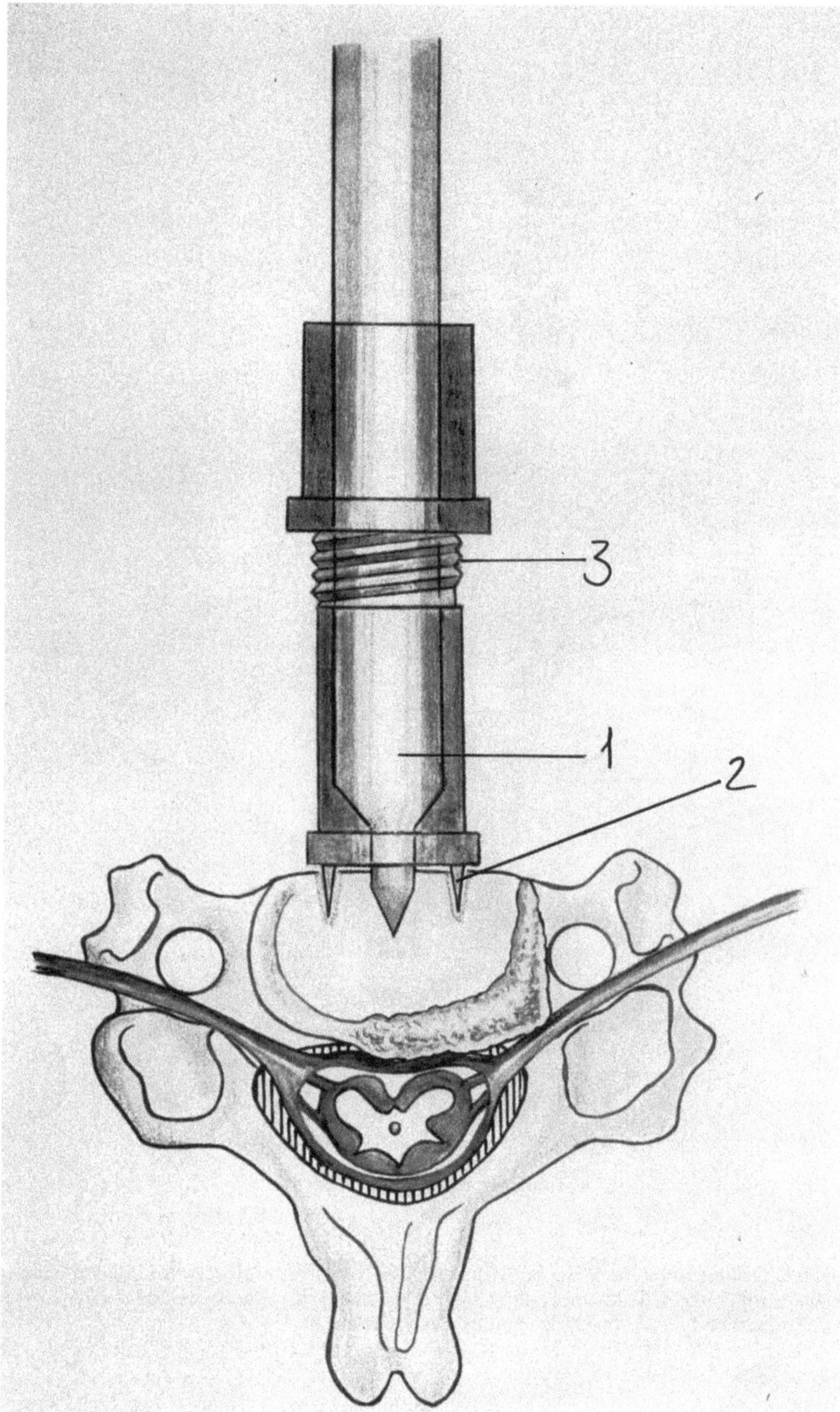

Fig. 9.5. Once the guide is in place within the disk space (*1*), the sleeve is slid forward to the margins of the bone and fixed by its four teeth (*2*). The threads (*3*) represent the mechanism by which the depth of drilling is monitored and gradually increased

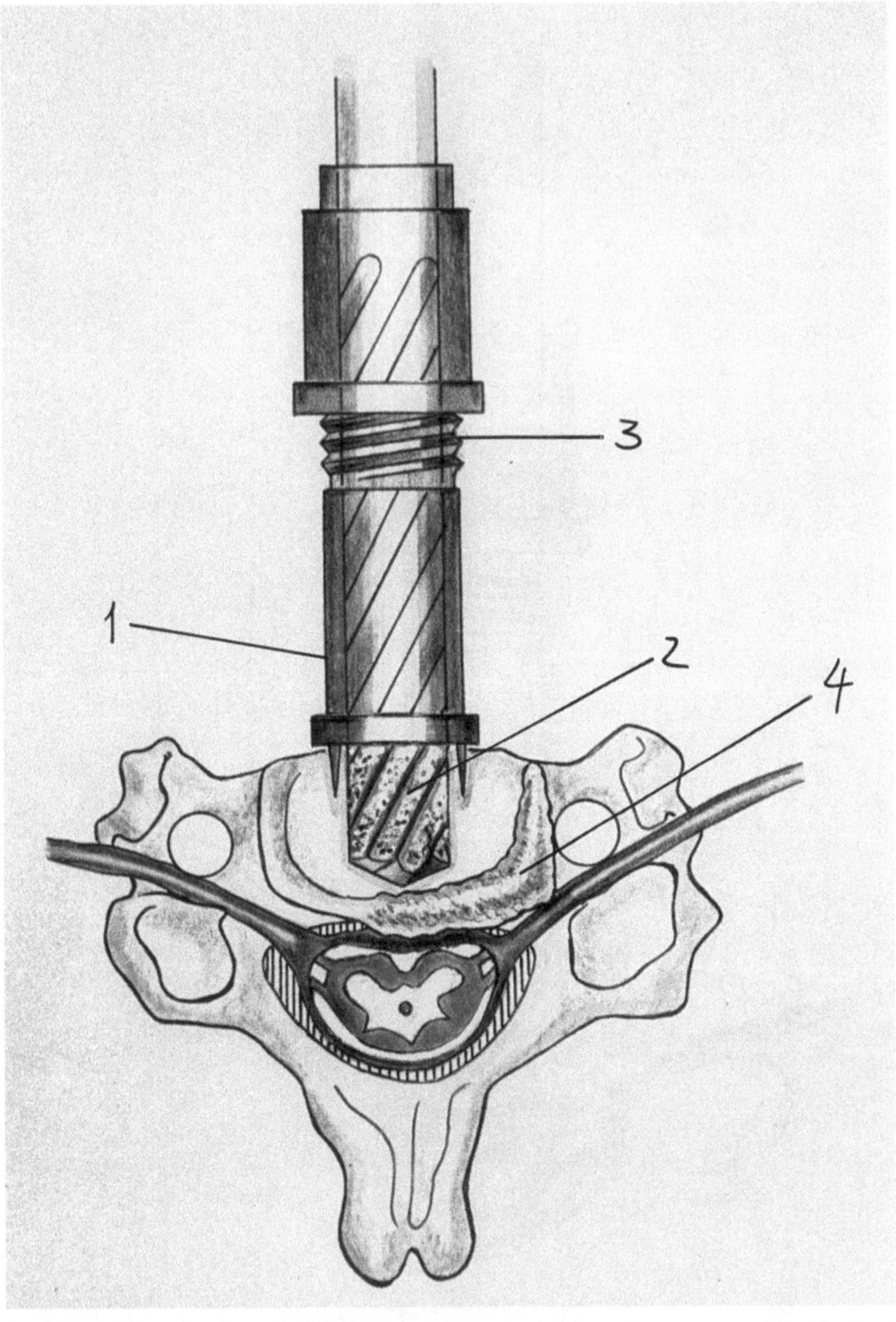

Fig. 9.6. Drilling of the vertebral body showing the sleeve (*1*) through which the drill advances (*2*) to the posterior wall of the vertebral body. Its progress is regulated by the gauge (*3*). Here a posterolateral osteophyte (*4*) is present and will eventually be removed

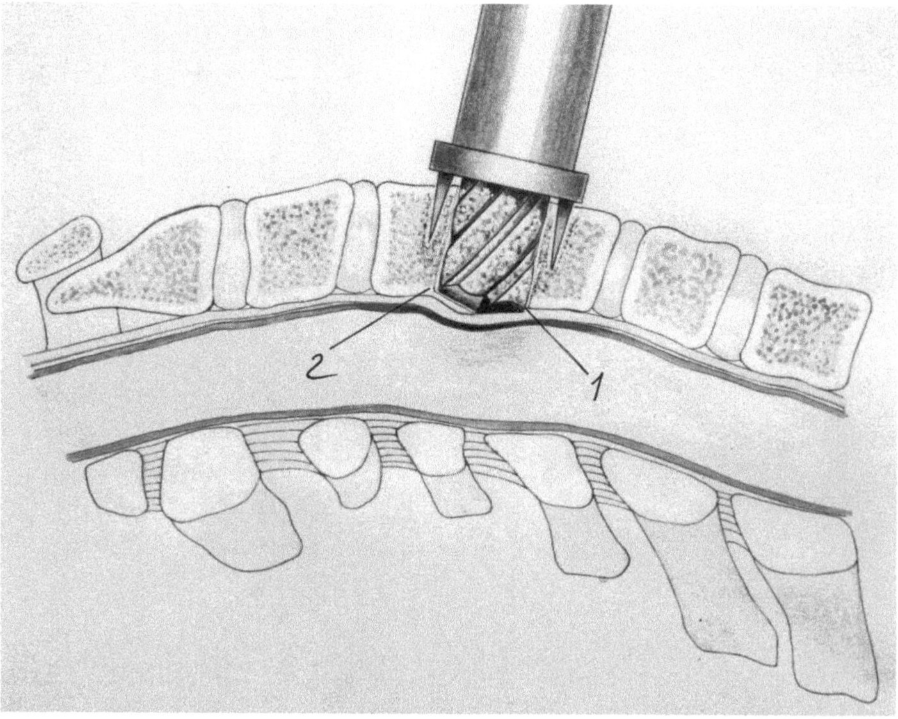

Fig. 9.7. The consequences of a malpositioned guide which is not perpendicular to the vertebral bodies. As it is advanced the drill follows an oblique path, reaching the posterior wall on one side (*1*), while the other side is still well within the vertebral body (*2*). In such circumstances, the surgeon feels that he is drilling bone, while in fact he may be injuring the soft tissues

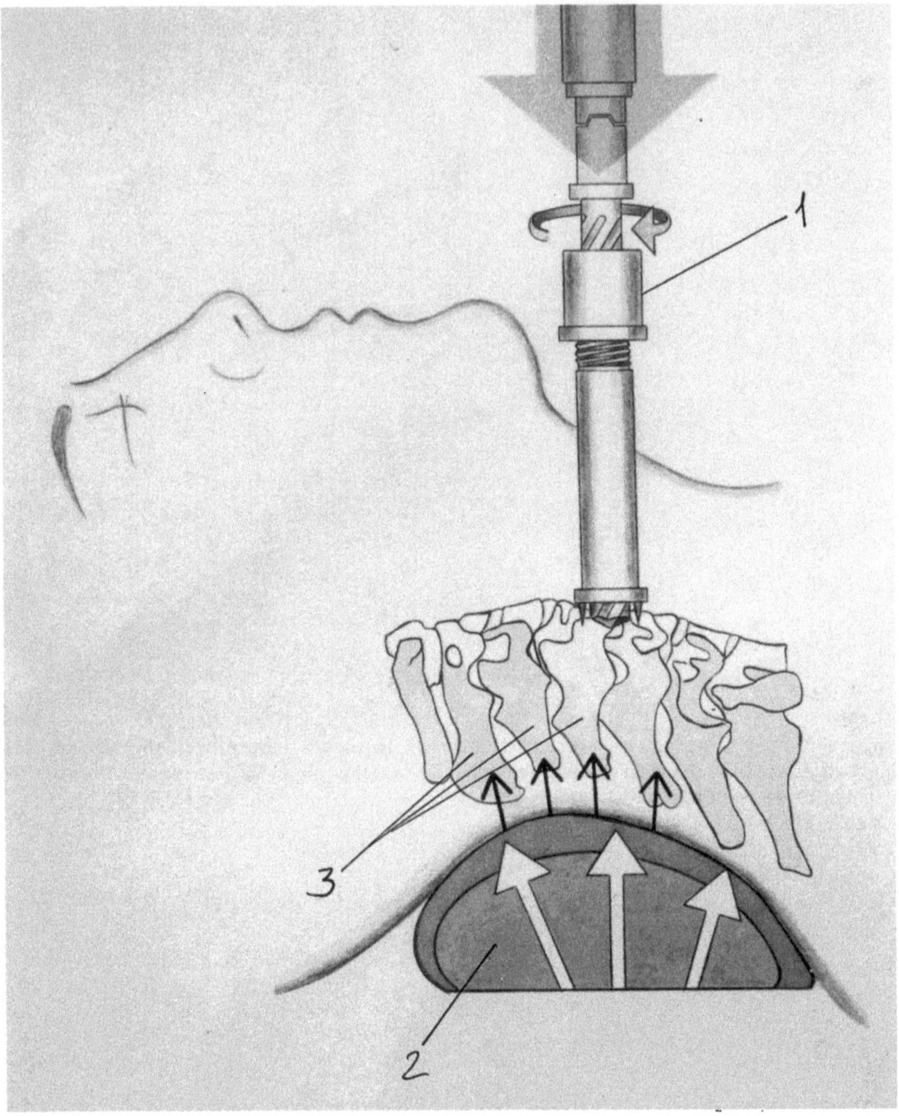

Fig. 9.8. Illustration of the value of the rigid support to the neck posteriorly (*2*) as part of positioning the patient on the operating table. As the Cloward drill (*1*) is advanced into the vertebral bodies, the support to the posterior elements (*3*) must be rigid enough to provide a counterbalancing support

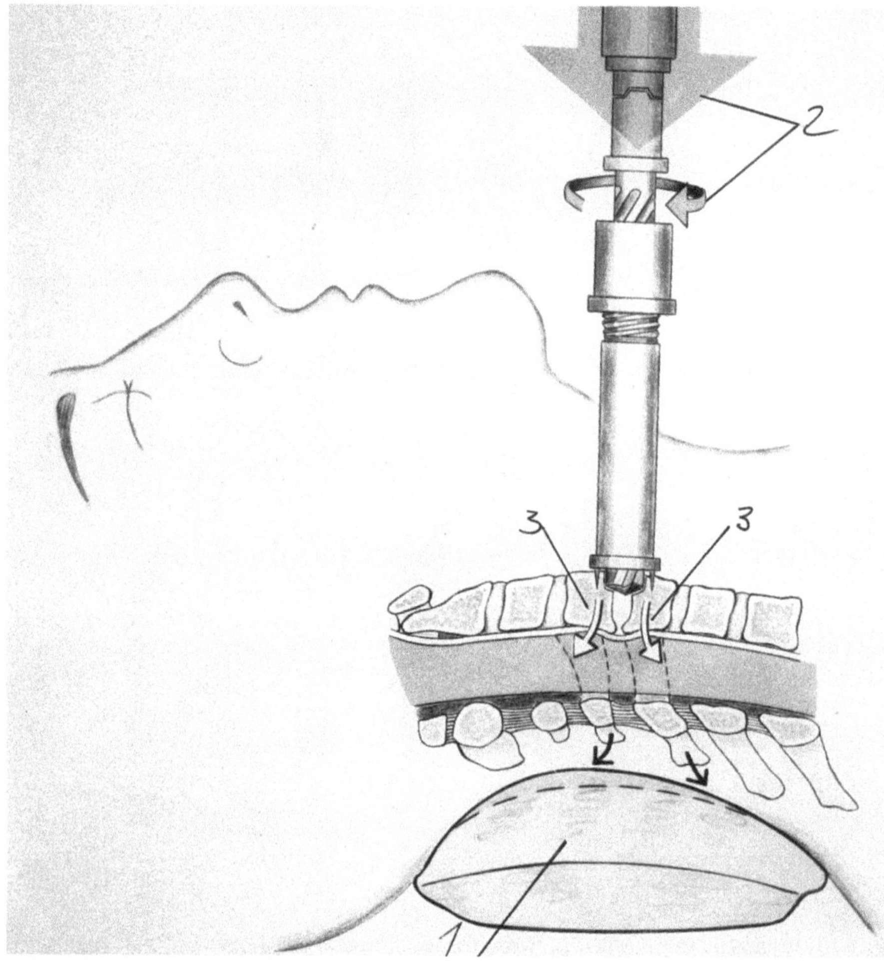

Fig. 9.9. The consequences of the absence of a rigid support for the spinous processes (*1*). The force of the drilling and the rotation (*2*) cause posterior dislocation of the vertebral bodies (*3*). This drives the osteophytes and any other fragments of the posterior wall of the vertebral body further into the cord with potentially serious consequences

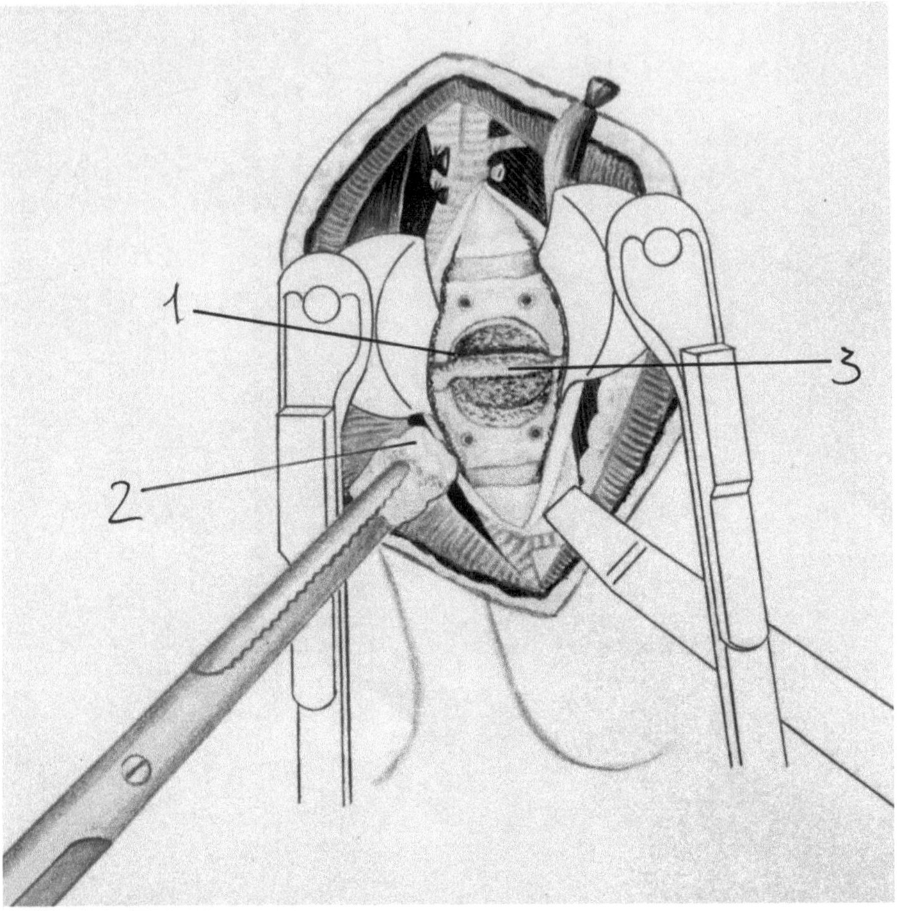

Fig. 9.10. When the drilling of the two adjacent vertebral bodies is completed (*1*), in the depths of the gaping hole there will be extensive hemorrhage from the richly vascular spongiosa. It is essential that the operative field be free of blood and, for this reason, the free use of bone wax (*2*) is important. It can be applied with a sponge held by a clamp and packed into the depths of the drill hole (*1*). The sponge (*2*) loaded with bone wax is a valuable instrument in keeping the drill hole clean and free of bleeding, in order to permit the surgeon to visualize the bottom of the drill hole and to gauge the depth of the remaining posterior wall (*3*)

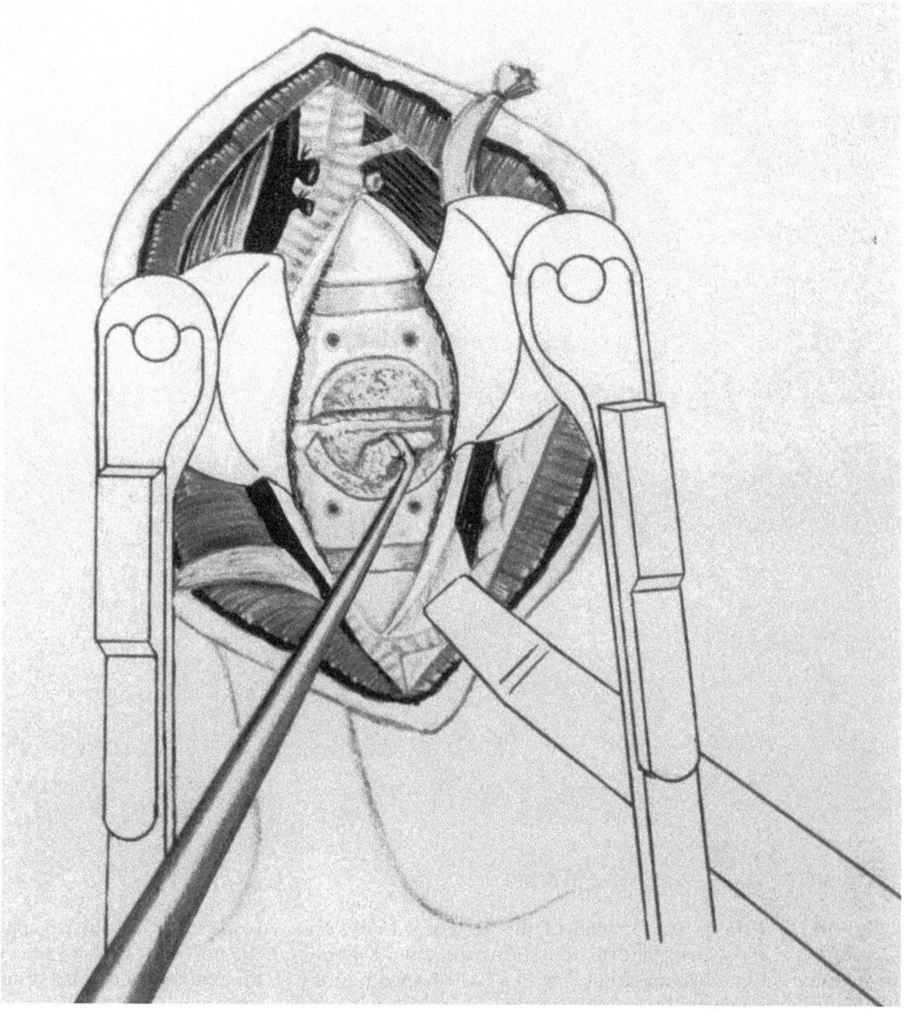

Fig. 9.11. A curved (45°)curet is used to remove the remaining bone and disk fragments. Evacuation of all the loose pieces allows the surgeon to assess the amount of remaining posterior wall that must still be removed

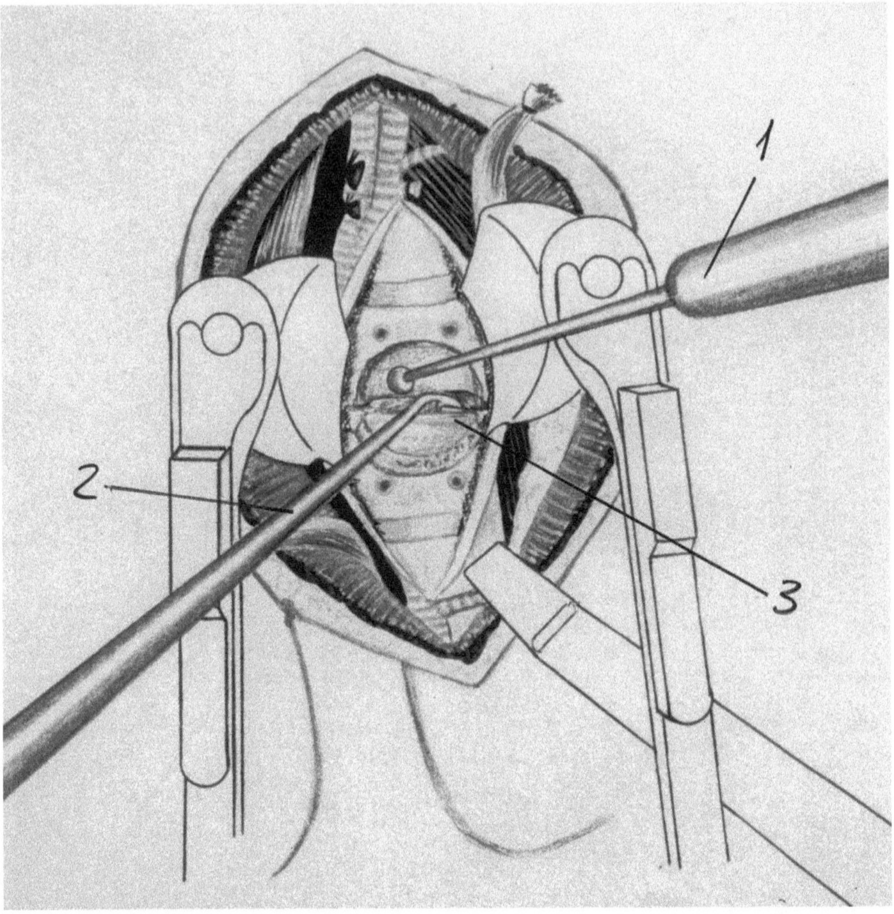

Fig. 9.12. At the posterior wall of the vertebral body, one cannot use the Cloward drill to remove reactive sclerotic osteophytic bone. An air drill (*1*) with a ball-shaped bit may be helpful in gradually extending the cavity towards the posterior longitudinal ligament. Curets may then be used (*2*) to clear the intradiskal space and to complete the removal of the posterior walls of the vertebral bodies (*3*). Obviously, the air drill minimizes the amount of effort required in the complete removal of the remnants of the posterior wall

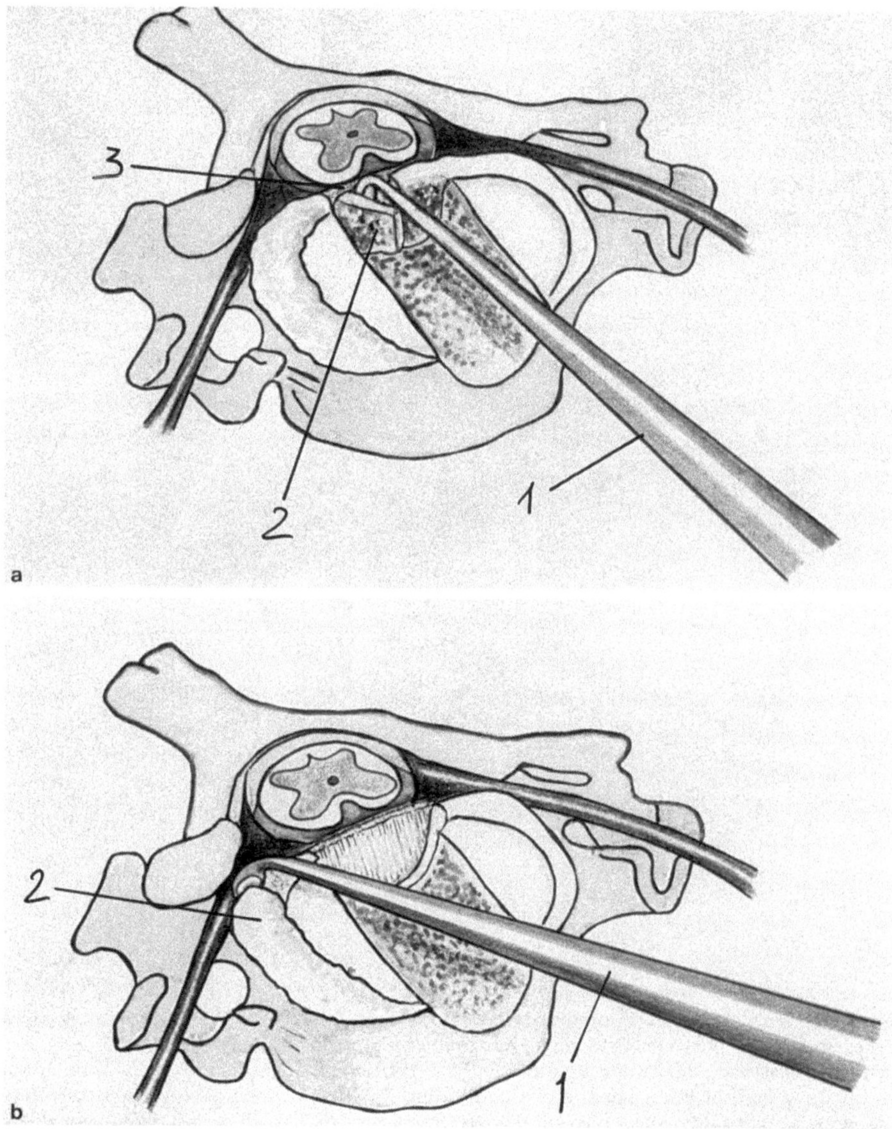

Fig. 9.13a, b. The horizontal plane of dissection. **a** The curved curet (*1*) scoops out the remnants of the posterior wall of the vertebral bodies (*2*), freeing them from the posterior longitudinal ligament (*3*). **b** The dissection is carried laterally with curved curets (*1*) to remove any cause of compression or obstruction of the nerve root canal that may be present in the posterolateral portion of the body (*2*).

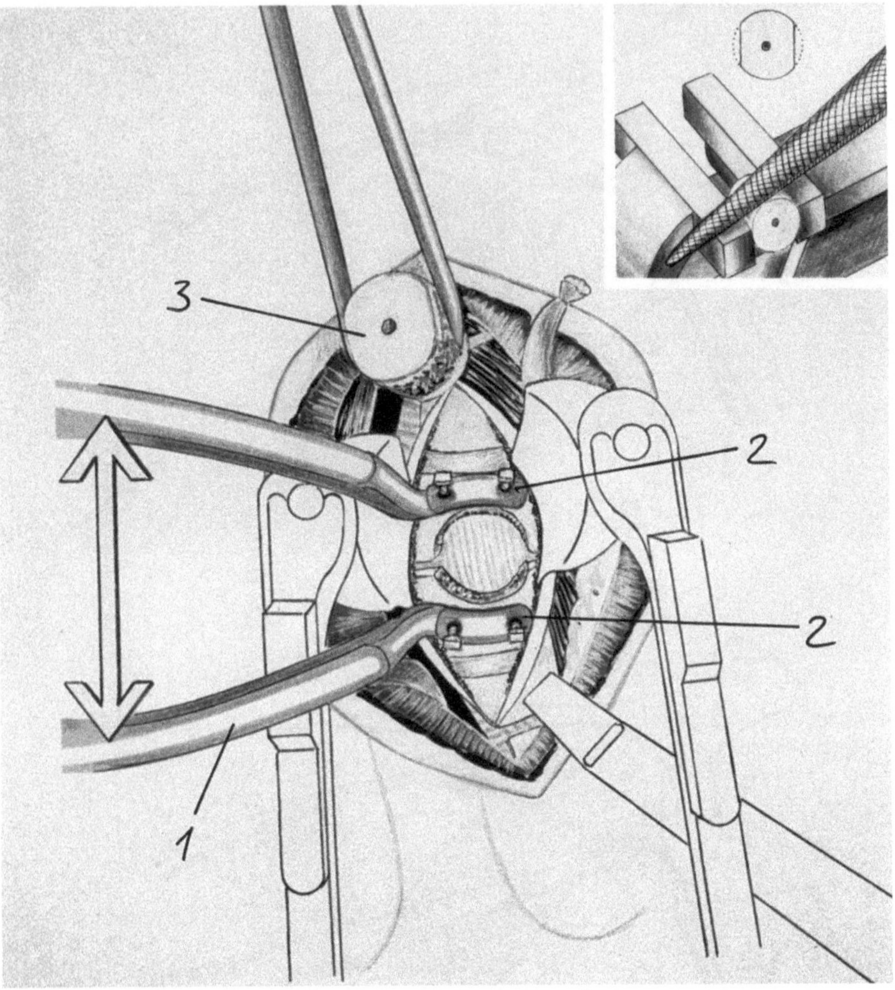

Fig. 9.14. Once the removal of the posterior walls of the bodies and of any posterior osteophyte has been completed, a specially designed distractor is applied (*1*). This instrument sits on the vertebral bodies just above and below the drill hole, with its foot plates shaped to conform to the outline of the drill hole itself. The foot plates are anchored in place with four self-tapping screws (*2*). A bicortical cylindrical graft (*3*) from the iliac crest, appropriately shaped, is then slotted into the drill hole being held apart by the distractors. The insert shows the use of a file in shaping the graft. The diameter of the graft is greater than that of the drill hole. The distractor will permit lengthening, but the side-to-side diameter remains constant. The lateral aspect must therefore be filed down in order to fit into the drill hole

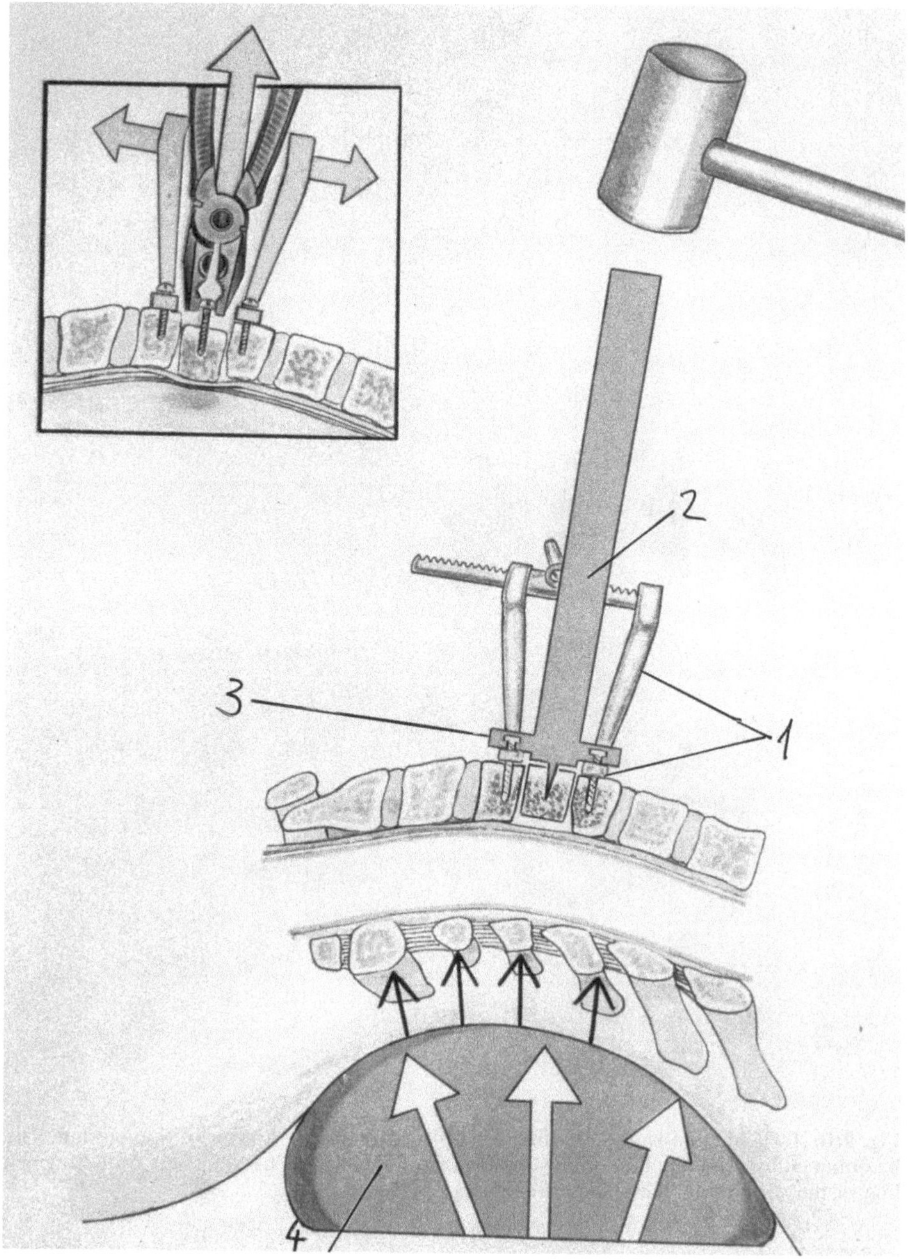

Fig. 9.15. The distractor is in place (*1*), fixed by self-tapping screws onto the vertebral bodies. Tapping on the instrument (*2*) specially designed for insertion pushes the graft into the grooves on the two opposing vertebrae. The wings (*3*) of the instrument will impinge on the foot plates of the distractor, limiting the advance of the graft so that it is not pushed in too far. If necessary, the graft can be tapped into position as long as the neck is firmly supported (*4*), as described above. The insert shows how the graft should be pulled back if it has been placed too deeply

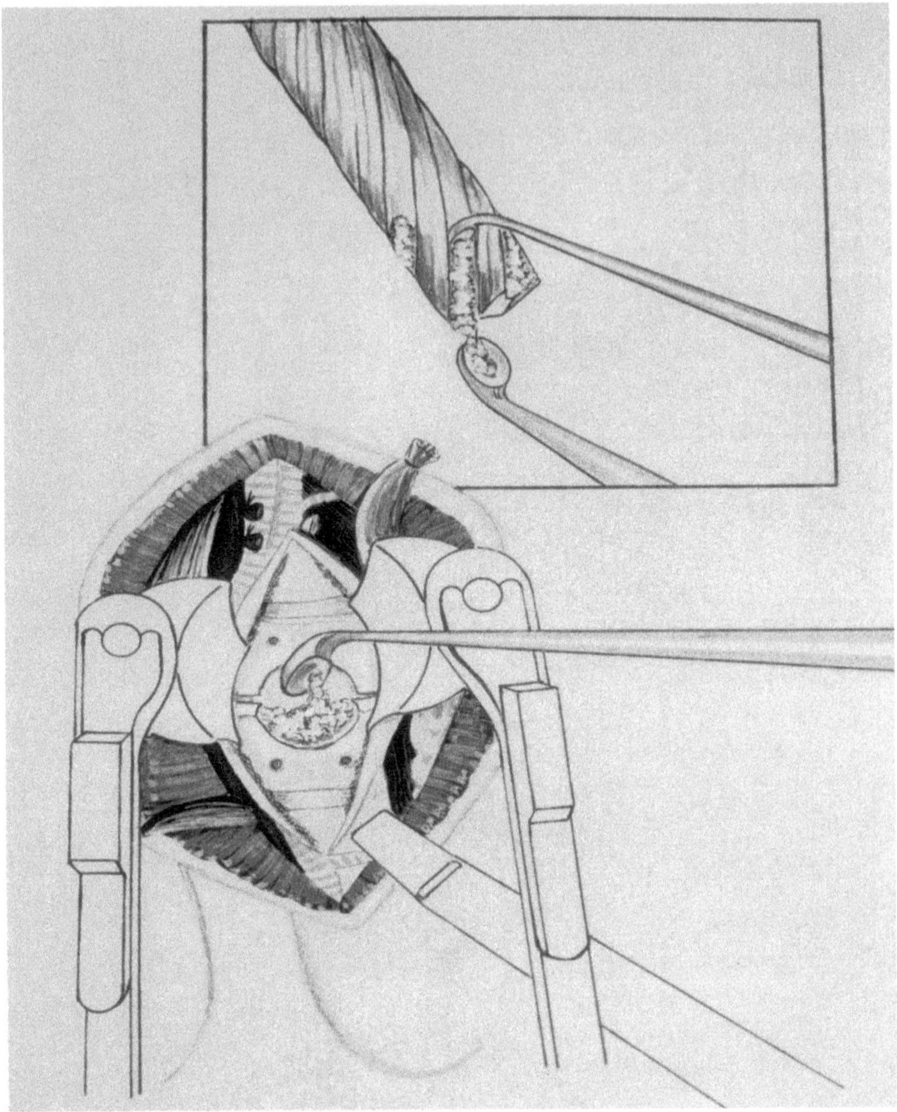

Fig. 9.16. If distraction is not essential, a simple fusion can be obtained by using the bone chips obtained from the drilling of the vertebral bodies. These fragments are placed on a layer of Spongostan. The insert shows a detail of the retrieval of the bony fragments from the drill bit

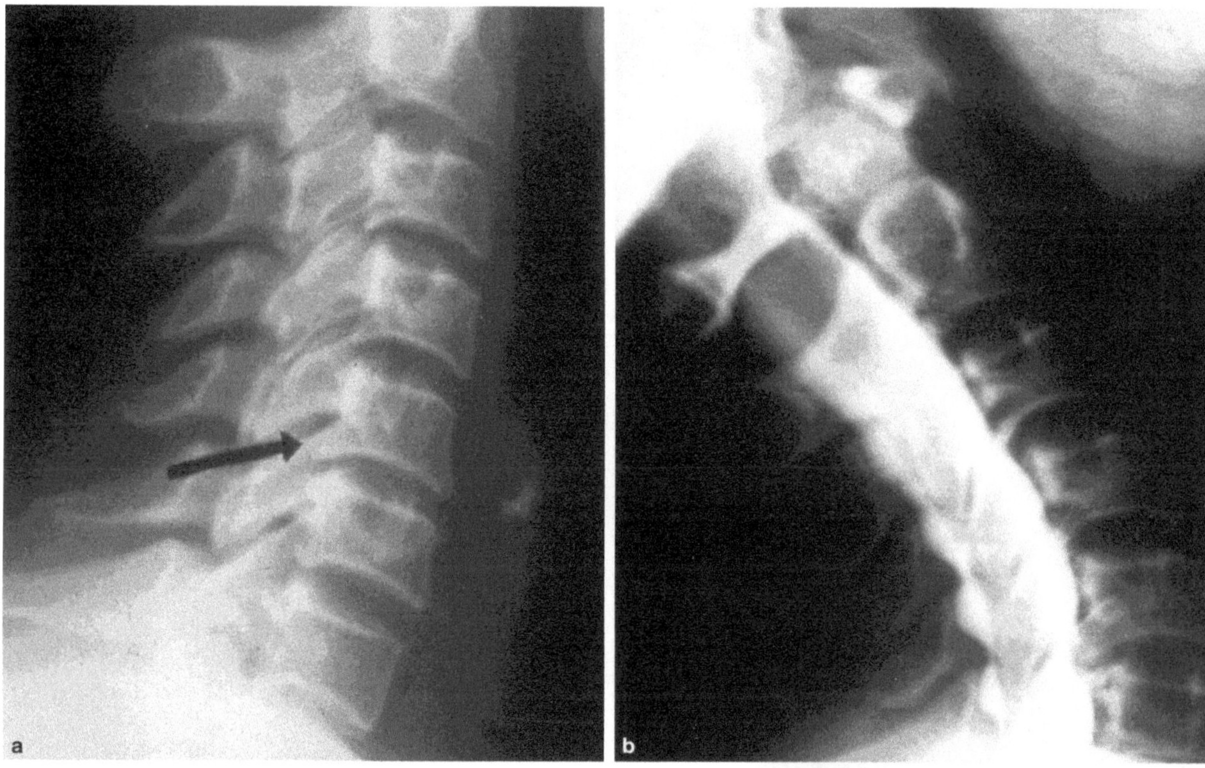

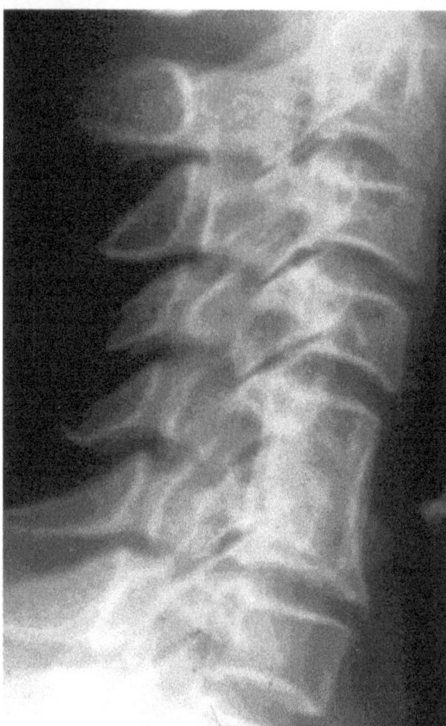

c

Fig. 9.17 a, b, c. Radiographs of a patient showing compression at the C5–C6 level (**a**). The C5–C6 level after anterior decompression using Cloward technique (**b**), and after 10-year follow-up (**c**)

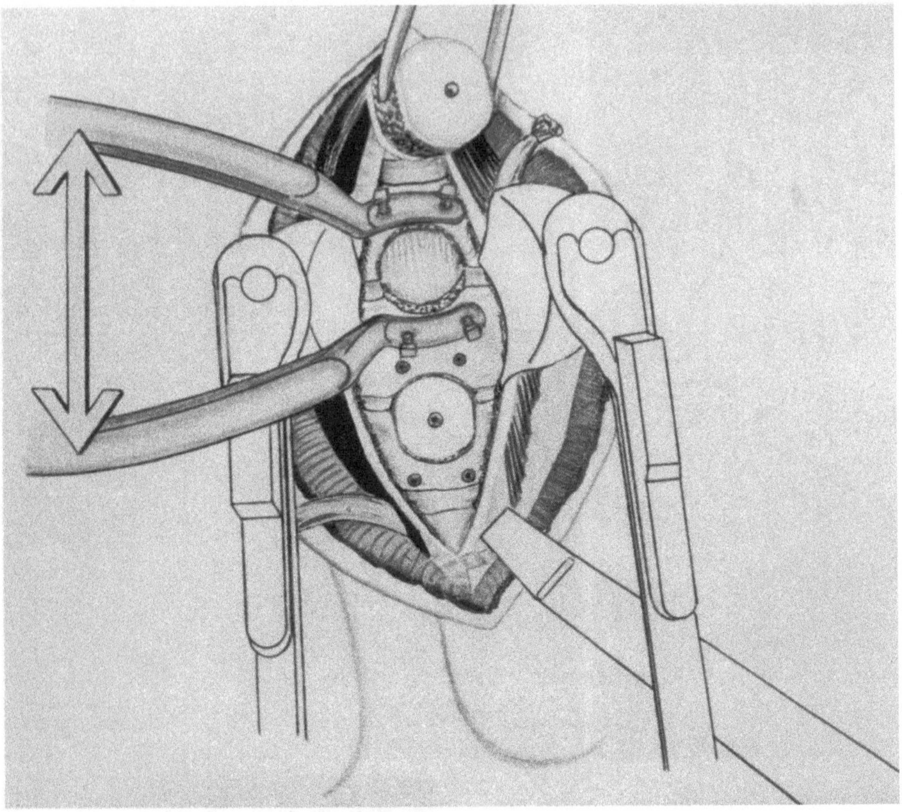

Fig. 9.18. The Cloward procedure carried out at two levels in an asymmetrical fashion. A bridge of bone remains in the middle of the vertebral body which is strong enough to provide good support for the two grafts on either side of it. The distractor is fixed above and below the drill hole with self-tapping screws. Please note that there is sufficient space in the vertebral bodies for the fixation of the distractor in spite of double drilling

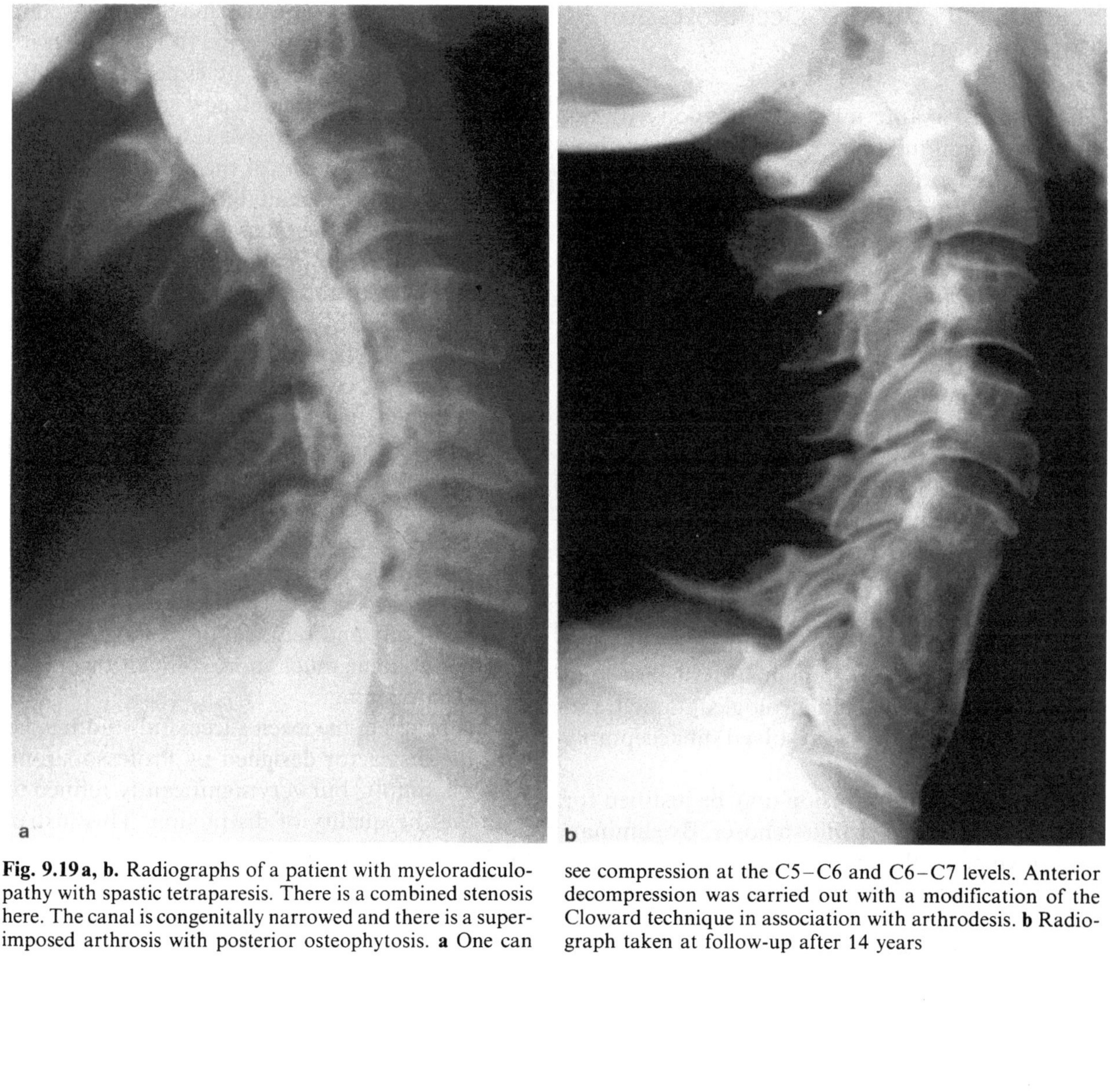

Fig. 9.19 a, b. Radiographs of a patient with myeloradiculopathy with spastic tetraparesis. There is a combined stenosis here. The canal is congenitally narrowed and there is a superimposed arthrosis with posterior osteophytosis. **a** One can see compression at the C5–C6 and C6–C7 levels. Anterior decompression was carried out with a modification of the Cloward technique in association with arthrodesis. **b** Radiograph taken at follow-up after 14 years

Transdiskal Anterior Decompression With Fusion

The transdiskal anterior decompression with fusion are techniques currently used in modifications of the original techniques described by Smith and Robinson, Dereymacher et al., and Baily and Badgley, involving simple fusion at one or more vertebral levels. In the past, transdiskal anterior decompression with fusion was used in the treatment of arthrosis in order to immobilize the involved segment or segments without removing the cause of the stenosis, which we now know to be posterior osteophytes. The thesis offered was that, with time, "these spurs may be resorbed after fusion by bone remodelling" (Robinson 1962). It may well be true that, with time, these bulging osteophytes remodel and decrease and the associated neuromedullary injury may be resolved. However, it cannot be ignored that this occurs so slowly that the cause of the injury remains for such a long period of time that the neurological deficit and the symptoms may be resolved unacceptably slowly.

This type of simple fusion may be justified for treating very early organic stenoses. By eliminating movement, the microtrauma and hence the irritation to the neuromedullary structures will be removed. Another possible indication is segmental instability with functional stenosis in association with severe distortion. The techniques currently used have been developed to treat the consequences of arthrosis by removing the specific causes of the resulting stenosis, i.e., the posterior osteophytes. The removal of the cause of the stenosis will require fusion of the operated levels with the use of osseous graft.

Technique

The approach should be a right presternocleidomastoid with the patient placed as described in Fig. 8.18. When dissection has advanced to the level of the spine, a check radiograph is taken to identify the spinal levels for purposes of orientation. The anterior longitudinal ligament and then the intervertebral disk which is to be resected are then incised. The disk may be removed in fragments with either hernia forceps or with straight or curved curets at either 45° or 90°. Under visual control, small curved curets can be used to successfully remove residual fragments of the posterior aspects of the annulus fibrosus.

This step may be facilitated by using an instrument that widens the intervertebral disk space – commonly, the Cloward distractor is used. It is placed either centrally or laterally on the vertebral bodies and, by separating them, provides a larger operative field with better visualization of the structures. Nevertheless, one must point out that although this particular instrument, once anchored to the anterior wall of the vertebral bodies, provides good separation of the bodies anteriorly, a severly limiting factor is its tendency, at the same time, to cause compression of the posterior portion of the intervertebral disk space (Fig. 9.20). Access to the posterior portion of the vertebral body and removal of the posterior osteophyte become much more difficult through a narrowed opening.

This problem has been successfully addressed with the distractor designed by Professor Boni, which is simply, but very significantly refined to improve the quality of distraction. This instrument is composed of four pins that deeply penetrate the vertebral bodies to be operated on. Its major disadvantage is that it must be applied with force; the pins must be tapped with a hammer. In some arthritic cervical spines with significant sclerosis and deformity of the anterior cortices of the vertebral bodies, the forced insertion with a hammer is far from easy. To avoid these difficulties, I and my colleagues have designed a distractor that can be applied on the vertebral bodies at the operative levels through self-tapping screws. This provides relatively easy anchorage and a firm grip on the vertebral bodies (Fig. 9.21). The screws penetrate to a level of 12–14 mm of depth, and their depth of penetration is calculated so as not to reach, let alone penetrate, the posterior cortex.

Once the screws are well anchored in the bodies, the distraction is achieved in such a way as to maintain the parallel relationship of the two adjacent vertebral bodies which are being pulled apart. This therefore allows better access to the posterior portion of the intervertebral disk space, and hence makes it much easier to accomplish posterior decompression more safely. Once the distractor is fixed in position, then the following definitive procedure can be started.

The cartilaginous end plate of the vertebral bodies in the central zone is removed. This is achieved with a 12-mm wide chisel (Fig. 9.22) with which serial portions of the vertebral body can be removed, a few millimeters at a time, above and below the disk space as far as the spongiosa below this end plate cortex. Removal of the end plate may be extended posteriorly to the posterior end of the vertebral body, producing a linear trough with a rectangular outline, comparable to the circular bed obtained with Cloward instrumentation. Using curved and thin curets and maintaining distraction of the vertebral bodies, one can then begin to remove the osteophytes from the posterior vertebral wall. The use of a dissecting microscope or magnifying glasses may be advantageous at this time in the dissection. The trough may be deepened and shaped as desired using an air drill. This can be carried right out to the posterior cortex, which is thinned out to the point where it is relatively easy to use a 45° curved curet to remove the remaining cortex and any osteophytes all the way out to the posterolateral uncal wall (Figs. 9.23, 9.24). The presence of this trough, in fact, just like the gap obtained with Cloward instrumentation, widens the operative field making the maneuvers easier. However, the use of a chisel to resect the end plates of the vertebral bodies can, at times, be technically difficult. Bone may be quite sclerotic. However sharp the chisels may be, the posterior osteophytes are jammed back with each blow of the hammer and may cause injury to the neuromedullary structures. This risk of injury can be avoided if an air drill is used for all of the dissection in forming the rectangular trough. This may be advisable in cases of post-traumatic stenosis or in cases of malunion where the dissection must be slowly advanced avoiding any undue stress on the disrupted vertebral body. At the same time, the use of Cloward-type drills and of chisels may be extremely dangerous, causing displacement of bony fragments which may damage the neuromedullary tissues. With the use of appropriately selected types and sizes of drills, the dissection may be more safely advanced towards the posterior wall of the vertebral bodies.

If the end plates of the vertebral bodies are not removed, decompression must be undertaken through the unmodified disk space. Although appropriate distraction provides additional space, facilitating this part of the procedure, this may not be sufficient in cases of severe stenosis with marked posterior compression (e.g., large osteophytic buttresses). In the following, however, a modification of the techniques is described, that addresses this difficulty in achieving decompression and removing the large osseous spurs. When the disk has been removed and with the distractor in place, a small drill is passed through the disk space to remove the posterior portion of the body and of the posterior surfaces of the end plate. The result is a conical space with its base lying posteriorly (Fig. 9.25). This first step permits the introduction of additional curets that can be used to remove the osteophytes and the posterolateral walls to the uncus (Fig. 9.26).

With the decompression completed, attention can be turned to the osseous graft. First of all, it must be of a rectangular shape in order to fit in the trough sculpted in the vertebral body. The graft is a solid tricorticated portion of the iliac crest, which is removed as described in the section "Bone Grafts" (p. 278; Figs. 9.27, 9.28). We must remember that the size of the graft must be such that it can only be introduced during distraction in order to retain a well-fixed position across the disk space. The graft must therefore be larger than the curetted space. It should be shaped right at the operative site in order to assure that it fits accurately and tightly into place.

The graft must be placed in position during distraction. In the literature there are descriptions of a method of applying a head sling preoperatively and using this from outside the sterile area of the operating table to apply traction during insertion of the graft. This is too inaccurate and unpredictable a procedure and it does not assure the distraction necessary for the appropriate impaction of the graft. It is therefore more reliable to use the distractor described above. When the desired level of distraction has been achieved, the graft is forcibly pushed into place. An appropriate instrument for this has been designed with a holder that facilitates positioning of the graft (Figs. 9.27, 9.28). The external cortical surface of the graft should match the anterior cortical surface of the vertebral bodies being operated on. This step will avoid any subsequent displacement of the graft. Postoperative immobilization can be adequately achieved with an orthopedic appliance such as the Somi brace, which provides proximal support for the occiput and chin and distal support on the shoulders. Incorporation and fusion should occur within 45–60 days postoperatively. This type of procedure can also be carried out at multiple levels.

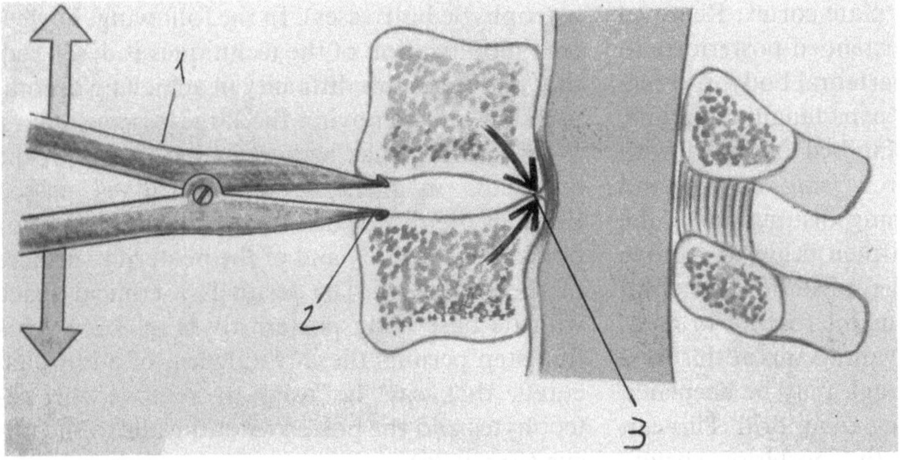

Fig. 9.20. The success of the procedure depends on the use of a distractor that separates the adjacent vertebral bodies in parallel. Cloward-type distractors (*1*) tend to separate the anterior end of the vertebral body (*2*) while at the same time include approximation of the posterior end (*3*). This would not provide the required exposure of the posterior disk space, and removal of posterior osteophytes would be much more difficult

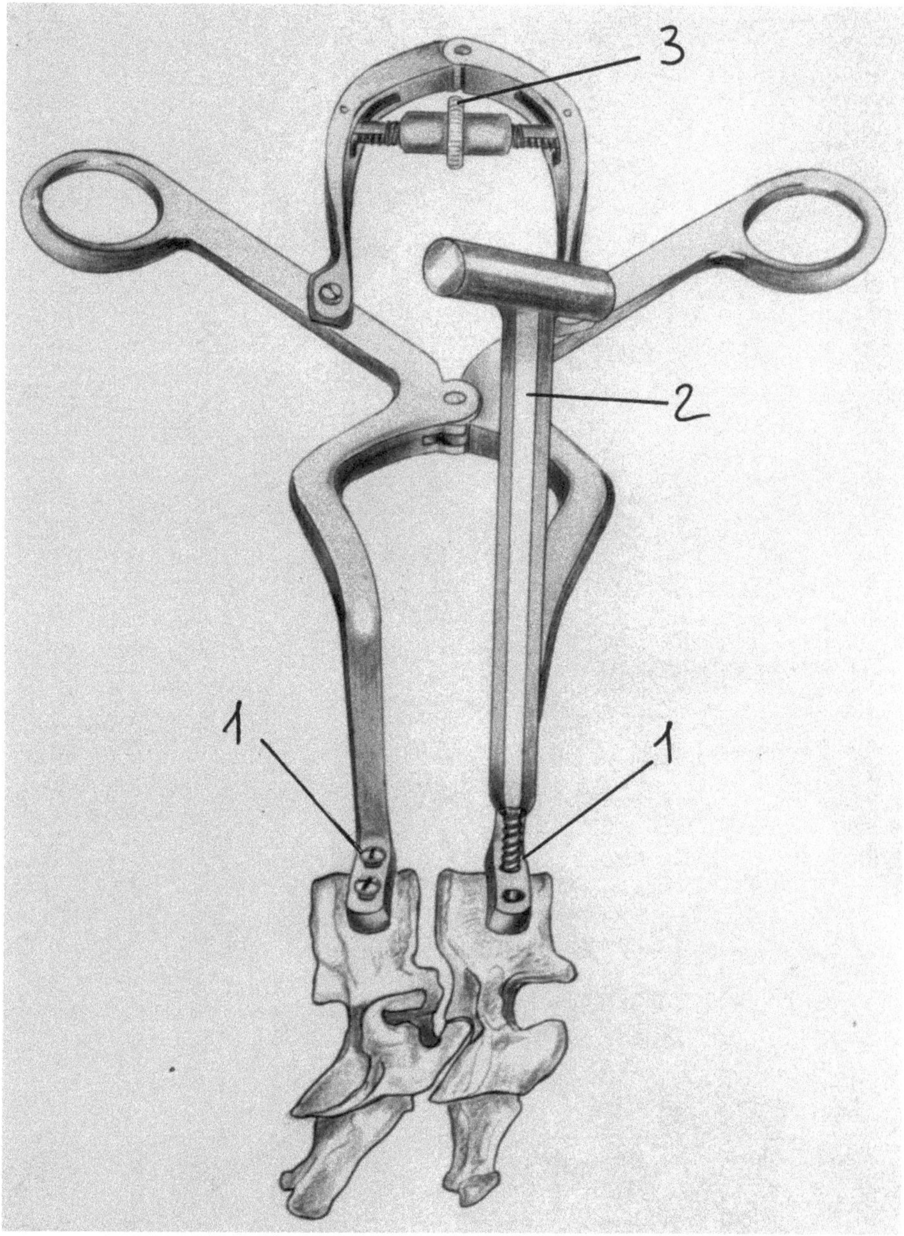

Fig. 9.21. Our distractor bridges the vertebral bodies and is held in place with self-tapping screws (*1*), which are inserted using an appropriate screwdriver (*2*). The degree of diastasis is controlled with the adjustable screw, which permits the required gradual and progressive distraction (*3*)

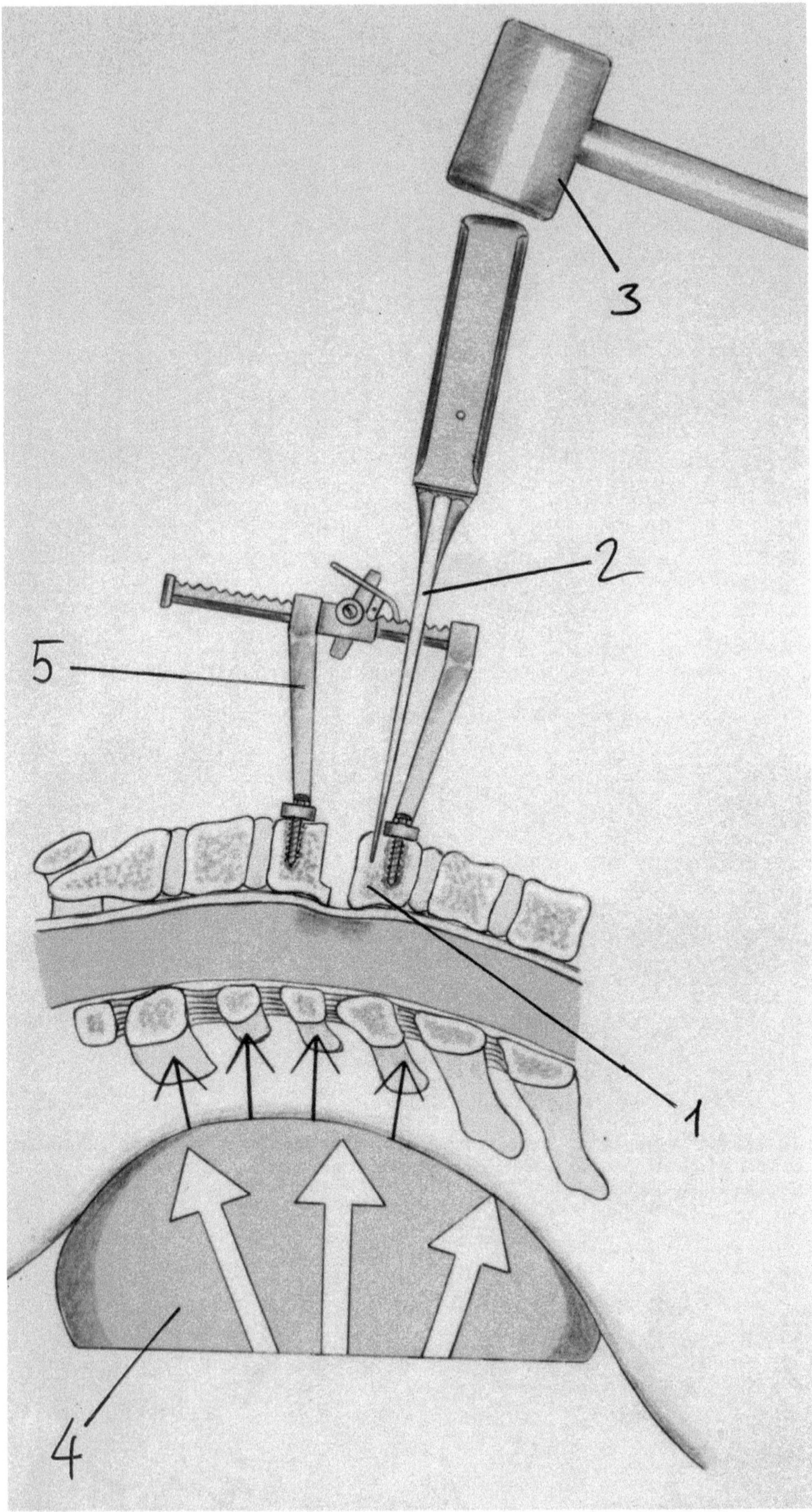

Fig. 9.22. The osteocartilaginous surface (*1*) of the two vertebral bodies adjacent to the disk is removed using a scalpel (*2*). The mechanics of the use of a hammer (*3*) require resistance (*4*), which is provided by the rigid support of the spinous processes. Also in place is the self-retaining distractor (*5*)

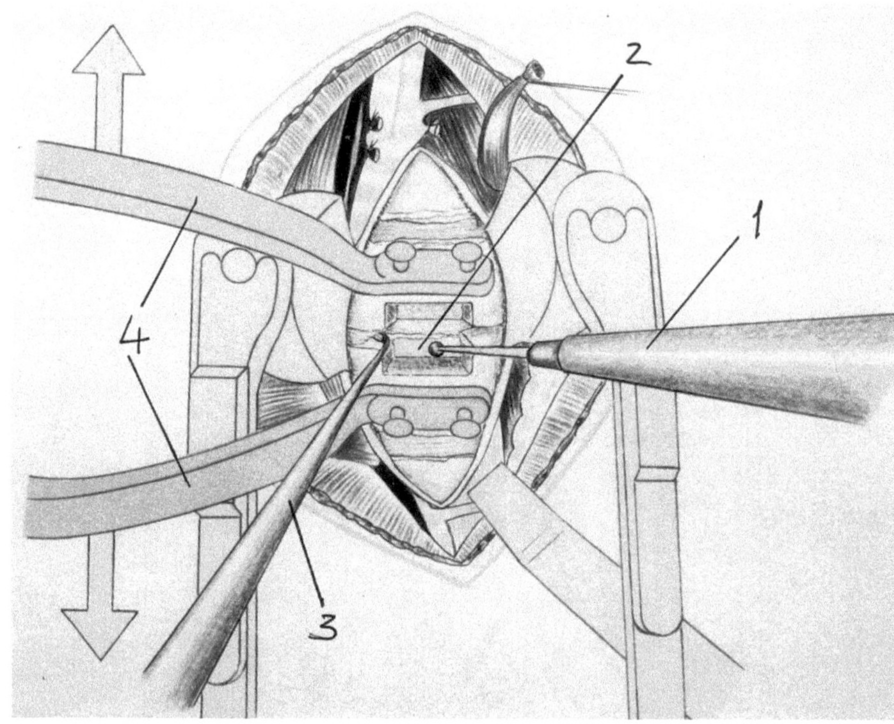

Fig. 9.23. Once the osteocartilaginous tissue of the adjacent bodies has been drilled out (*1*), the dissection is extended towards the posterior cortex of the bodies (*2*). Curets (*3*) are used to remove any remaining disk tissue. The dissection in the deep hole is facilitated by the use of a distractor (*4*)

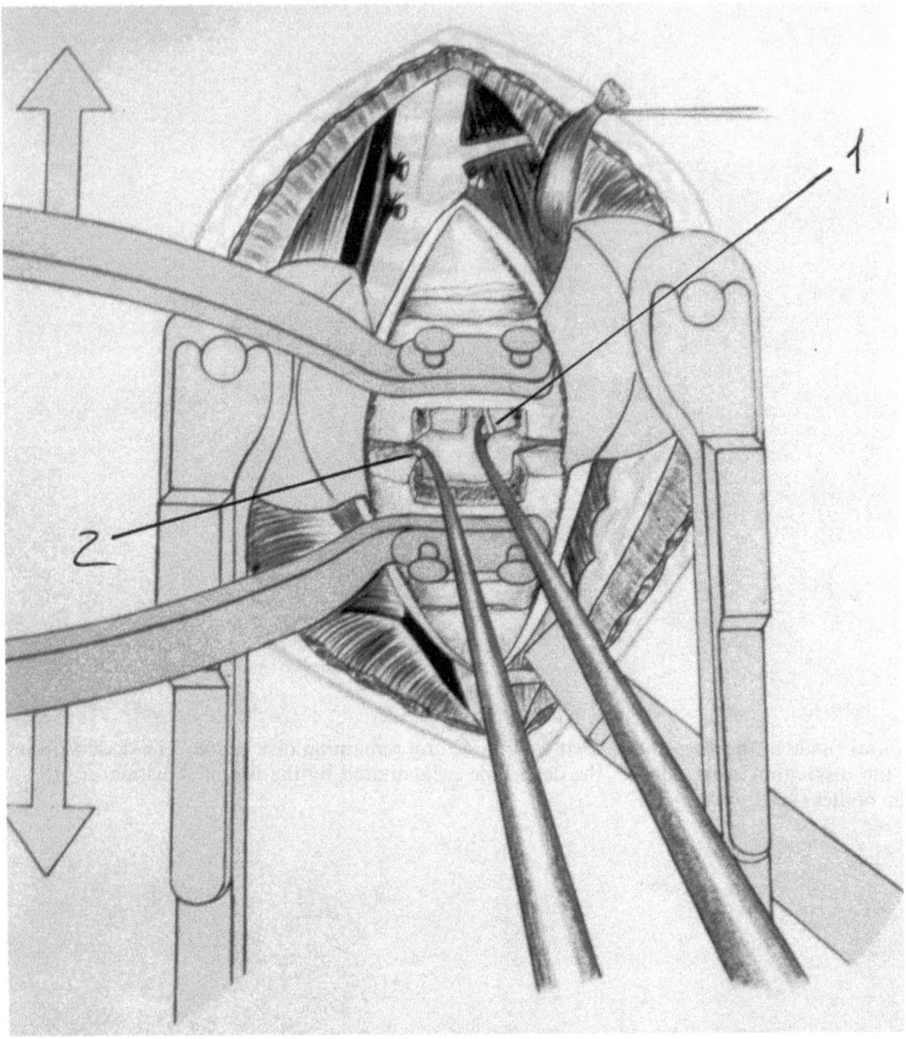

Fig. 9.24. With adequate distraction, one can reach the posterior wall of the bodies (*1*) as well as the posterolateral uncal portion (*2*)

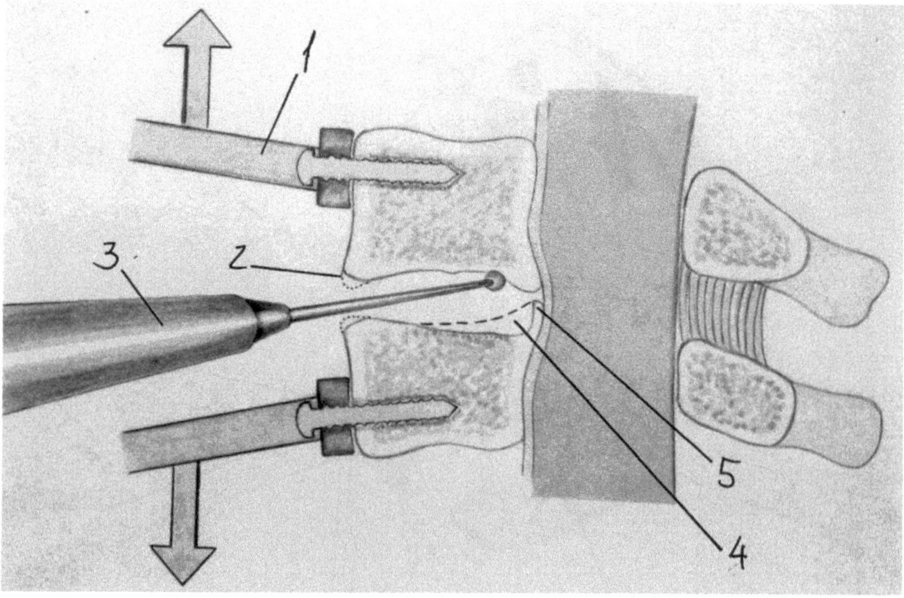

Fig. 9.25. Removal of posterior osteophytes through the disk space. The distractor is used to widen the disk space (*1*). Once diskectomy has been completed, the anterior osteophytes may be removed (*2*). Using an air drill (*3*), the posterior portion of the apposing vertebral bodies can be removed (*4*) right up to the posterior cortex and the posterior osteophytes (*5*)

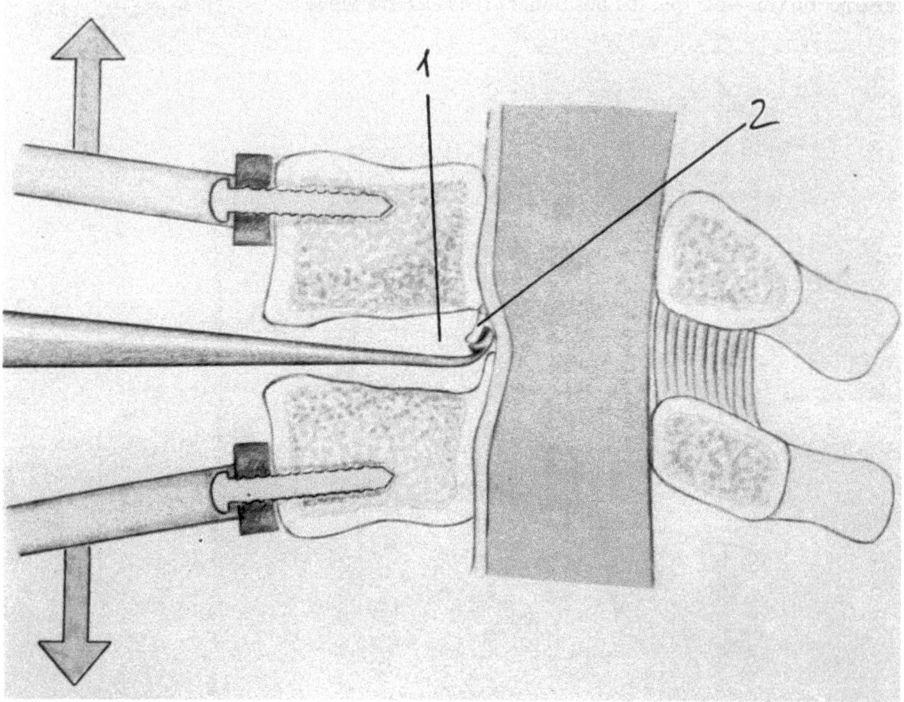

Fig. 9.26. Completed evacuation of the disk space posteriorly (*1*). The curet now removes the residual posterior wall and the osteophytes (*2*) from the superior vertebral body

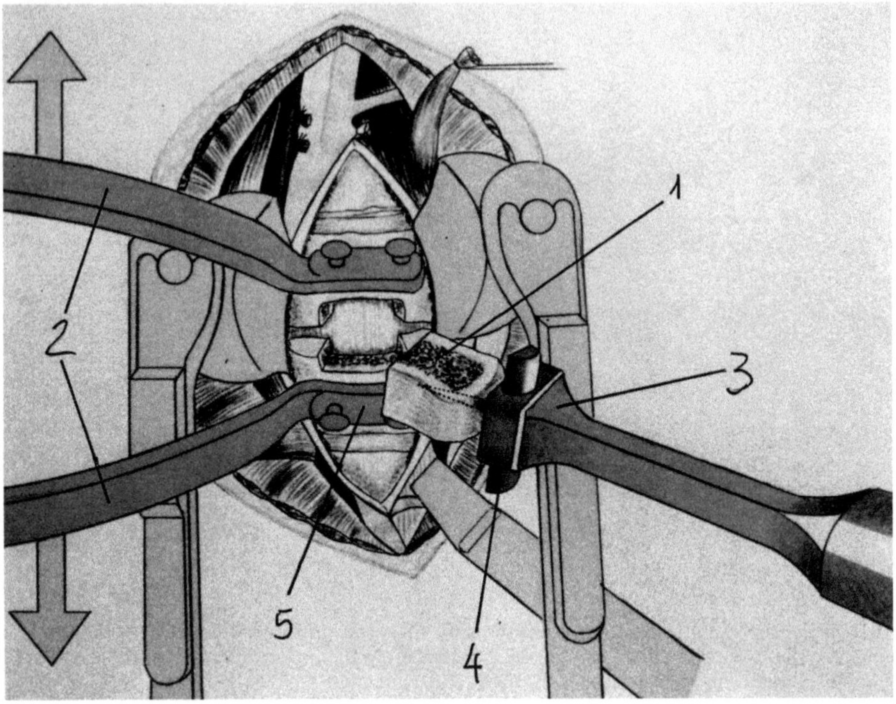

Fig. 9.27. Tricortical graft (*1*) with a rectangular shape and slightly larger than the prepared host bed is inserted with distraction (*2*). Note that the positioner (*3*) has lateral wings (*4*) that will act as markers (*5*), limiting the progression of the positioning of the graft

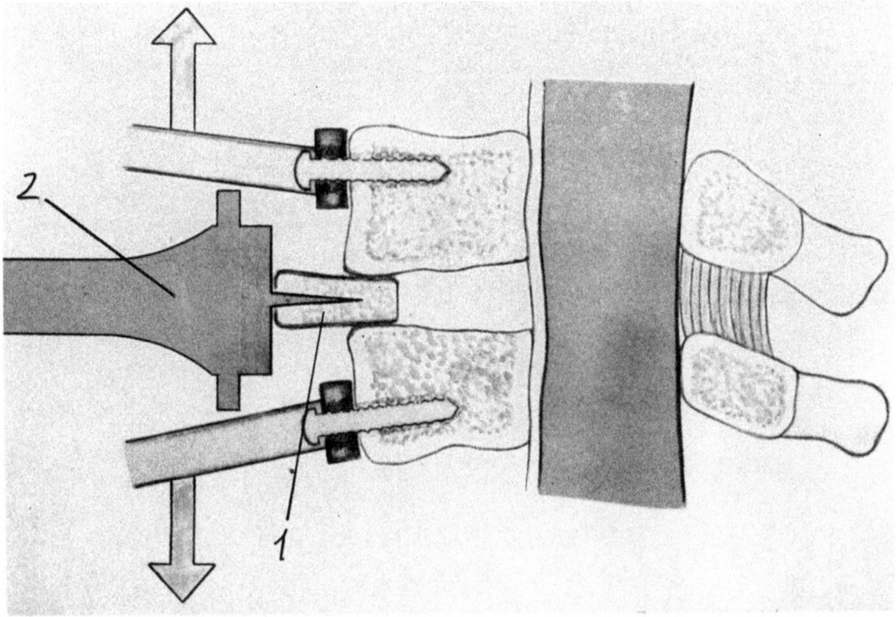

Fig. 9.28. The tricortical autograft (*1*) is inserted into the distracted disk space using the appropriate applicator (*2*)

Transdiskal Anterior Decompression Without Fusion

It is possible, in some cases, that once decompression of the cord has been achieved, the patient may not require fusion across the disk space at the level of operation. In other words, once the large protruding posterior osteophytes have been removed and the cord and roots decompressed, the surgical intervention is completed. It is easy in these cases to appreciate the advantages of avoiding the procedure needed for harvesting the graft and the time required for shaping and inserting the dowel graft. As a result, the operative time and the potential difficulties and complications that may arise from harvesting the graft are avoided, with an improved postoperative course for the patient.

Personal experience has shown, however, that this option can only be successfully pursued in cases in which there is decreased movement at the intervertebral joints at the level of operation, as demonstrated by dynamic preoperative radiographic assessment, in other words, if there is stiffness or rigidity. Fusion is unequivocally indicated if the level of operation is not rigid and is either as mobile as or more mobile than normal. This would be the case, for example, in cases of disk herniation or degenerative spondylolisthesis in spinal arthrosis, circumstances in which there would be an element of instability. If fusion is not performed in such cases, then it is to be expected that a segmental kyphosis with persistence of the patient's symptoms or a segmental instability with signs of spinal and hence neck malfunction will result shortly after the operation. Eventually, all of these circumstances necessitate supplementary surgery to achieve fusion at the involved spinal level.

In the presence of joint stiffness or rigidity at the level of surgery, then fusion may not be necessary; this would be the case in severe spinal arthrosis associated with rigidity and loss of movement. In the cases without fusion, one should expect a limited but detectable degree of segmental kyphosis to result. This will eventually develop into further rigidity at the level of operation. If the surgical disk level is one of the normally more mobile levels of the inferior cervical spine, i.e., at the levels of C5–C6 and C6–C7, then, with time, the stresses of normal function may result in a superadded element of instability that leads to persistence or recurrence of the symptoms that were relieved by the simple decompression. This indicates that, although in some cases one might be inclined to undertake a simple decompression without fusion, it is often wise to take steps that will encourage spontaneous fusion at the decompressed level. This can be easily achieved during the Cloward procedure for decompression of the cord. All the tissue obtained from the drilling should be harvested. Once appropriately minced, this tissue can be laid on a bed of Spongostan so that it will act as a stimulus to eventual fusion at the level of operation (Fig. 9.16).

Anterior Decompression with Multiple Subtotal Corpectomies

By using anterior decompression with multiple subtotal corpectomies, the cord may be freed at multiple levels with a true widening of the cervical canal anteriorly. This technique was developed by Professor Mario Boni in Pavia in 1969. Since then the basic technique has been enriched by a series of modifications that have improved and simplified it, while avoiding identifiable and predictable problems.

Technique

The surgical approach that provides wide and easy access for all the definitive surgical procedures and the one recommended here is the right presternocleidomastoid approach. Once the approach has been completed and the spinal levels have been clearly identified, the procedure is begun at the lowest disk level. Once the procedure has been completed at that level, it is repeated at the next proximal level.

This technique is indicated in stenosis involving two, three, four, or, rarely, even as many as five disk levels. A modified Cloward instrumentation is used. The preparation and surgical steps are similar to those described for the

Cloward procedure. One then proceeds with the following steps:

- Incision of the anterior longitudinal ligament.
- Removal of the intervertebral disk.
- Drilling of the disk space with a Cloward drill with a diameter of 12 mm (Fig. 9.29). The method of drilling of the vertebral bodies is exactly as has been described on page 140 (Figs. 9.5–9.9).
- Gradual deepening of the space that has been drilled at each disk level right up to the posterior wall of the vertebral bodies. Remember to keep the operative fields as free of blood as possible in order to permit accurate visualization of the procedure at all times.

Finally, the posterior wall of the vertebral body and any posterior osteophytes that might be present are removed and the posterolateral aspect at the uncal region cleared of any osteophytic tissue.

This may be particularly difficult and even dangerous in cases of calcification of the posterior longitudinal ligament or with massive posterior osteophytes that protrude into the canal, producing a localized compression of the cord. This is often the case in severe degenerative arthrosis of the cervical spine. Here, one should drill carefully so as to just reach the level of the posterior wall of the vertebral bodies. The wall may then be removed more easily once the drilling is completed at each of the levels selected. Once the osseous buttresses and spurs have been removed, a wide trench is created as the drilled spaces are joined and the intervening bone removed. This can often be easily achieved with the use of rongeur-type bone forceps. Following removal of these osseous bridges, the walls are then smoothed out by using an air drill and augmenting the dissection with angled curets (45° or 90°) until the decompression of the posterior longitudinal ligament and of the posterolateral or uncal portion of the vertebral bodies has been completed, according to the requirements of the Cloward method (Figs. 9.30, 9.31).

This is a very important and delicate part of the procedure which must be undertaken with extreme caution. The operative field must be as bloodless as possible. This can be achieved by using bone wax, Spongostan, and sponges soaked with coagulants. The surgeon should always pause at regular intervals during the procedure in order to lavage and pack the operative site. This will encourage him to work with good visual control of the operative field, thereby avoiding the danger of injury to the neurospinal structures. Great care must be exercised in removing the posterior osteophytes or the massive calcification that might be present in the posterior longitudinal ligament. The surgeon should always proceed with caution and very gradually in removing the osteophytes with curets. It is important to avoid sudden collapse of the posterior structures caused by the excessive use of force.

Heavy bleeding may result from the removal of the posterior osteophytes or from the curettage removal of the posterior longitudinal ligament. The use of a bipolar microcoagulator will facilitate careful and complete coagulation in the deep-seated dissection. Often one is dealing with blood vessels within the calcified posterior longitudinal ligament that may not be amenable to coagulation and hence will require packing with Spongostan and coagulants. When coagulation is difficult, continous aspiration may be used to complete the decompression. Once the offending osteophytes have been removed, one is in a better position to achieve hemostasis by packing the operative field with Surgicel or Spongostan and with the use of warm sponges dipped in coagulants. The instrumentation available in these steps is variable and should be specifically selected to facilitate the procedure and hemostasis, such as a 50°-angled Kerrison punch (either cutting or blunt) and a selection of curved curets. The high-speed air drill can be used effectively to smooth out the contour all along the extent of the bony trough that has been dissected (Figs. 9.30, 9.31). It is important to be particularly meticulous in this. The posterior wall and the osteophytes all the way up to the most lateral portions of the posterior aspect of the vertebral body must be fully removed. One must avoid leaving even the smallest fragments of bone in the lateral recesses. This may extend operative time, but it is important that the evacuation be scrupulously completed so that no fragments are left in the lateral aspects of the posterior wall of the vertebral body or in the region of the root canal.

Once neuromedullary decompression has been satisfactorily completed, the next step is to prepare the bed for the autograft from the iliac crest (Fig. 9.32). Remembering that the graft must be firmly embedded like a dowel, then one can appreciate the importance of the drilling and how important it is to be careful to drill immediately behind the anterior vertebral wall in order to perfectly shape the bed for the graft (Fig. 9.33). We can now turn to the harvesting of the bone graft, which must be tricortical (Figs. 9.117–9.119) and preferably should be obtained from the iliac crest. The surgeon should be forewarned that the skin incision, parallel to the crest of the ilium has to be long. This may be associated with a number of difficulties in healing including hematoma, pain, and esthetically poor scar healing.
However, if a graft greater than 4 cm in length is required, the surgeon has no choice but to make such a long incision to be able to harvest a graft. Obviously, smaller grafts only require the shorter incision and this usually means fewer problems postoperatively. The removal is carried out with chisels. In order to avoid necrosis of tissue as a result of heat, a bone saw should be avoided (Fig. 9.117).

The graft should be 5–10 mm longer than the trench cut in the vertebrae. It should be shaped and it must be placed so as to interlock rigidly with the host bed in the operated vertebral bodies. The graft should be placed during distraction (Fig. 9.32). This is essential and can be achieved by using the distractor fixed to the vertebral bodies which have been operated on. The distractor used in multiple corpectomies is similar to that already described, with two points of attachment of the vertebral body, above and below the levels of operation. Fixed with four screws to the vertebral bodies, it is then used to extend the trench created in the host bed for the graft. Placing the dowel-type graft with distraction not only aligns the vertebral body and favors the restoration of a physiological lordosis, but also widens the root canals (Fig. 9.33). The curvulinear outline of the iliac crest also helps to restore the physiological lordosis. The tension under which the graft is inserted as well as the way it is modelled to fit as a dowel favor compression of the graft and therefore its incorporation, which should be achieved between 60 and 90 days postoperatively.

This type of surgical procedure with arthrodesis will require the use of a reliable orthopedic equipment in the postoperative period. Experience has shown that the best and the safest way to provide protection in such cases of corpectomy and massive graft is the halo jacket or an orthopedic appliance made of leather and aluminium, which should be prepared preoperatively. The use of minerva-type plaster immobilization must be very carefully constructed if it is to be closely adherent. In our experience, alternative braces (Somi brace, Philadelphia brace, etc.) do not provide postoperative stability and the movement that they permit results in prolongation of the healing process and of the fusion of the graft.

When following this technique of graft preparation and insertion during spinal distraction, we have found that, unlike published reports, the use of plates or other additional steps for internal immobilization is not necessary. Consolidation is assured by the compression of the graft if it is inserted during appropriate distraction with the distractor described. Postoperative immobilization, however, remains essential in maintaining stability and encouraging incorporation of the graft. It must also be pointed out that using plates, screws, etc. for internal immobilization precludes the opportunity to follow the patient during the postoperative period with CT and MRI; metal rules out the use of these diagnostic modalities in the assessment of the decompression achieved surgically and in the sequential following of the healing process at the operative levels of the spinal canal (Fig. 9.34).

We do not commonly use the fibula as a graft, since it is hard, cylindrical, and composed primarily of cortical bone. Its straight-line configuration is not easily modified to maintain the physiological cervical lordosis. Even in the cases where surgery extends across several vertebral bodies, it tends to put the operated portion of the neck into a more erect position. The incorporation time is also longer than that of the corticocancellous graft from the iliac crest. This is not to say that the fibula would not provide a mechanically more solid type of graft, but, in our experience, this is only needed if one wishes to achieve an immediate mechanical stabilization in patients with trauma or tumor. It is in these cases that a fibular graft, well anchored by the appropriate internal stabilization, will provide the best probability of mechanical stability immediately postoperatively.

Multiple Subtotal Corpectomies Without Massive Graft

Some forms of organic stenoses, particularly those associated with rigidity of the spine, can be treated successfully using the techniques described by Senegas. The degree of rigidity can be determined by preoperative dynamic radiographic investigation. In such cases, the cord is first decompressed and then, instead of a massive graft, the bone reamings harvested from the drilling of the vertebral bodies are used. A layer of Spongostan is placed on the posterior longitudinal ligament (Fig. 9.35). It will separate the ligament from the bony reamings which are used as graft. This is a most useful technique. Within a period of 30 days, arthrodesis will be achieved in the segments which were already hypomotile or rigid preoperatively. We emphasize that this procedure can only be utilized in selected cases with the typical, well-documented rigidity of cases of organic fixed stenosis. This surgical method has a number of important advantages.

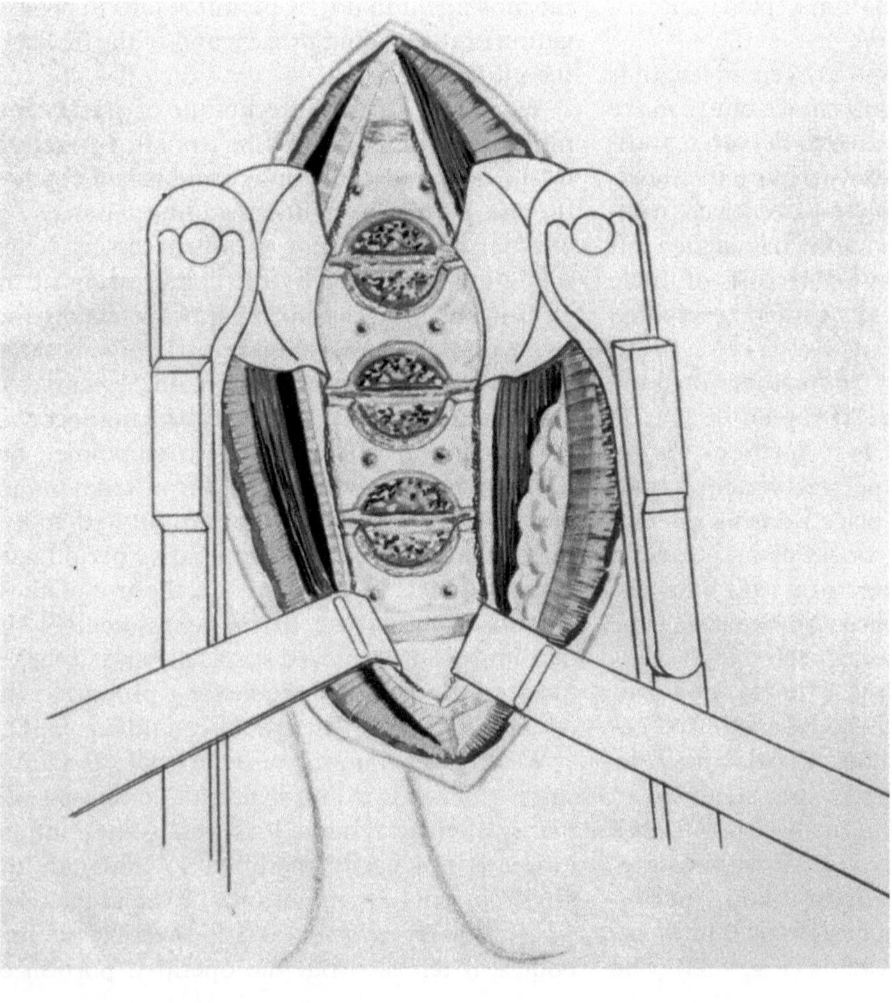

Fig. 9.29. In order to relieve stenosis at multiple levels of the canal using anterior decompression, a method similar to that described by Cloward is followed (in other words, as many holes are drilled with the instument described by Cloward as there are levels to be operated upon). This is described in Figs. 9.7–9.10

The operating time is reduced by half in that the need to harvest a graft is avoided. It is a well-known fact that when a large graft has been obtained from the iliac wing, it is necessary to close the wound in multiple layers, a time-consuming procedure, which, however, is essential if dehiscence of such a large wound is to be avoided. In addition, the time required for preparing the host site and for the careful shaping of the dowel graft, along with the technical time needed for distracting the graft site to insert the graft are saved.

In cases where an iliac crest graft is obtained, the patient often complains more of the hip wound than of the neck wound following surgery. This is often a cause of delay in mobilizing the patient immediately post-operatively. All of this can be avoided by using this surgical technique. The patient cannot only be mobilized, but may actually walk in the first postoperative day. The necessity for total immobilization is also avoided; there is no need for halo traction, plaster cast nor for the associated limitations to postoperative patient activation. A Philadelphia or Shanz-type simple collar is often all that is required for adequate support postoperatively. The patient is usually ready to be discharged by the fifth postoperative day, by which time retraining has already begun (Figs. 9.36, 9.37).

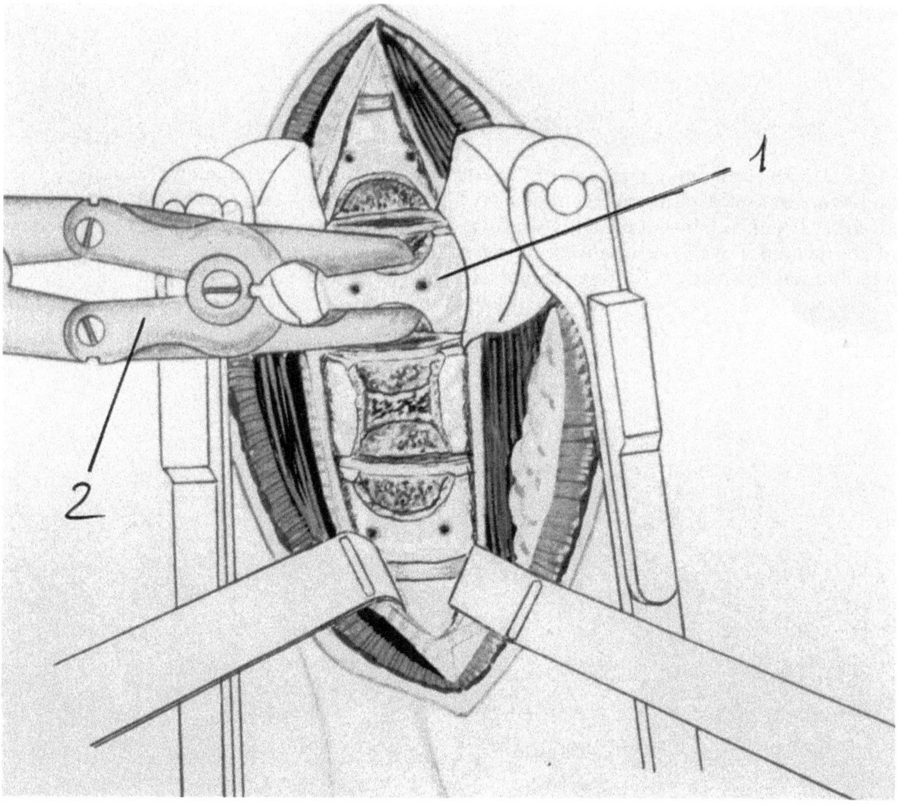

Fig. 9.30. Using large rongeurs (*2*), one removes the osseous bridges (*1*) that remain between the drill holes

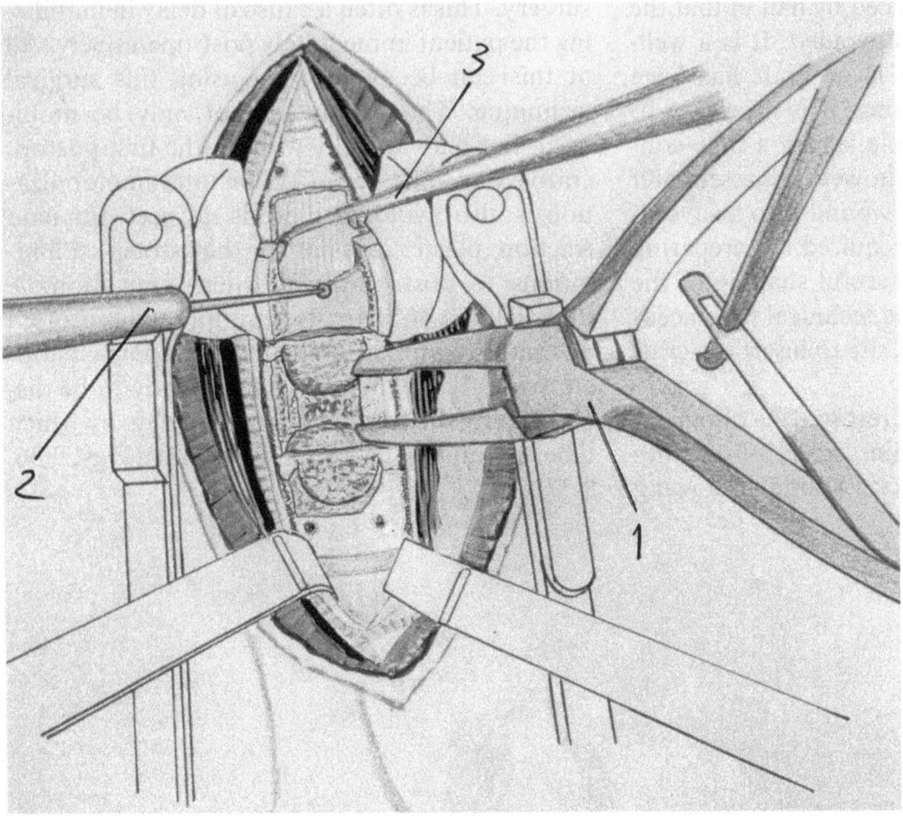

Fig. 9.31. The remaining portions of the lateral walls of the bodies are removed with smaller rongeurs (*1*). Next, using an air drill (*2*) with ball bits of differing sizes, the final fragments of the posterior wall are removed to expose the posterior longitudinal ligament. The final stages of removal of the remaining fragments of the posterior wall are carried out manually with curets (*3*). With a curved curet (with a 45° angle) and a wide opening, it is easily possible to remove osteophytes in the posterolateral area of the body

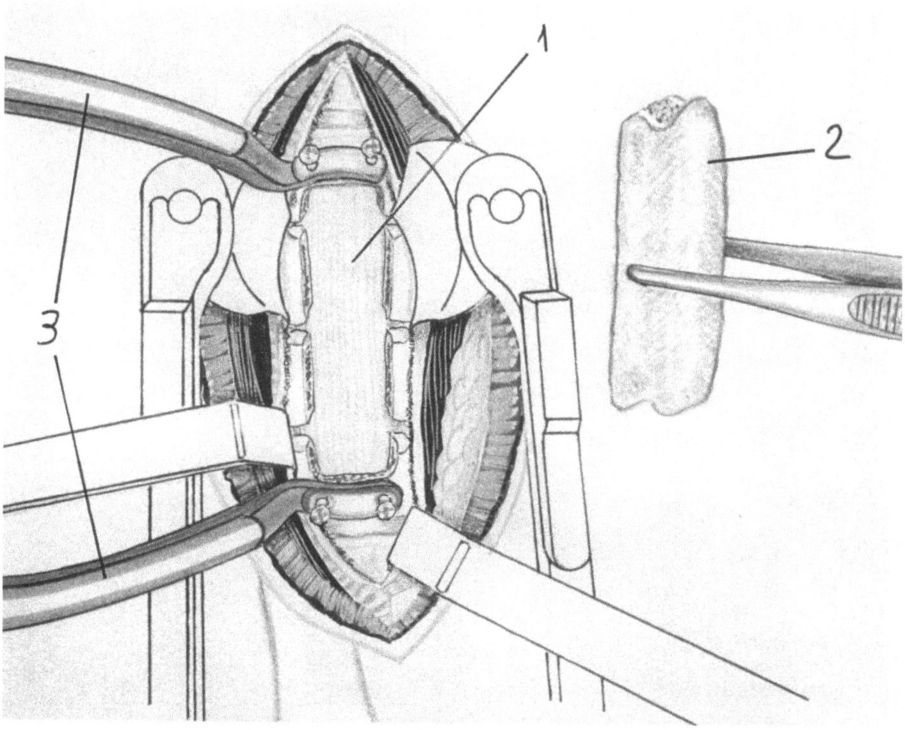

Fig. 9.32. The bony trough is prepared. The posterior longitudinal ligament (*1*) is free. Posterolateral osteophytes have been removed. The next step is the retrieval of a tricortical bone graft from the iliac crest (*2*). The graft is then modeled into the shape of the slot into which it must fit in such a way as to interlock with the two adjacent vertebral bodies, which will then hold it fast in place from above and below. The graft can only be put in place while the vertebral bodies are being distracted (*3*)

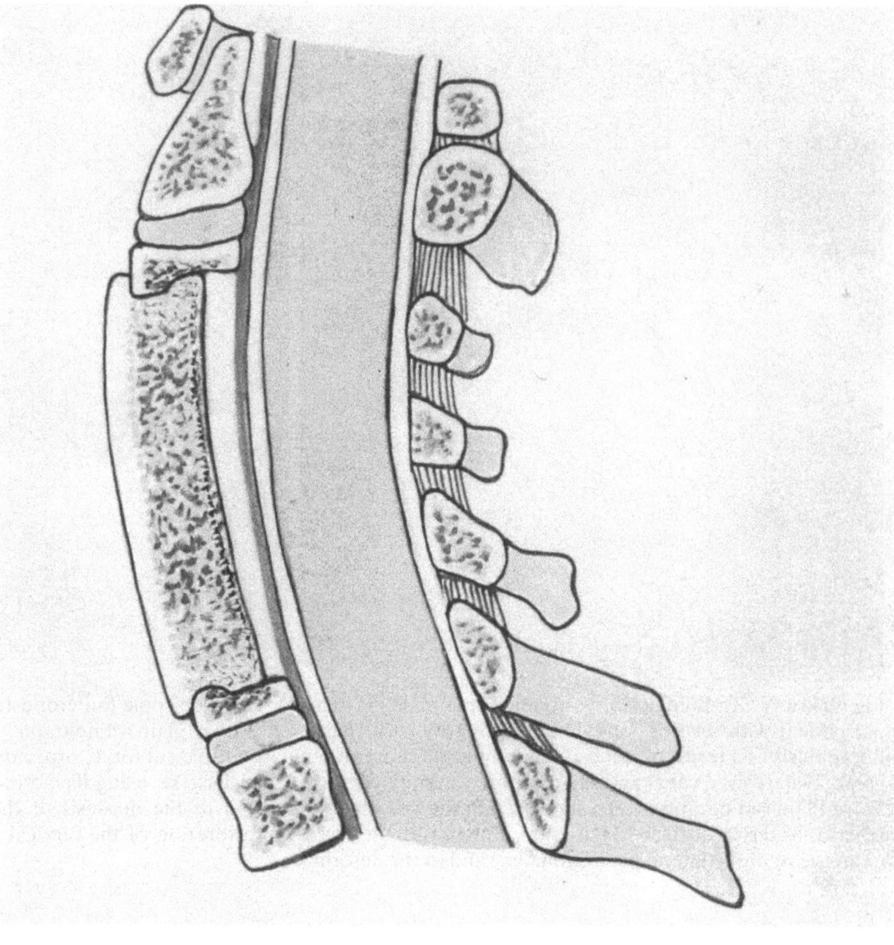

Fig. 9.33. Lateral view of how the graft is positioned and held in place. There is an interlocking tongue and groove effect at the interface between the graft and the vertebral body. For this reason adequate distraction during insertion of the graft is required

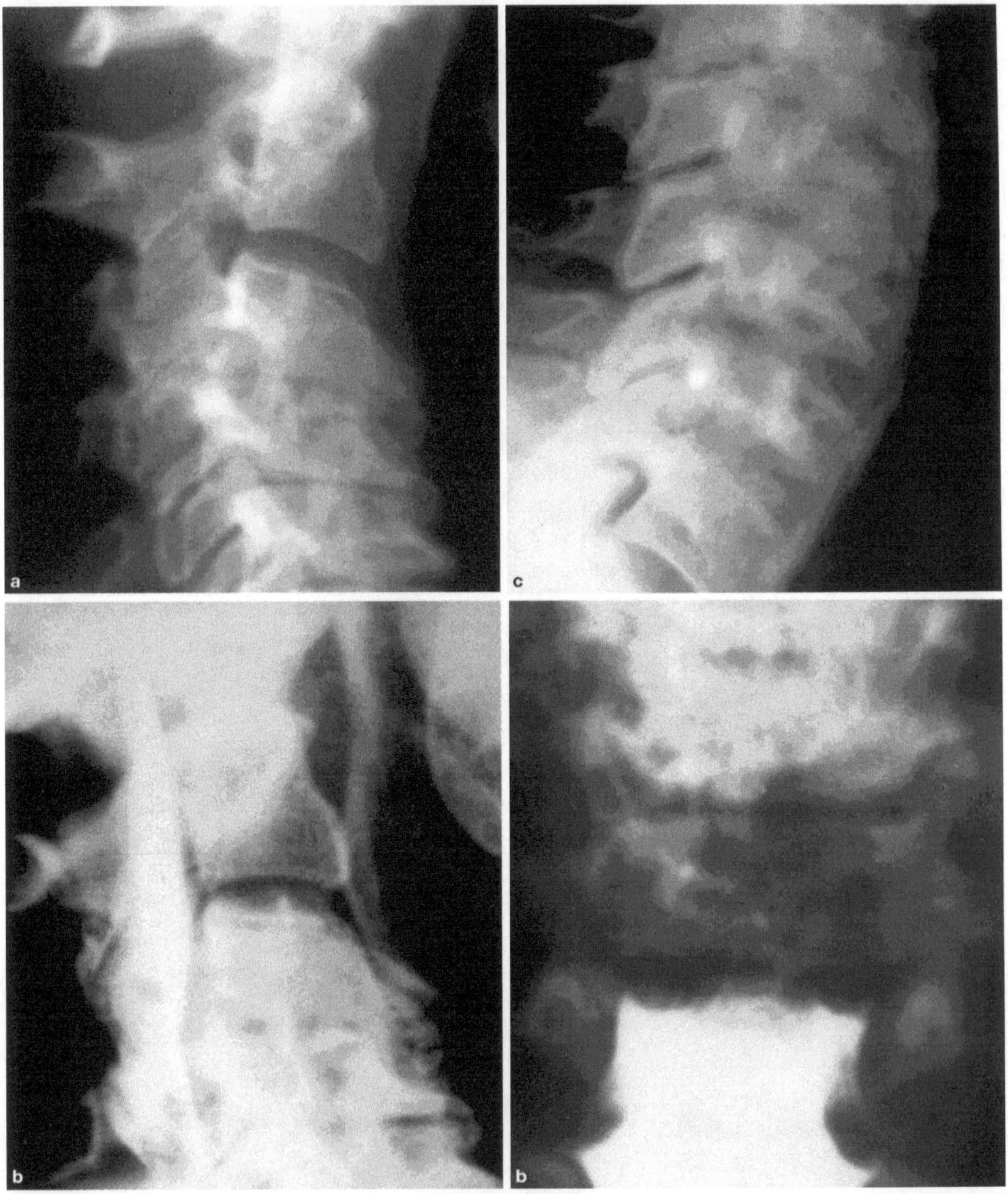

Fig. 9.34 a–c. Radiological investigation in a male, 51-year-old patient with severe spondylitic myelopathy with spastic tetraparesis as a result of stenosis from multiple causes (congenitally narrowed canal and superimposed spondyloarthrosis). **a** Plain radiograph in lateral projection showing marked reversal of the lordosis. **b** Myelograms illustrating the severity of the stenosis (lateral projection, *left*) and of the deformity of the spine (anteroposterior projection, *right*). **c** Postoperative plain radiograph in a lateral projection following multiple subtotal corpectomies carried out with arthrodesis in diastesis using iliac crest autograft. To be noted in addition to the diastesis of the vertebral bodies is the partial restoration of the cervical lordosis

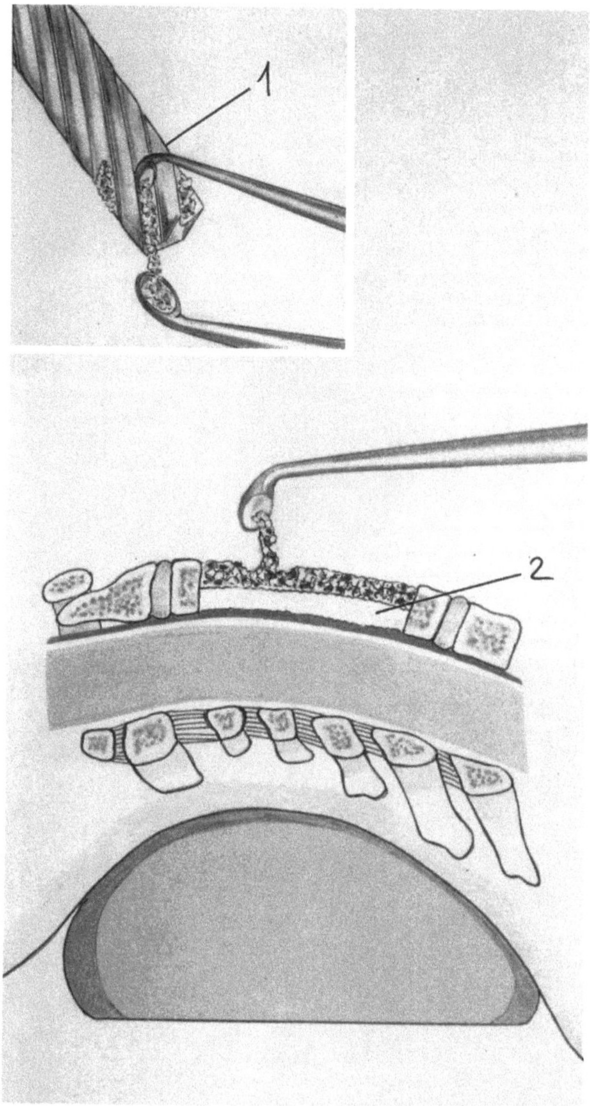

Fig. 9.35. Fusion with only the graft obtained from the Cloward drill. The graft retrieved from the drill bit (*1*) is laid on a bed of Spongostan (*2*). This method (described by Senegas) is useful in cases with already rigid spinal segments. Fusion can be achieved while avoiding the problems associated with the more formal graft harvesting from any of the donor sites

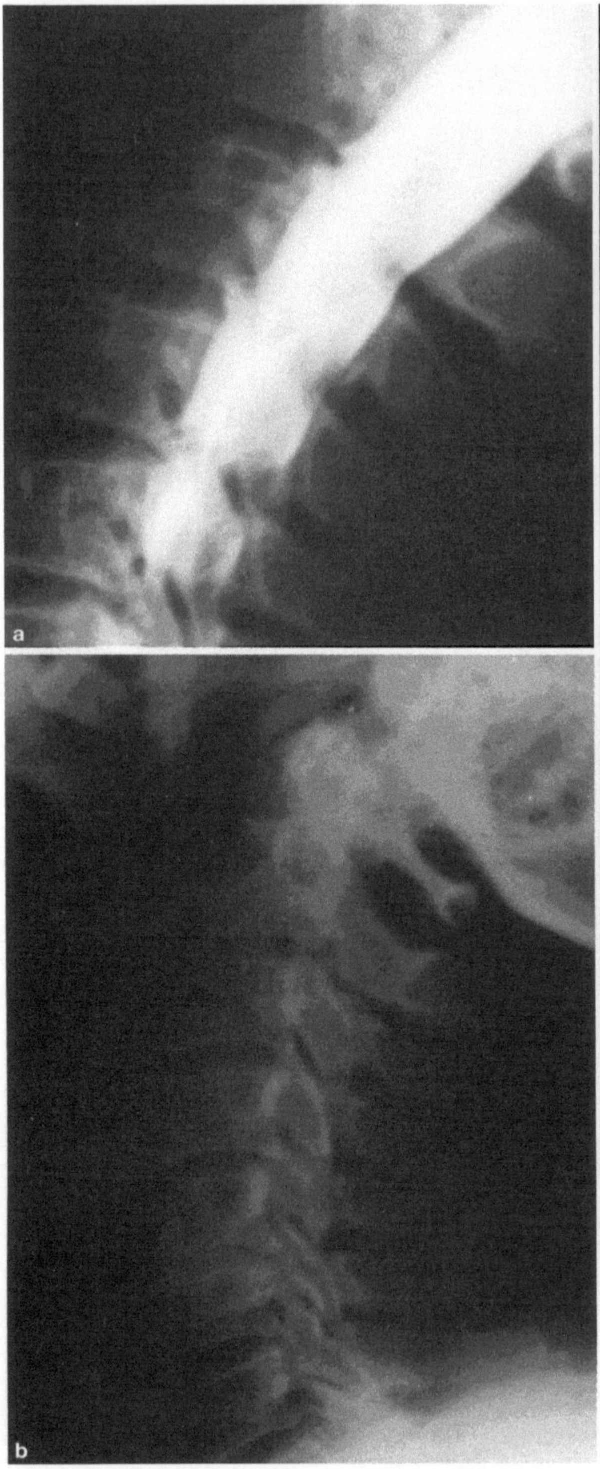
a
b

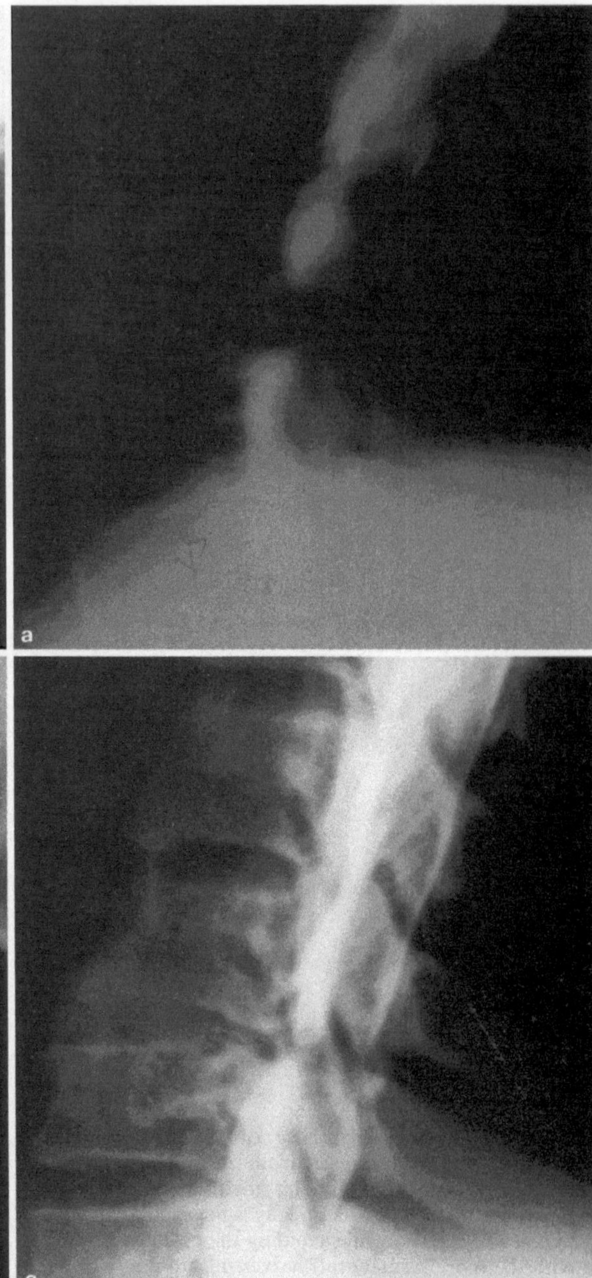
a
c

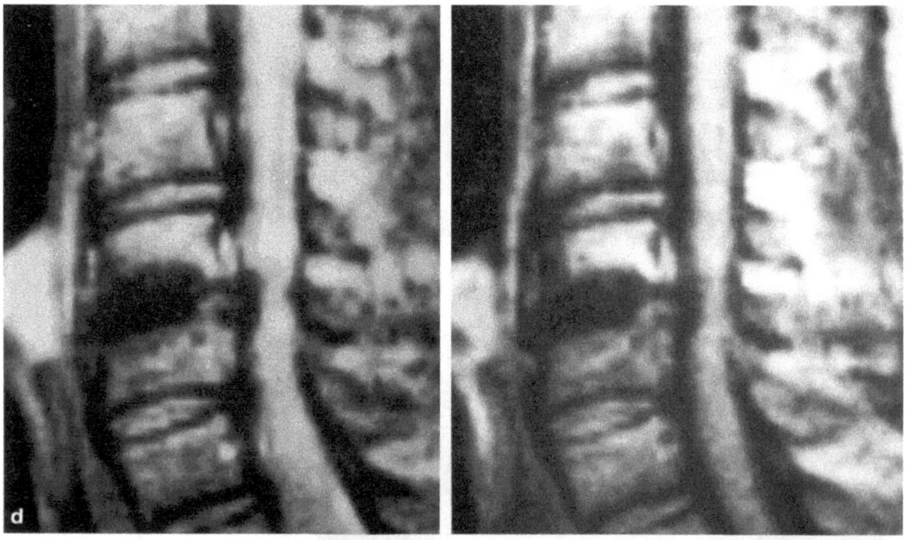

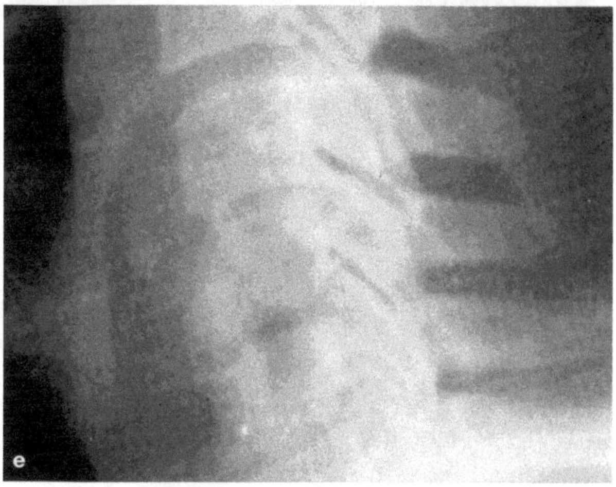

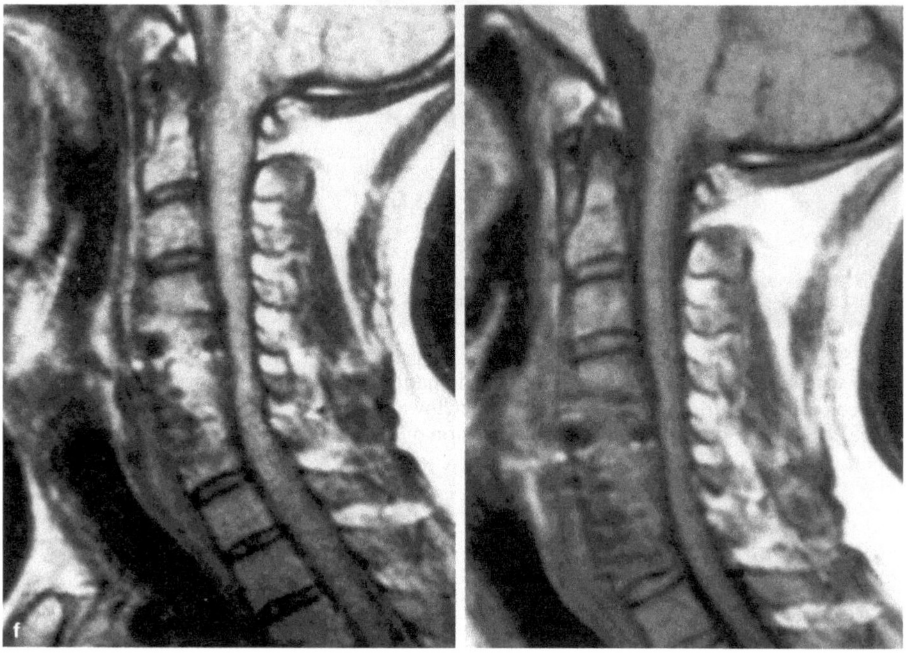

Fig. 9.36 a–f. Radiological imaging of a male, 54-year-old patient with spondylotic myelopathy with tetraparesis at the C5–C6 level. **a** Two preoperative myelograms. **b** Radiograph taken after the patient had undergone intersomatic arthrodesis according to Smith-Robinson procedure using acrylic cement. Note cement and posterior osteophytes. **c** Symptoms persisted and a subsequent myelogram showed spinal cord compression, roughly as severe as that observed preoperatively. **d** MRI taken prior to second operation showing persisting compressions. **e** Plain radiograph taken after the second operation showing anterior decompression was carried out, with removal of cement and osteophytes in C5–C6 and C6–C7. **f** MRI showing completed decompression after the second operation

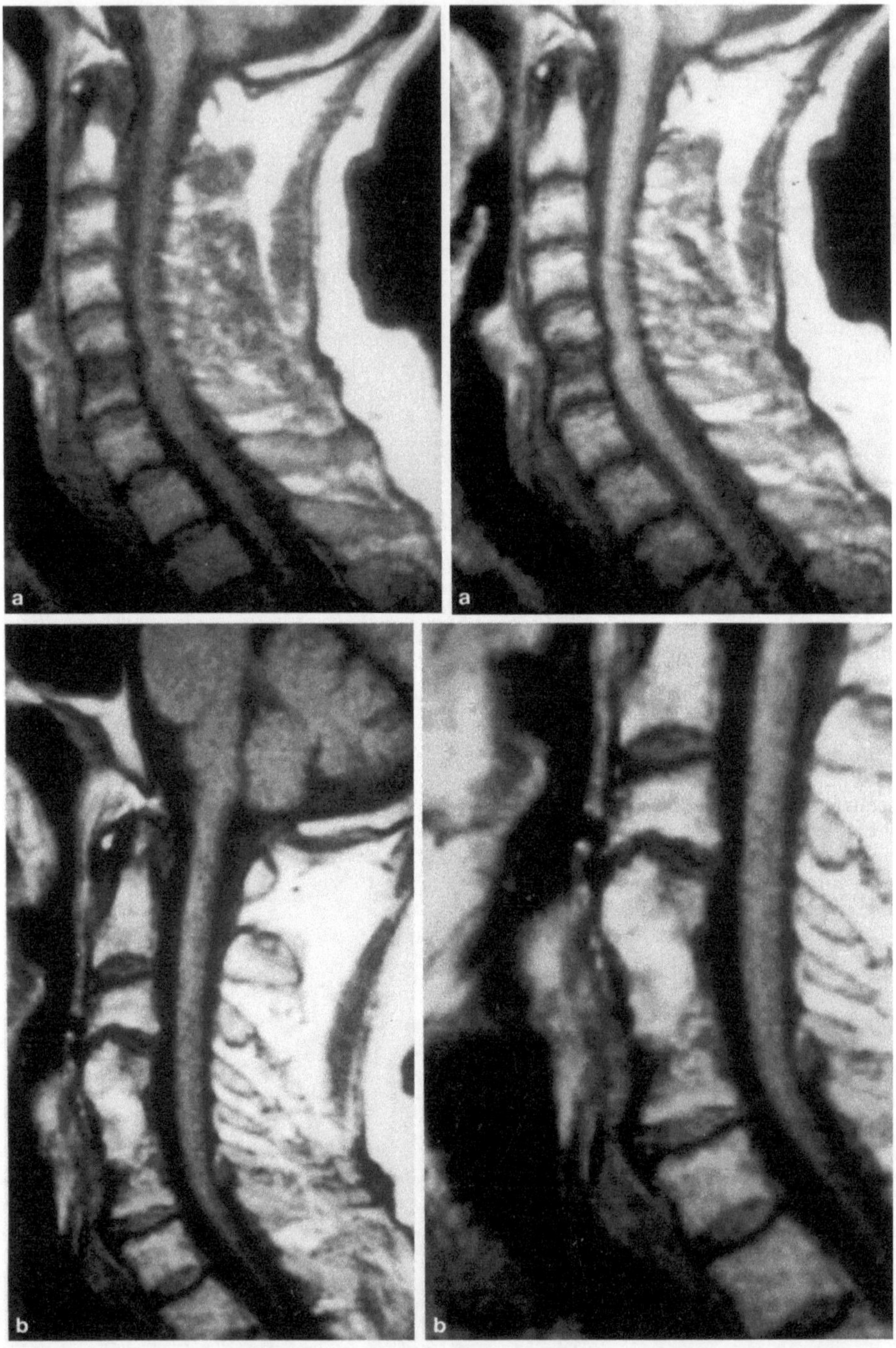

Fig. 9.37 a, b. MRI investigation of a male, 54-year-old patient with severe spondylotic myelopathy, who had previously been treated at the level C5–C6 using the Cloward procedure. **a** The graft has collapsed and compression of the spinal cord is still present. **b** Postoperative MRI after multiple corpectomies and autograft. The spinal cord has been relieved from compression and the canal appears enlarged

Anterior Decompression in Post-traumatic, Neoplastic and Infectious Causes of Stenosis

Post-traumatic Stenosis

Post-traumatic stenosis is associated with deformed vertebrae and displaced malunited fragments of bone that protrude into the canal. In such cases, it is not advisable or indeed possible to use the techniques described that employ drilling or Cloward instrumentation. Drills can be particularly dangerous in these cases. First of all, it is not possible to accurately place the guide in position for the drill, because the vertebral bodies to be drilled are misshapen and difficult to orient. Secondly, the tissues may be injured and weakened to the extent that they do not provide a solid base for placing the guides and drills. Finally, the risk of further displacement of nonunited, malunited or deformed bony fragments by the drill should be a major consideration. These fragments may in fact be driven by the drill into the cord and nerve roots with severe consequences (Fig. 9.38). In such cases, the use of a high-speed air drill is advisable. The drill bits can be appropriately selected for the purpose: a selection of pointed or ball-shaped bits should be available. These will permit the accomplishment of all the necessary dissection in preparing a slot for the graft. Their careful use will permit the avoidance of injury to neurological structures, and the shaping of the contour of the dissection can be completed with a selection of curets and forceps such as Kerrison's.

The initial step of the actual dissection at the spine should be to identify the disk spaces adjacent to the fractured bodies. The extent of the lesion and hence the extent of the decompression must be carefully assessed. As always, the first step in this procedure is the evacuation of the disk space, with removal of all soft tissue and of any fragments of the disk still remaining in situ (Fig. 9.39). A pointed drill bit is suitable as a saw and may be used to outline the margins of the graft bed across the area of decompression (Fig. 9.40). This dissection may be safely extended into the bone for a distance of 10 mm from the anterior surface. Rongeurs or other suitable forceps can be used to remove any fragments that might be encountered in this part of the dissection. A drill with a ball-shaped bit can be used to remove larger or more firmly fixed fragments of various sizes (Fig. 9.41). By utilizing drills, straight and curved curets, Kerrison forceps and hernia forceps, etc. for these steps, the decompression of the cord is achieved. One should proceed slowly and very carefully, ensuring that the progression is gradual since this is a very delicate and important part of the dissection (Fig. 9.42).

Following decompression, fusion is achieved with a massive dowel autograft that is shaped and put in place with the spine in diastasis using the distractor as described in the previous section (Fig. 9.43). There is rarely a need to use plates and screws for internal fixation in addition to the bony graft. These should only be necessary when the graft is less than optimal in quality, size, or shape, or where residual segmental instability does not permit the dowel graft to be placed with sufficient distraction to fix it in such a way as to remove all mobility and instability from the operated site (Figs. 9.42, 9.43).

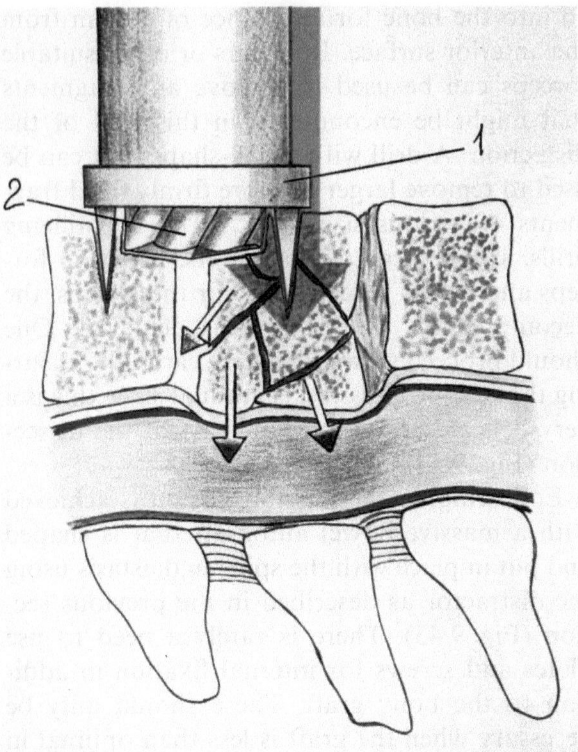

Fig. 9.38. At this stage of decompression, the use of the Cloward instrumentation is to be categorically avoided. The foot plate of the sleeve (*1*) would rest on an unstable as well as uneven surface. As the drill (*2*) is advanced posteriorly, it runs the risk of driving bone fragments posteriorly, producing cord injury

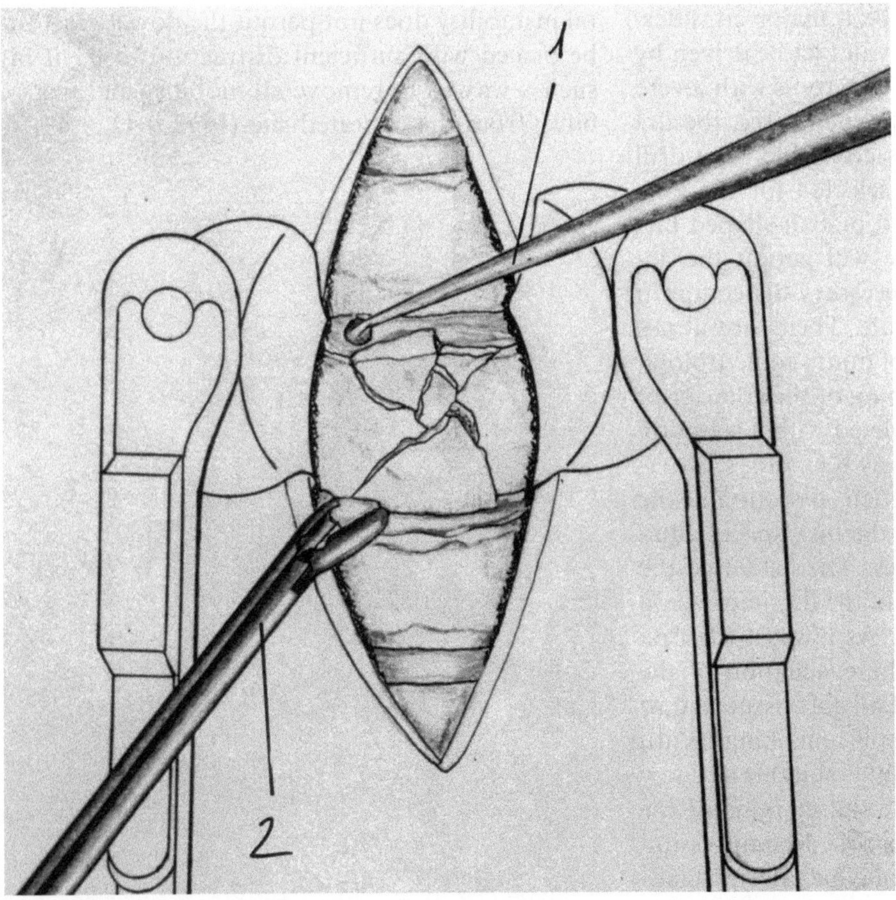

Fig. 9.39. The first stage of anterior decompression. The disk spaces are identified and the involved ones are emptied with curved curets (*1*) or with hernia forceps (*2*)

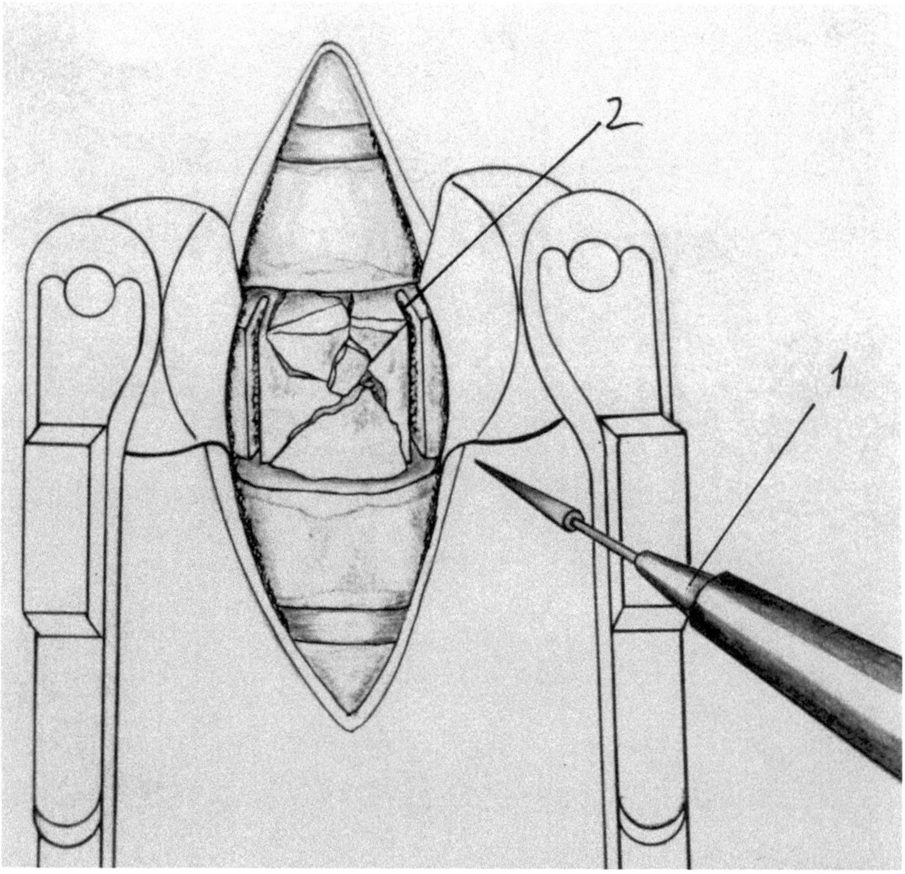

Fig. 9.40. This shows the use of an air drill with a pointed bit (*1*). It is advanced from the side (*2*), until it reaches the posterior wall of the body

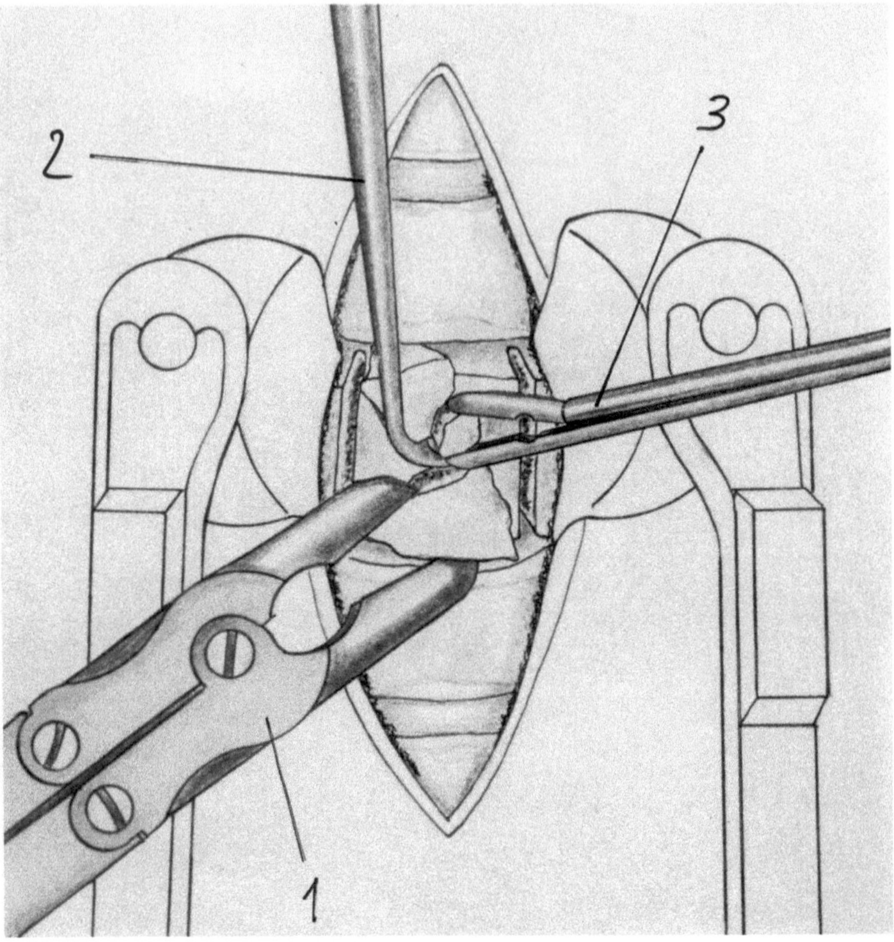

Fig. 9.41. The most superficial fragments of the disrupted body are removed with rongeurs (*1*), curved curets (*2*), or hernia forceps (*3*)

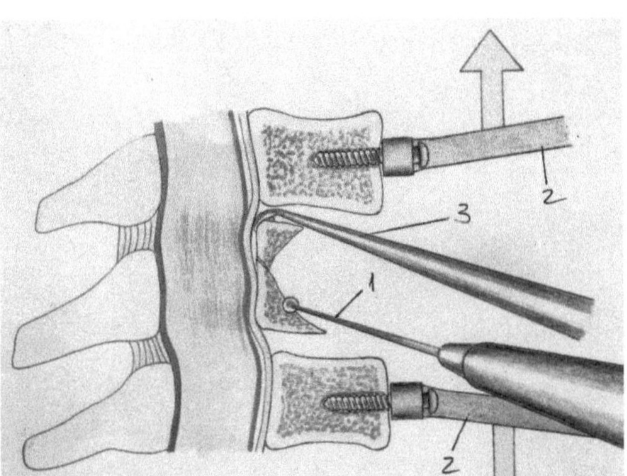

Fig. 9.42. This shows the final stages of removing the deep-seated fragments of bone with gradual thinning out of the wall using drill bits (*1*) of specially adapted shape and size. The vertebral bodies are separated from each other by the distractor (*2*), which is anchored on the vertebral bodies above and below the level of resection. Remaining fragments of the posterior wall are removed manually using curved curets (*3*)

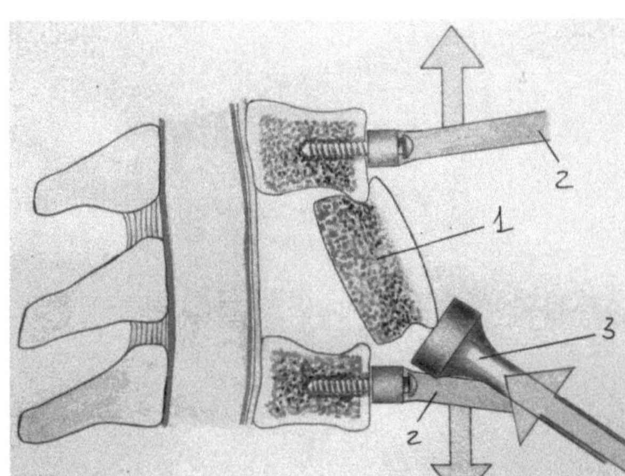

Fig. 9.43. The graft is shaped to interlock with the host bed (*1*). It is tapped (*3*) into place with appropriate distraction (*2*) of the operative site

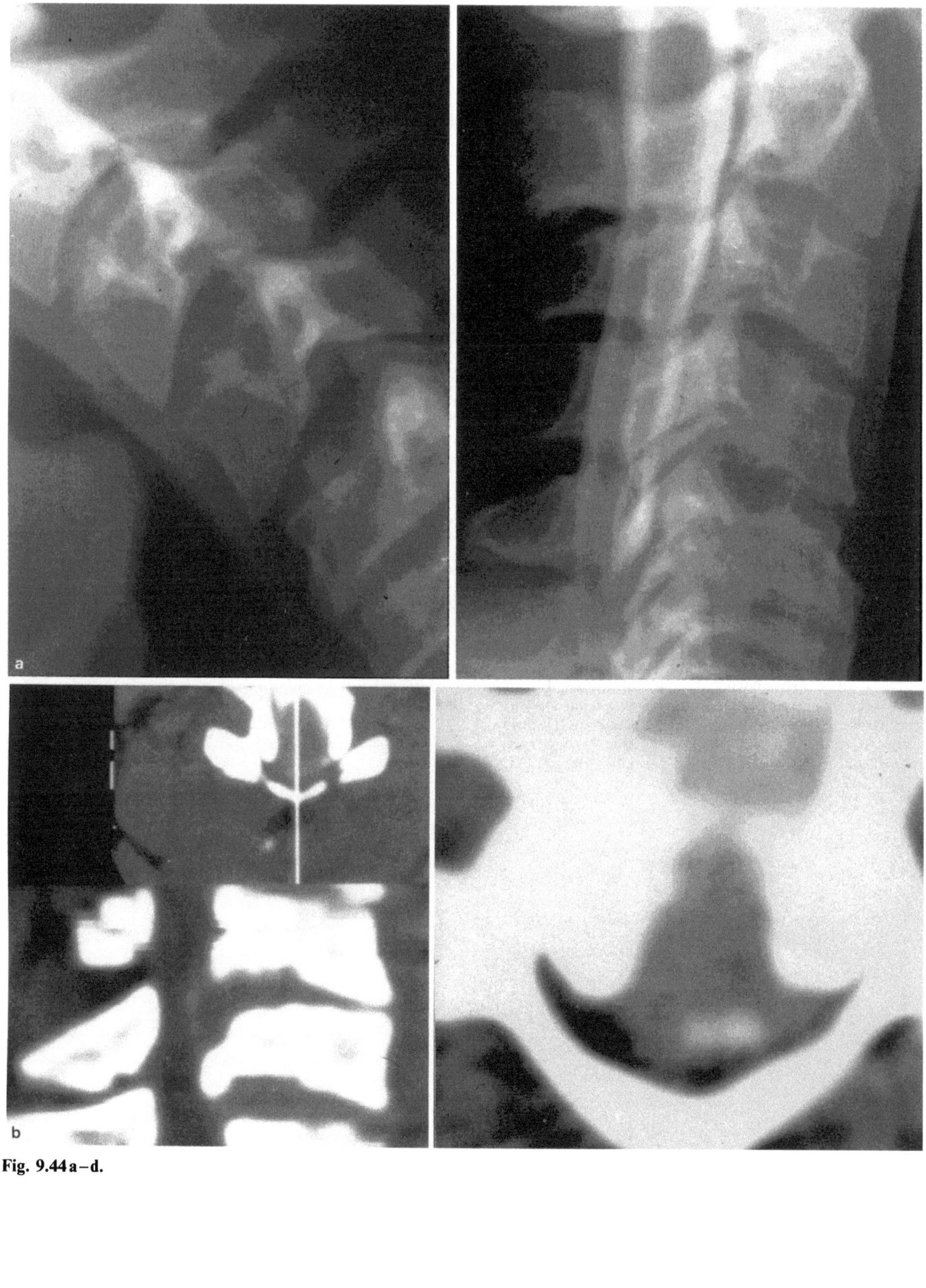

Fig. 9.44 a–d.

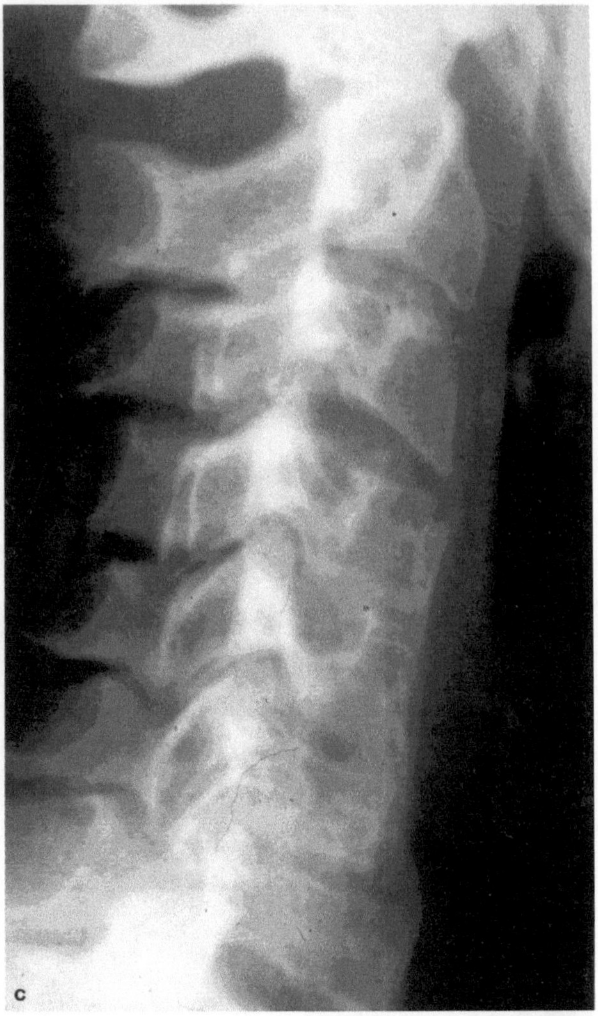

Fig. 9.44 a–d. Radiological imaging in a 32-year-old male patient. **a** Plain radiograph and myelogram in the lateral projection showing vertebral body compression and deformity with segmental stenosis at the C5–C6 and C6–C7 levels. **b** Computed tomograph with longitudinal reconstruction demonstrate well the various combined causes of the stenosis including a congenitally narrow canal, the posterior protrusion of a fragment of the posterior wall of C6, and the presence of a soft hernia at the C5–C6 level. **c** Plain radiograph taken after anterior decompression had been carried out with an extensive corpectomy and autograft. **d** Comparative pre- (*left*) and postoperative (*right*) computed tomographs show, both in horizontal cuts and in longitudinal reconstruction, that the cause of the stenosis has been removed and that the canal is now actually enlarged

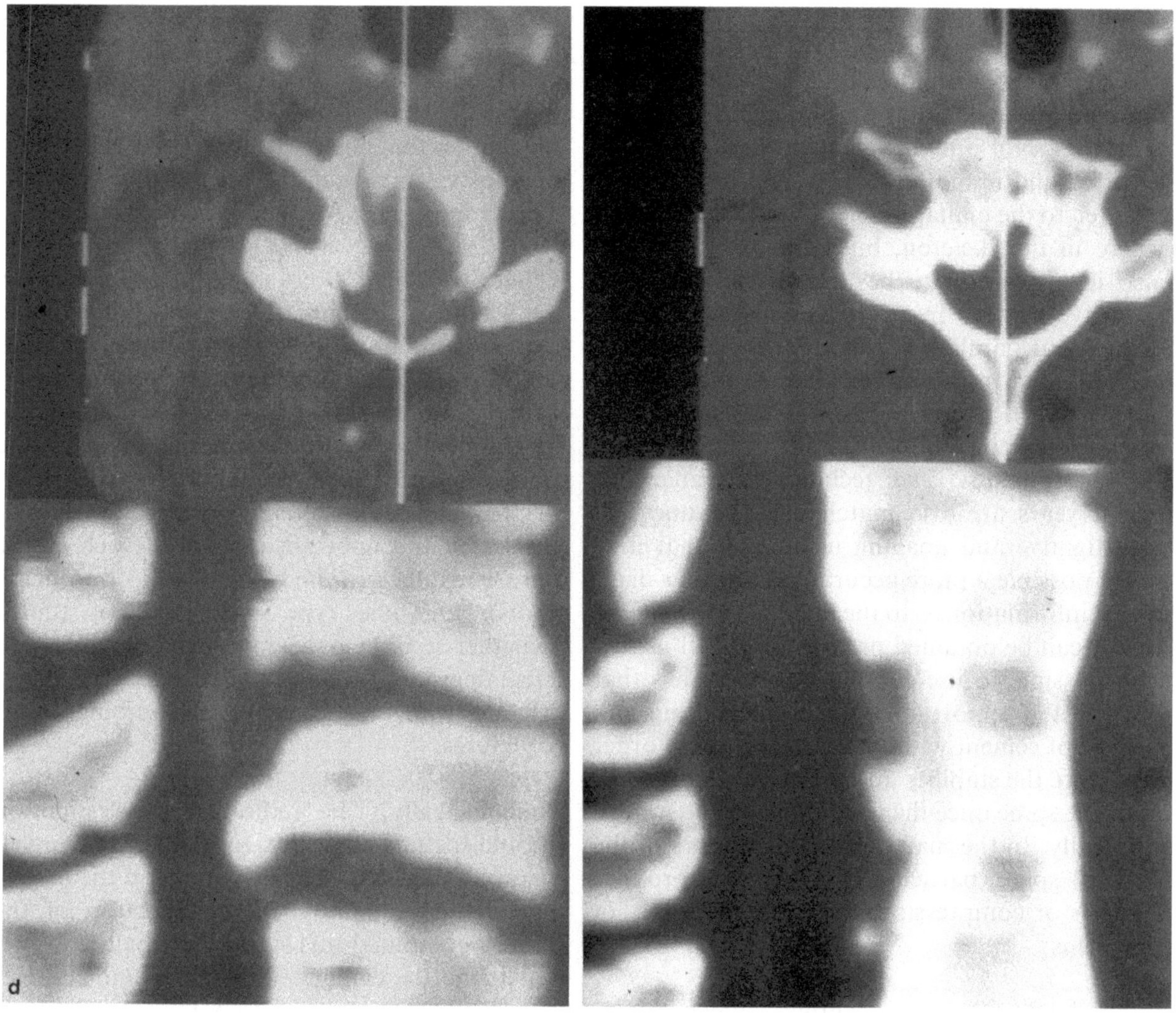
d

Neoplastic Stenosis

The treatment of tumors of the cervical spine has undergone considerable development in the last few years. Not only have chemotherapy, radiotherapy, and immunotherapy significantly contributed to the management of these tumors elsewhere in the skeleton, but surgeons are today also in a position to be able to remove large extensive tumors from the cervical spine to a degree that parallels the management of tumor in the limbs. In the cervical spine, once the tumor has been removed, one obviously must undertake steps to produce stabilization of the affected segments. The technical advances of recent years are also matched by advances in investigative and imaging techniques that now make possible a more accurate and earlier diagnosis; information as to the aggressiveness of the tumor can be obtained preoperatively. It is now also possible to use combined approaches that provide the opportunity for bone grafting and the use of cement with internal fixation in order to restore the stability and the structural integrity of the spine once the tumor has been removed surgically. In the management of tumors of the cervical spine, particularly when they produce stenosis or compression, there are two types of problems:

- The need for aggressive surgery, which is associated with a high degree of difficulty in reaching and resecting the tumor. Multiple approaches may be required as is often the case in the upper cervical spine. In these areas one has to be aware at all times of the various vascular and neurological structures during the approach.
- The surgical procedure extends the dissection to an area near the cord and neuroradicular structures, which must be protected and saved from injury.

As stated above, a tumor at this level of the spine that has been deemed completely benign histologically may, nevertheless, represent a very significant threat to the structures within the canal. Destruction of parts of or of entire vertebrae, regardless of the benignity of the cause, will have very severe consequences on the cord and nerve roots. In addition, when a tumor invades the canal, compression of the cord results, regardless of the state of the skeletal tissues. The first precaution that one must always take is a careful diagnostic survey of the area of involvement. This is important for the following reasons:

Clinically. There is no simple classification or definition of the clinical pictures that patients can present, because of the multiple variables that interact. One variable is the point of origin of the tumor (whether it is situated high or low in the cervical spine, whether it involves the body, the lamina, or the pedicles, or whether it destroys the entire vertebra). The relationship of the lesion to important structures (such as the cord, medulla – in the higher levels – and nerve roots), and the type and grade of tumor (whether it is benign or malignant) will, to a great degree, reflect its destructive potential and its ability to invade, grow, and impinge onto structures.

Radiologically. The radiological investigation should include clinical X-rays, CT, MRI, myelography (which is primarily useful in the assessing changes due to dynamic function of the spine), computed myelography (which will better define the extent of the tumor and its relationship to the surrounding bony and soft tissue, e.g., meningeal dissemination), angiography of the tumor (to determine the degree of vascularization and the necessity for preoperative embolization – this is most important particularly in dealing with vascular neoplasms, where the degree of vascularity must be diminished in order to be able to dissect completely without interference from massive bleeding), and isotope scans which will define not only the localization and invasiveness of a tumor, but will also help to identify satellite lesions or other foci of dissemination).

Biopsy. The most important diagnostic step is probably biopsy. It will not only identify the lesion, but represents a direct approach to the early diagnosis of a lesion. Based on the histologic findings, the approach and the surgical techniques necessary for dealing with the lesion surgically may be determined. Biopsy can be then performed with a needle aspiration technique or through a more formal surgical approach to the lesion. Needle aspiration biopsy is the simpler, faster, and less complicated approach to histologically diagnosing a tumor. For lesions in the higher cervical spine, particularly C1 and C2, needle aspiration biopsy can easily be carried out through the mouth. Indeed, the only structure to be crossed in order to reach the spine with a needle for biopsy is the posterior wall of the pharynx. Biopsy can be carried out after local anesthesia with a long needle through the open mouth. One should use radiological control such as CT to ensure access to the lesion by the needle. This approach permits biopsies of the cervico-occipital region, the arches, lateral masses, and bodies of the atlas and the axis, and the body of C3 (Fig. 9.45).

For lesions in the lower spine between C3 and C7, needle aspiration biopsy should be performed through the anterolateral approach. The needle should be guided to pass in front of the neurovascular bundle of the neck. The bundle can easily be identified and protected by placing the examining finger in front of the sternocleidomastoid muscle. The pulsation of the carotid artery can be felt in the bundle, and this is a feature that helps identify it. If the needle is passed in front of the bundle, its tip can be safely advanced to the surface of the vertebral bodies. Under radiological guidance, one proceeds to the area of involvement where the tissue sample is obtained (Fig. 9.46). Open biopsy is necessary if the needle biopsy is inconclusive or does not provide adequate tissue for diagnosis. In these cases, one may need to confirm the tissue sampling by frozen section whenever possible. Calcified tissue must be decalcified prior to histologic processing, and thus it may take several days before it can be assessed.

Indications

In cases where there is direct compression of the cord as a result of tumor invasion into the canal or directly into the neural tissues themselves, or in cases where there is indirect compression of these structures, caused by the collapse of the osseous structure as a result of tumor invasion, the indications for surgical management are characterized by a multiplicity of factors.

The indications will obviously depend on the type of tumor present. In aggressive, invasive malignant neoplasms and, in particular, in metastatic neoplasms of the spine, it may not be possible to expect a surgical intervention to result in a total removal of the tumor, nor should this be a serious consideration in view of the poor prognosis. By contrast, in tumors of low-grade malignancy or those that are of local aggressiveness only, prognosis is obviously better and therefore complete tumor removal should be carefully undertaken.

The patient must be physically able to with stand any aggressive or extensive surgery. Particular attention must be paid to the neurological status and to the type of neurological deficit that is present and whether any or all of the deficit can be expected to recover after surgery. The current availability of instrumentation and materials permits the restoration of stability to the involved portion of the cervical spine, whether it be through the anterior or posterior approach and whether the involvement is high or low in the cervical spine.

The Experience of the Surgeon

One very important determining factor is the amount of experience the surgeon has. In dealing with these patients, one cannot generalize or standardize the type of surgical procedure to be undertaken. Each patient is a very individual and specific case and must be dealt with accordingly. The surgeon will therefore be required to call upon all his experience and expertise in surgery of the cervical spine. He must adapt the surgical procedure to the requirements of the individual. The approach and the actual surgical instrumentation and management must be specifically developed for each individual case.

Under these conditions, it is not possible to provide a description of the specific techniques that should be used, but only the general principles to be followed in the approach to these cases can be expressed. Removal must be complete when the location permits and the specific indications for removal of the tumor are present. Often the need for multiple approaches that will permit the surgeon to complete the total removal of a lesion that can otherwise not be removed by a single approach must be anticipated.

Once the removal of the lesion is complete, reconstructive surgery may well be necessary. In dealing with benign tumors or localized forms of reticulendotheliosis that affects younger patients who are still growing, reconstruction following removal of the tumor from the vertebral structure can only be performed with dowel-type osseous autografts for stabilization; it is not possible to utilize implants for internal fixation. In the postoperative period, stabilization and immobilization must be maintained with a halo vest or halo cast.

In malignant tumors, particularly those with a poor prognosis, one should aim at solid grafts that provide immediate stabilization and fusion (graft from tibia or fibula) or the use of cement and internal fixation. The use of cement requires a special precaution: the high temperature reached in the heat-generating reaction which occurs during polymerization of methylmethacrylate may be harmful to the bone. This is not a significant problem in posterior immobilization where the laminae have been preserved but in anterior reconstructions there is a very real risk of injury to important structures such as the cord. A technical step which has been found to be useful is to protect any exposed or immediately subjacent tissues such as nerves or cord with Spongostan. Also, whenever possible, a plastic sheet (such as the bag containing the cement monomer) may be used, as a barrier between the cement and the subjacent tissues. It should be shaped to fit across the base of the area of reconstruction. The combination of the plastic sheet and the layer of Spongostan protects neurological structures from the heat of polymerization when the cement is applied. Once the cement has set, with or without immobilization by plates and screws, the plastic sheet can be removed early in the polymerization stage, creating a line of separation between the cement and the underlying nerve tissues, which are therefore protected.

In cases of malignant tumors where it is neither desirable nor possible to completely remove the tumor, methods of immobilization must be used which still permit the architectural stabilization of the involved segments. In the occipitocervical region it is easy to see that internal immobilization only serves to provide enough support to relieve the symptoms, such as pain, that result from functional deficiency in the neck's ability to support the head. Internal immobilization is also intended to maintain the stability of the head, thereby avoiding progressive collapse that would increase neurological deficits which, in extreme cases, could have fatal consequences.

Cement or bone graft should be regarded only as part of the internal immobilization. Without them, any surgical procedure will be destined to fail because of the inherent instability of any procedure that avoids their use. The anchoring of metal implants will be subject to loosening because the bone tends to be weakened or osteoporotic and therefore does not assure the permanence of the immobilization that can be achieved. Stabilization must be secure and solid, particularly when there is total or subtotal absence of the vertebral body following removal of the lesion. Immobilization and stabilization may need to be carried out both anteriorly and posteriorly.

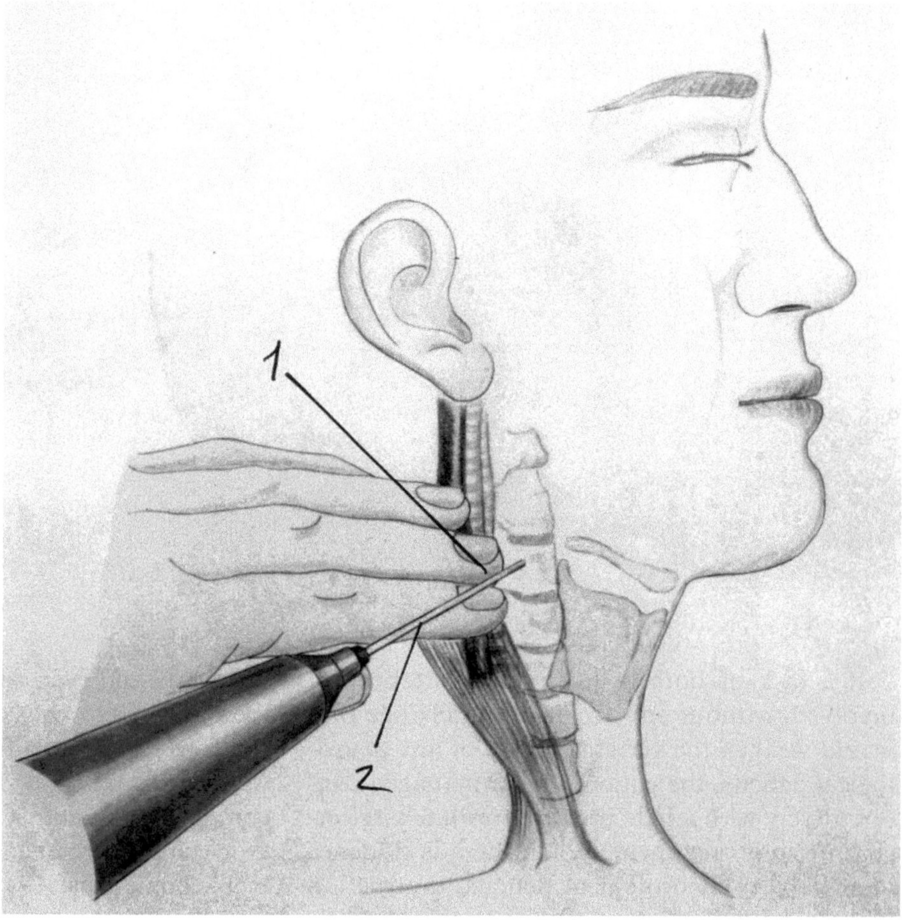

Fig. 9.45. A fine-needle biopsy (*1*) through the transoral route under local anesthesia. This method gives access to the levels C1–C3. A tongue depressor (*2*) and a retractor applied on the teeth (*2*) help to maintain visual access to the posterior wall of the oropharynx. The drawing also shows how, through a posterior approach (*4*), the lamina and the lateral masses of the cervical vertebral bodies may be reached

Preoperative embolization of the supplying vessels to the lesion is a very valuable step that facilitates the removal of the tumor mass, while at the same time minimizing intraoperative bleeding. Complete clean out of a tumor includes by definition extension of the dissection to the surrounding normal tissue. It is advisable to begin the dissection from the normal tissue and then proceed towards the tumor so as not to disseminate the tumor or miss marginal tumor extension (Figs. 9.47–9.50).

Inflammatory Stenosis

The problems are quite different in inflammatory types of stenosis due to infection. The inflammatory tissue not only extends into the canal, but may produce collapse of the bony structures leading to stenosis. The classification of cervical infections was discussed in Chap. 2 (p. 10). Obviously the initial step in deciding on appropriate management is, as with tumors, performing a biopsy to establish that it is an infection and to identify the specific causative agent.

As described above a needle aspiration biopsy at the level of C1 or C2 may be performed transorally, and, at the levels of C3–C7, it should be carried out through the presternocleidomastoid approach (Figs. 9.45, 9.46). The approaches are described in Chap. 8. The success of the management will depend on early diagnosis and on undertaking an appropriate combination of medical management, using antibiotics, the necessary orthotic support, and surgical intervention. Obviously the indications determining the management will depend on the clinical situation and on the degree of tissue destruction that has occurred.

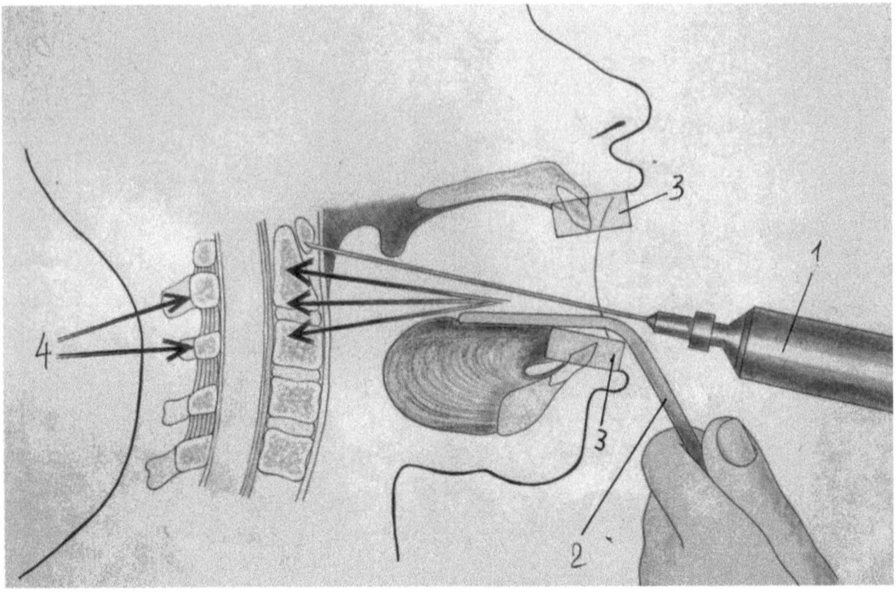

Fig. 9.46. The anterior approach for needle biopsy to reach the levels C3–C7. The neurovascular bundle is protected and pulled aside by the hand (*1*). The needle (*2*) is advanced in front of the hand under full visual and fluoroscopic control

If a disk or both a disk and a vertebra are involved, without any architectural change that would weaken the vertebral body or any neurological deficits, the patient can be managed conservatively with a halo and appropriately selected antibiotic treatment. When there is evidence of instability, neurological deficits, destruction with or without collapse of the vertebral bodies, or any combination of these, then immediate surgical management is indicated.

The first step should be to restore the alignment of the spine and the maintenance of the stability of the involved vertebrae. The immediate institution of halo traction is essential at this point. The surgical management should aim to evacuate any abscess cavities and remove any loose osseous fragments in order to decompress any involved neural structures. There should be careful and complete evacuation of any involved tissue right out to the normal, uninvolved, surrounding bone. This will require the use of a variety of instruments such as high-speed air drills, straight and curved curets, and bone forceps such as Kerrisons or Rongeurs. Keeping in mind the important anatomical relationships, it is obvious that any posterior fragments that are in contact with the posterior longitudinal ligament must be completely removed. Furthermore, granulomatous tissue may blend with the ligaments and even with the anterior surface of the dura mater; in such cases, one must dissect carefully in order to find a line of cleavage that will permit removal of this abnormal tissue as completely possible. One cannot overemphasize the need for care in lateral dissection; the instruments come close to the vertebral veins and arteries, and, because these structures are associated with increased vascularity and hyperemia, bleeding can be a significant problem.

When the surgical clean out is completed, the margins of the involved tissue defined, the wall

Fig. 9.47 a–f. Radiological imaging in a 23-year-old male patient. **a** Transoral view of C2 with lytic lesion characteristic of giant cell tumor. **b** Arteriogram to define relationship of the vertebral artery to the tumor. **c** Computed tomograph showing very clearly the bony destruction and the extent of the tumor. **d** Radiograph showing the operative procedure completed in stages. Using an anterior approach (high presternocleidomastoid), a wide corpectomy was carried out to remove the tumor, and the vertebral body was reconstructed with autograft and metal plates. Then, with the patient in halo traction, posterior fusion was undertaken using massive iliac crest autograft, metal wire with cerclage of the arch of the atlas anchored with wires to the cranium superiorly and to the lateral mass of C3 inferiorly. After radiotherapy (3 500 rad) bone resorption continued and the plates and the screws loosened. A second course of irradiation was followed by deposition of new bone. Radiographs taken at this time in maximum flexion (**e**) and maximum extension (**f**) show regeneration of the bony tissue

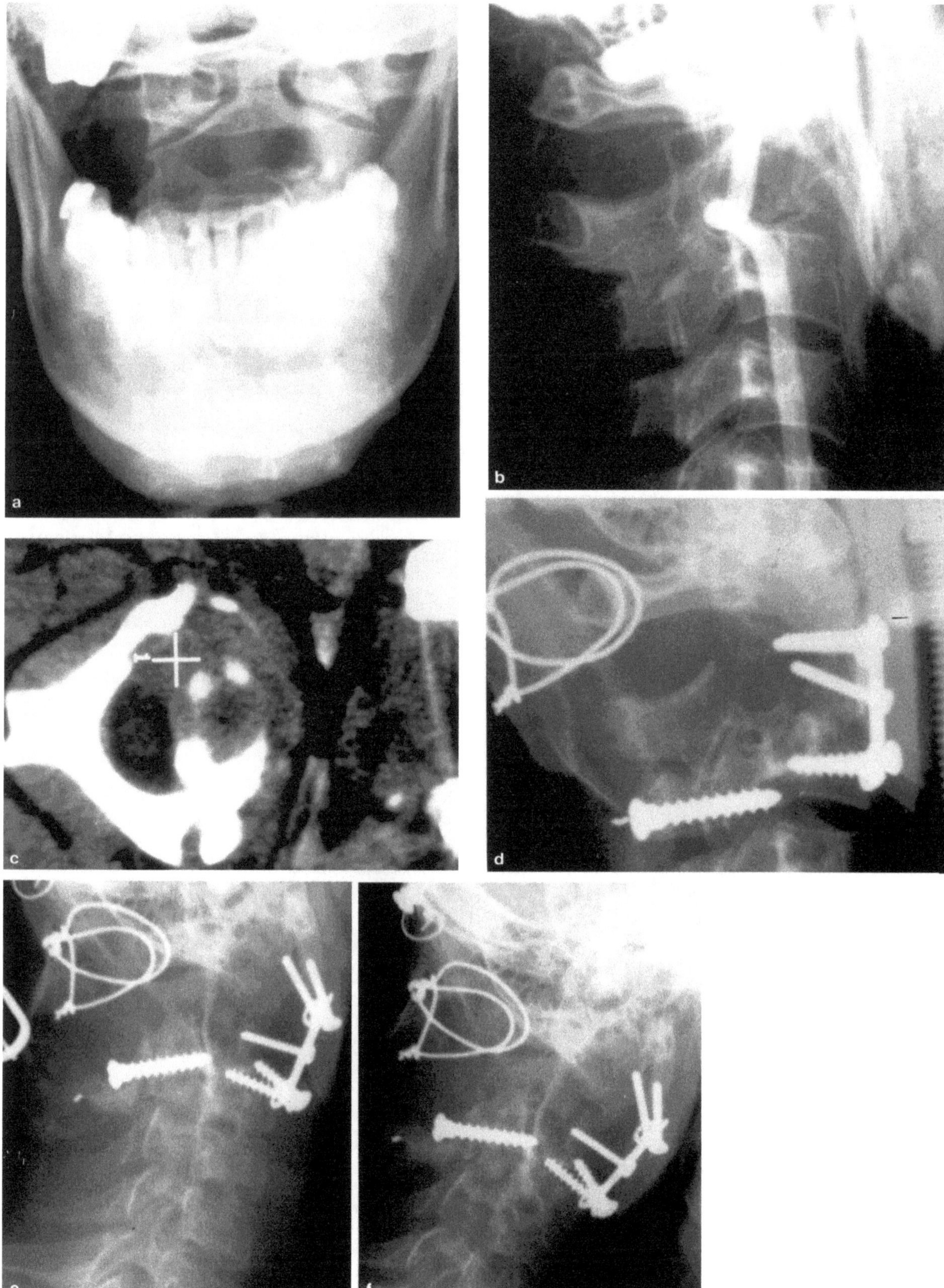
a
b
c
d
e
f

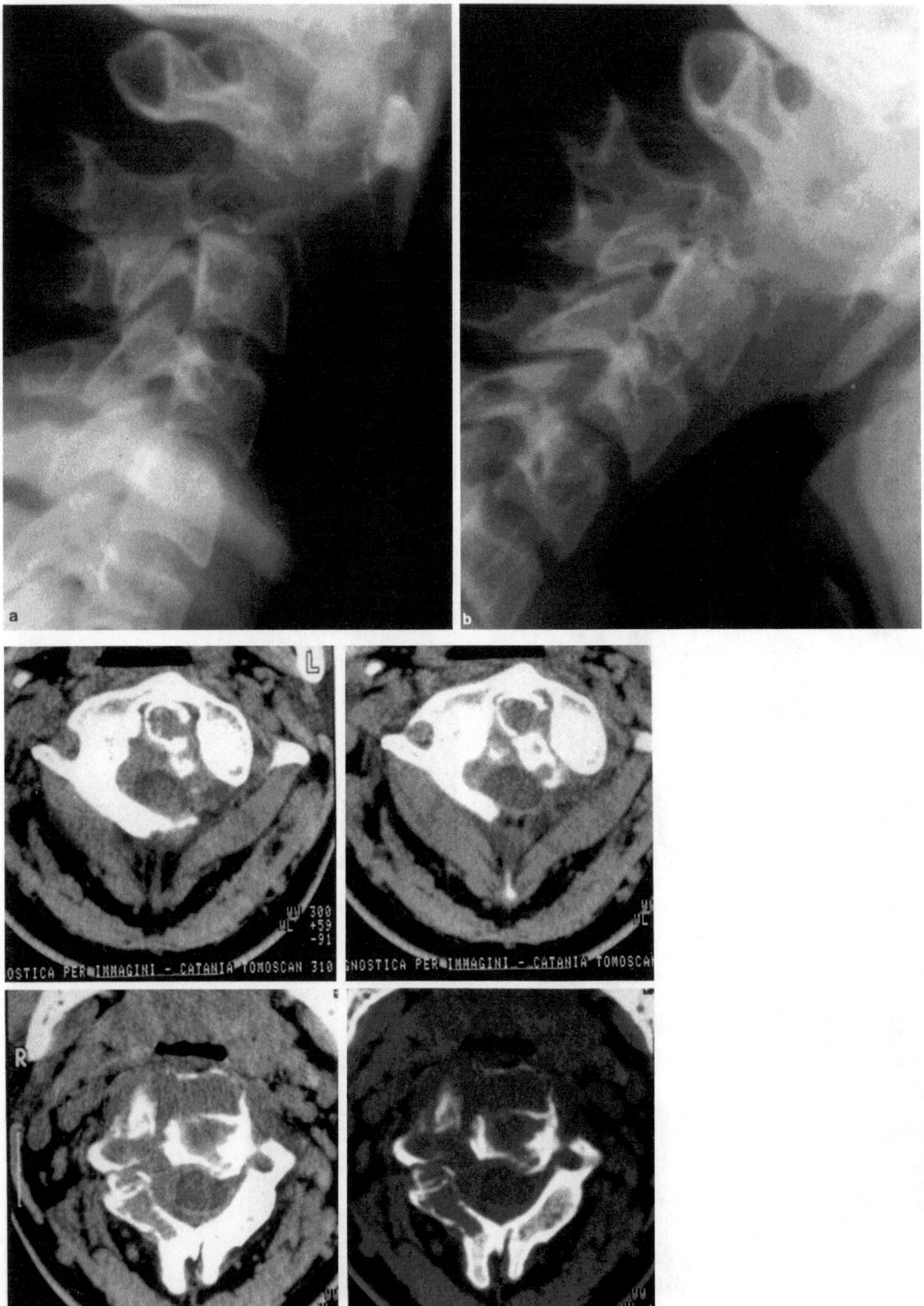
a
b
L
WW 300
WL +59
-91
OSTICA PER IMMAGINI - CATANIA TOMOSCAN 310
GNOSTICA PER IMMAGINI - CATANIA TOMOSCAN
R
c

Fig. 9.48 a–c.

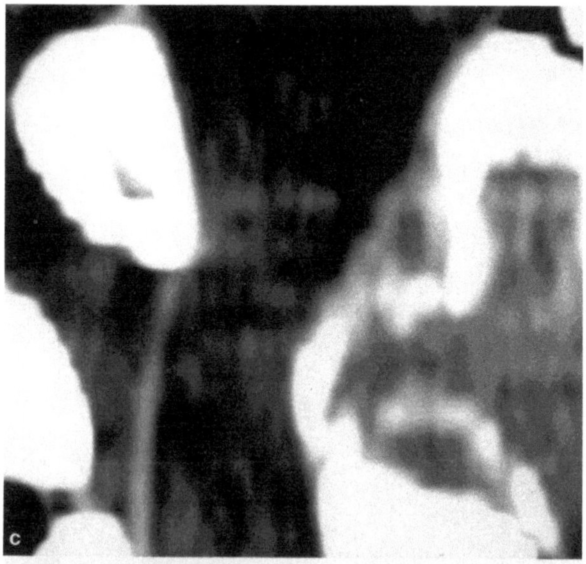

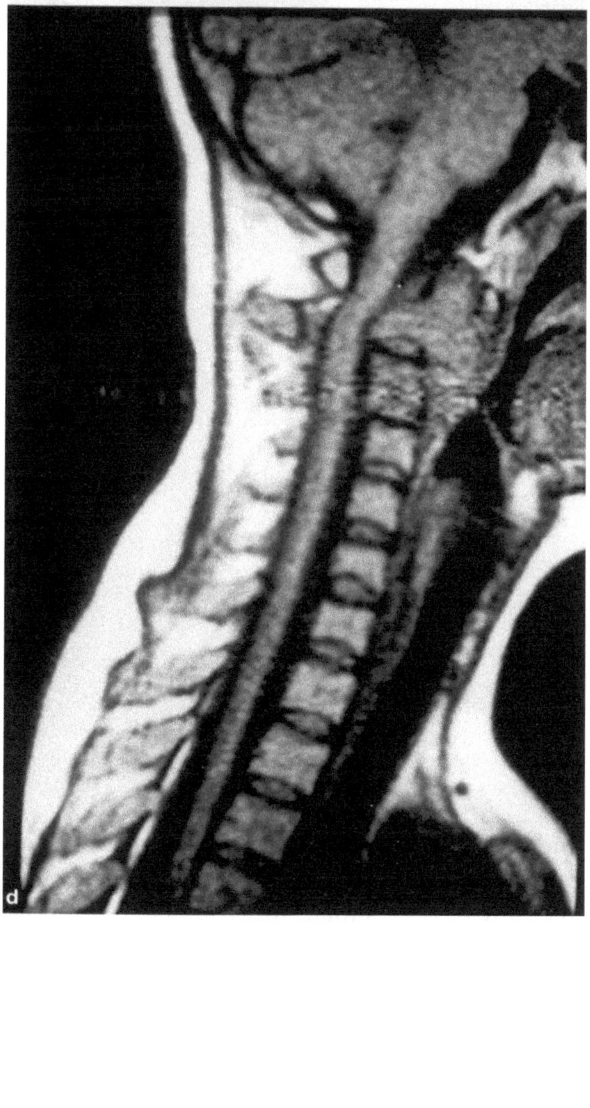

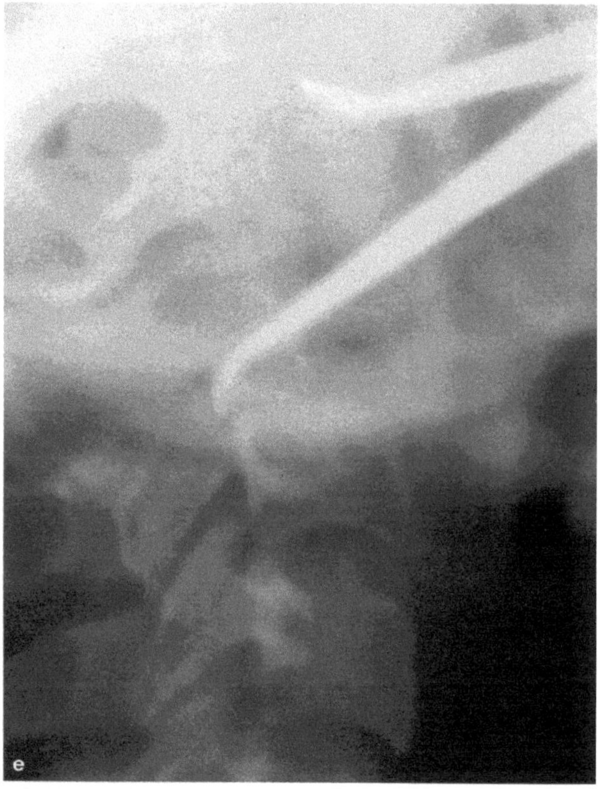

Fig. 9.48 a–h. Radiological imaging in a 21-year-old female patient with a giant cell tumor of C2. Radiographs taken in maximum flexion (**a**) and maximum extension (**b**) show involvement of the entire vertebral body right up to the apex of the odontoid process. **c** Computed tomographic cuts with longitudinal reconstruction demonstrating the involvement of the vertebral body posteriorly all the way to the laminae and anteriorly as far as the apex of the odontoid process. **d** MRI scan demonstrates that the tumor mass has produced anterior and posterior bulging with cord impingement. **e** Intraoperative and **f** postoperative radiographs of the first surgical procedure which was performed through the transoral approach and during which the tumor mass was removed. Stabilization with arthrodesis was achieved through autograft. **g** Postoperative radiograph after the second surgical procedure, which was carried out posteriorly and consisted of a massive autograft from the iliac crest for arthrodesis to supplement the consolidation achieved through metal cerclage of the atlas. **h** Radiographs which show deposition of new bone following radiotherapy. Fusion of the arthrodesis had already occurred 6 months after the operation, with stabilization in both flexion (*right*) and extension (*left*)

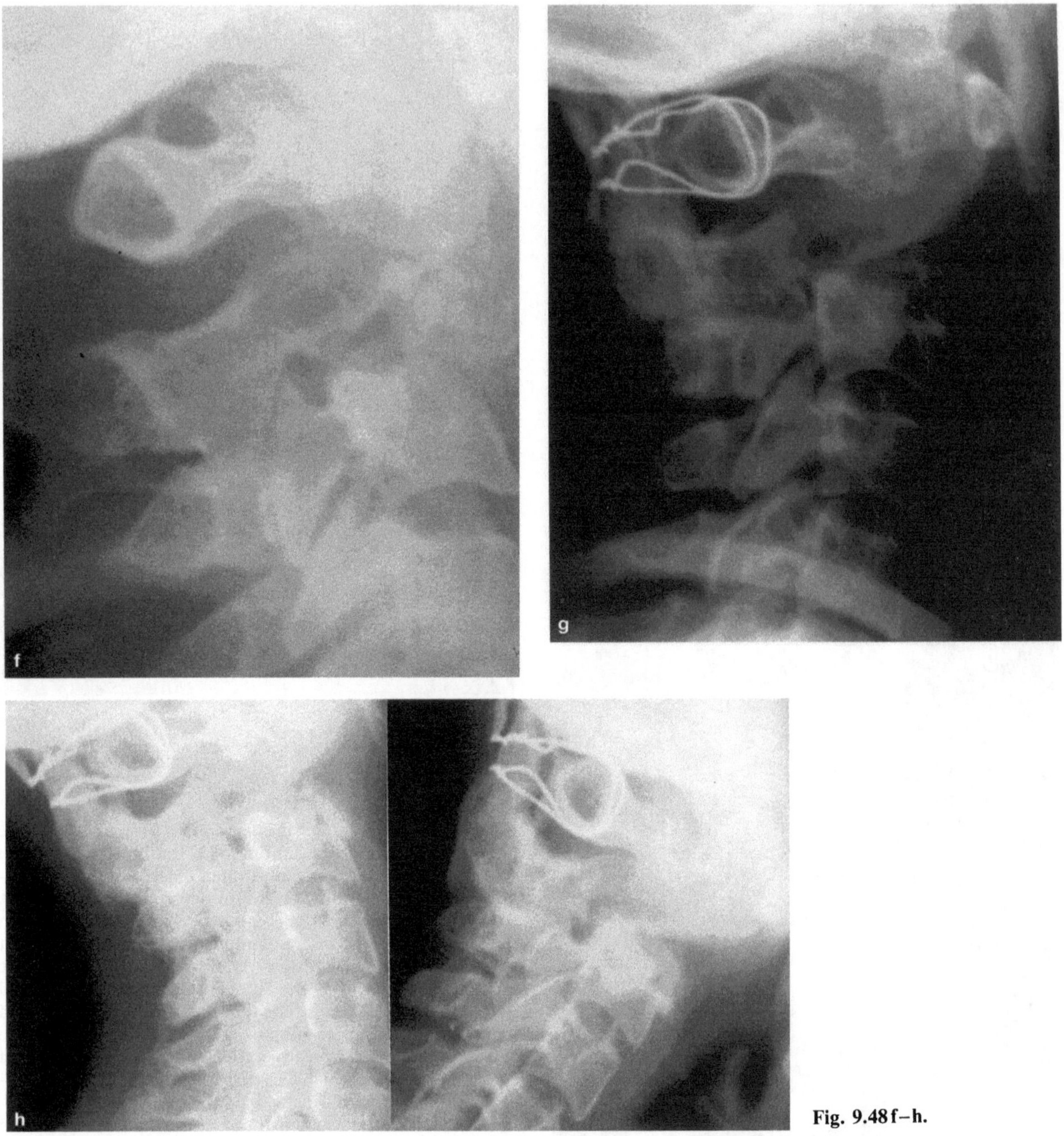

Fig. 9.48f–h.

of the lesion composed of the surrounding normal tissue remains. At this point, the destroyed vertebral bodies must be reconstructed and stabilized. A bony graft (autograft, if at all possible) that is shaped and placed in position without the need for additional immobilization by plates or screws should be used. The use of implants for internal fixation favors the infection and may not prevent collapse since they are susceptible to loosening as a result of poor anchorage into the subjacent osteoporotic bone (fig. 9.52). The combination of specific and appropriate antibiotics together with the surgical management described should be successful in dealing with the problem (Denaro and Kehr 1989).

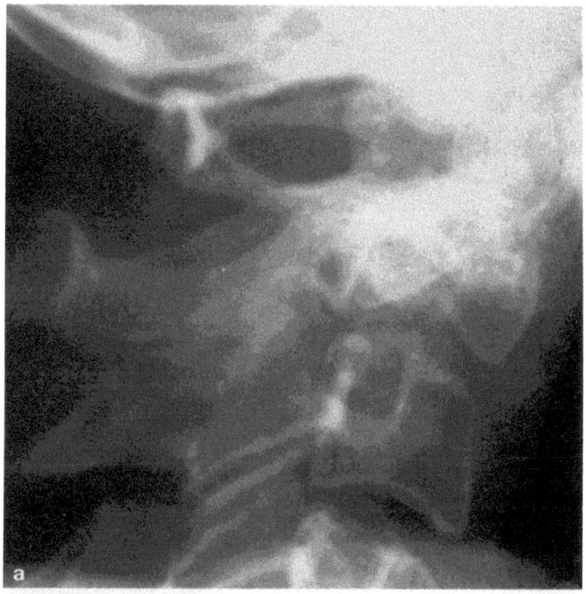

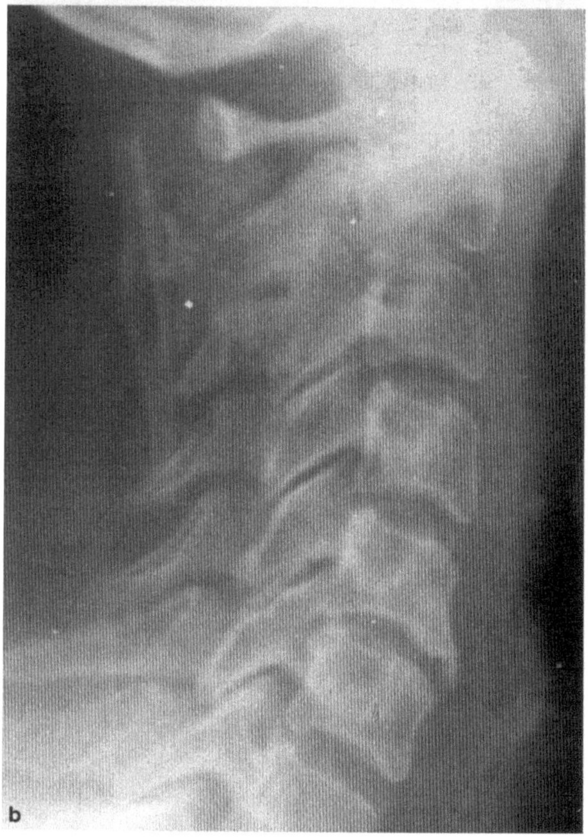

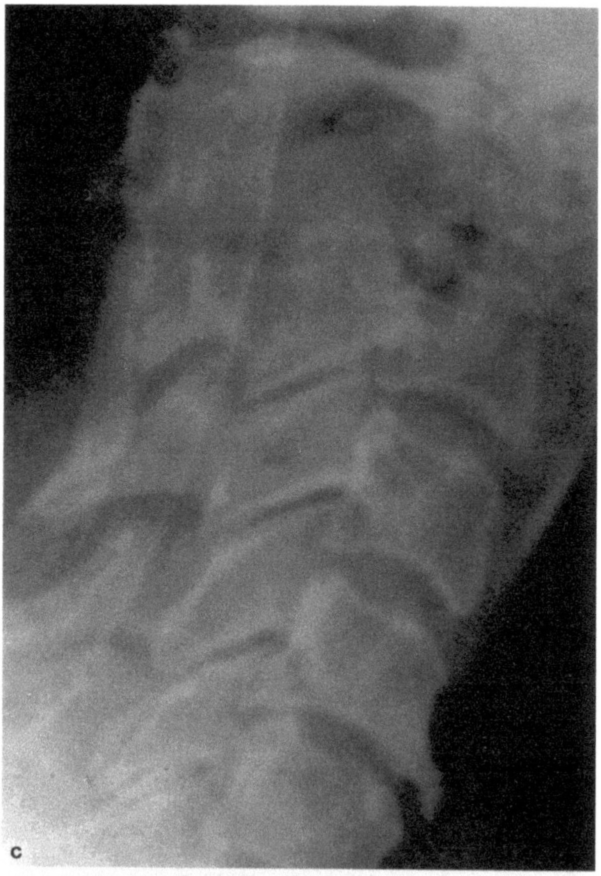

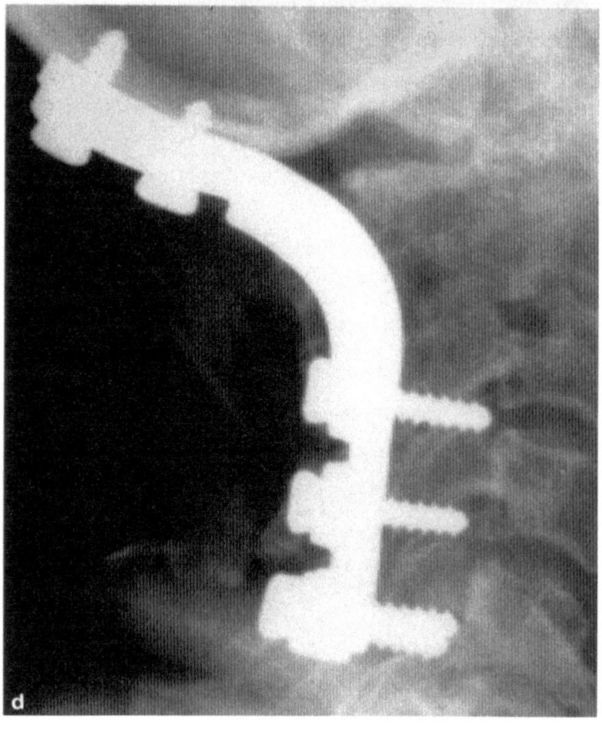

Fig. 9.49 a–f. Radiological imaging in a 56-year-old female patient with a giant cell tumor at the C1–C2 level. It was diagnosed by needle biopsy and the patient treated with radiotherapy prior to referral. Because of the degree of instability and the worrisome appearance, posterior stabilization with arthrodesis and nonmetallic wires was first performed.

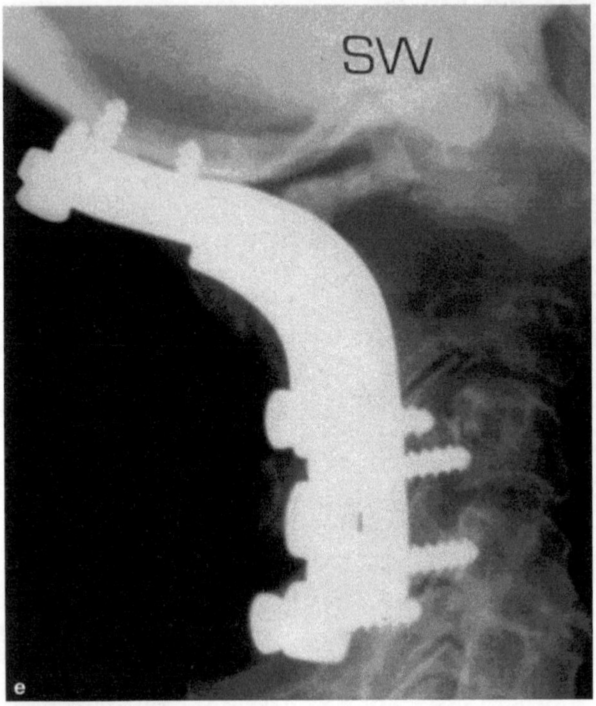

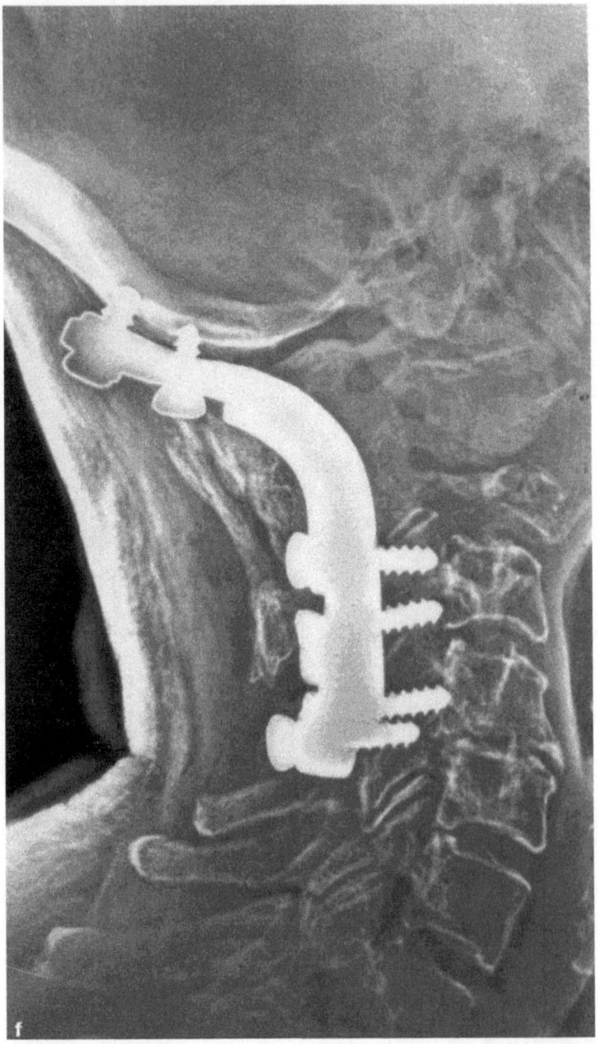

Radiographs in the lateral (**a**) and anteroposterior (**b**) projections. **c** The tumor recurred and, as seen in the radiograph, completely destroyed the body of C2. The stability of the spine was thereby weakened. **d** At the second operation, with the patient in a halo, an occipitocervical fusion was obtained using two premodeled Roy-Camille plates augmented by abundant corticotrabecular bone graft in bars. This was followed by courses of radiotherapy. **e, f** The tumor recurred again 2 years later, destroying the entire C1 and C2 segments. The tumor was now causing tetraparesis and was extensive enough to require tracheostomy. The patient died 3 years after the first operation

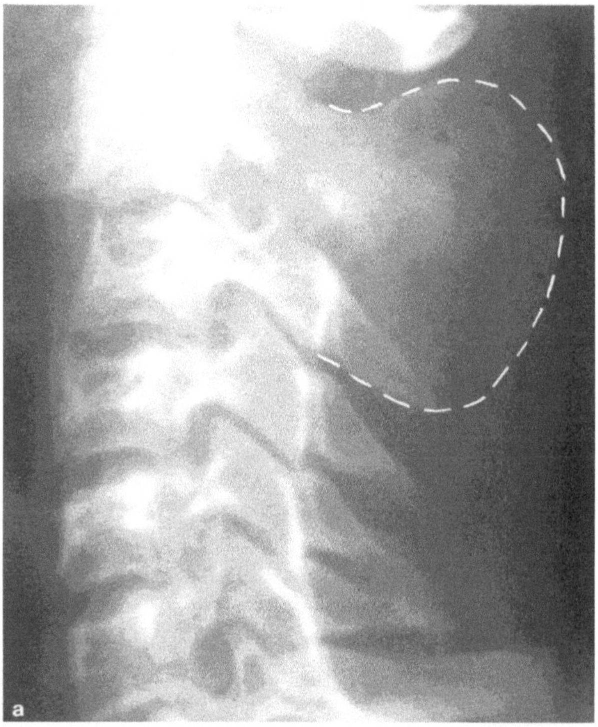

Fig. 9.50 a–h. Surgical procedure and radiological investigation in a 16-year-old female patient. **a** Radiograph showing a tumor involving the lamina and the spines of C2, giving them a lucent appearance. **b** Computed tomograph showing that the cortex is lost in several places. **c** MRI scan shows the tumor producing compression of the dural sac laterally. **d** Stages of arteriography during embolization. **e** Macroscopic appearance of the tumor mass. **f** Postoperative radiograph following laminectomy and arthrodesis at the C1–C3 levels. **g** Intraoperative view showing fusion of the C1–C3 levels achieved with autograft and non-resorbable sutures. **h** Postoperative MRI scan shows that the tumor has been completely removed

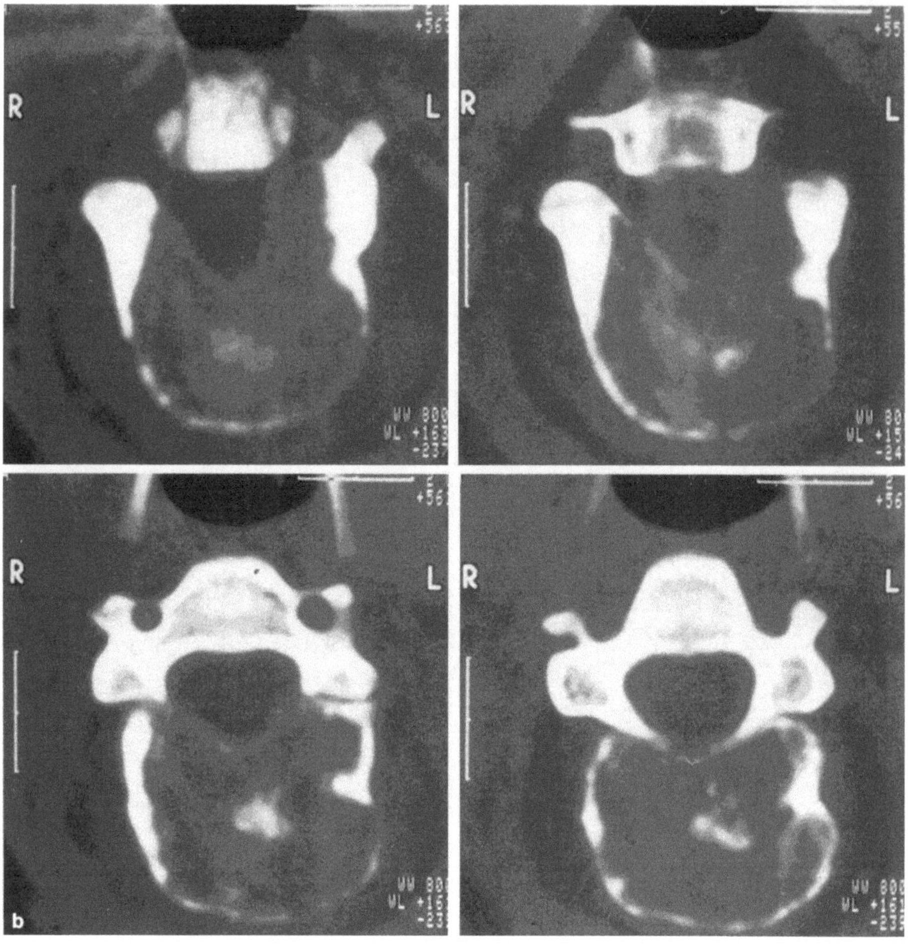

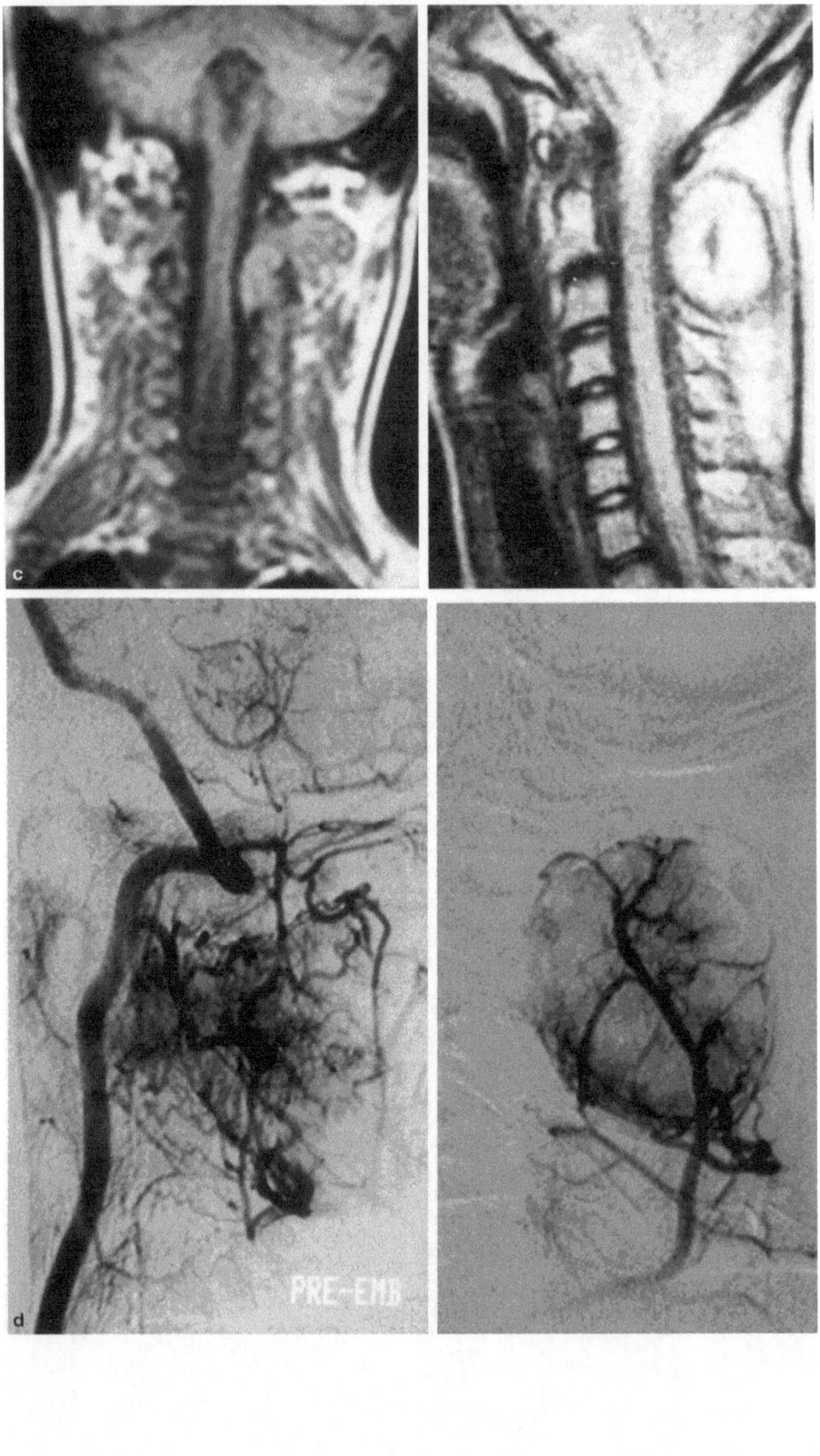

Fig. 9.50 c, d.

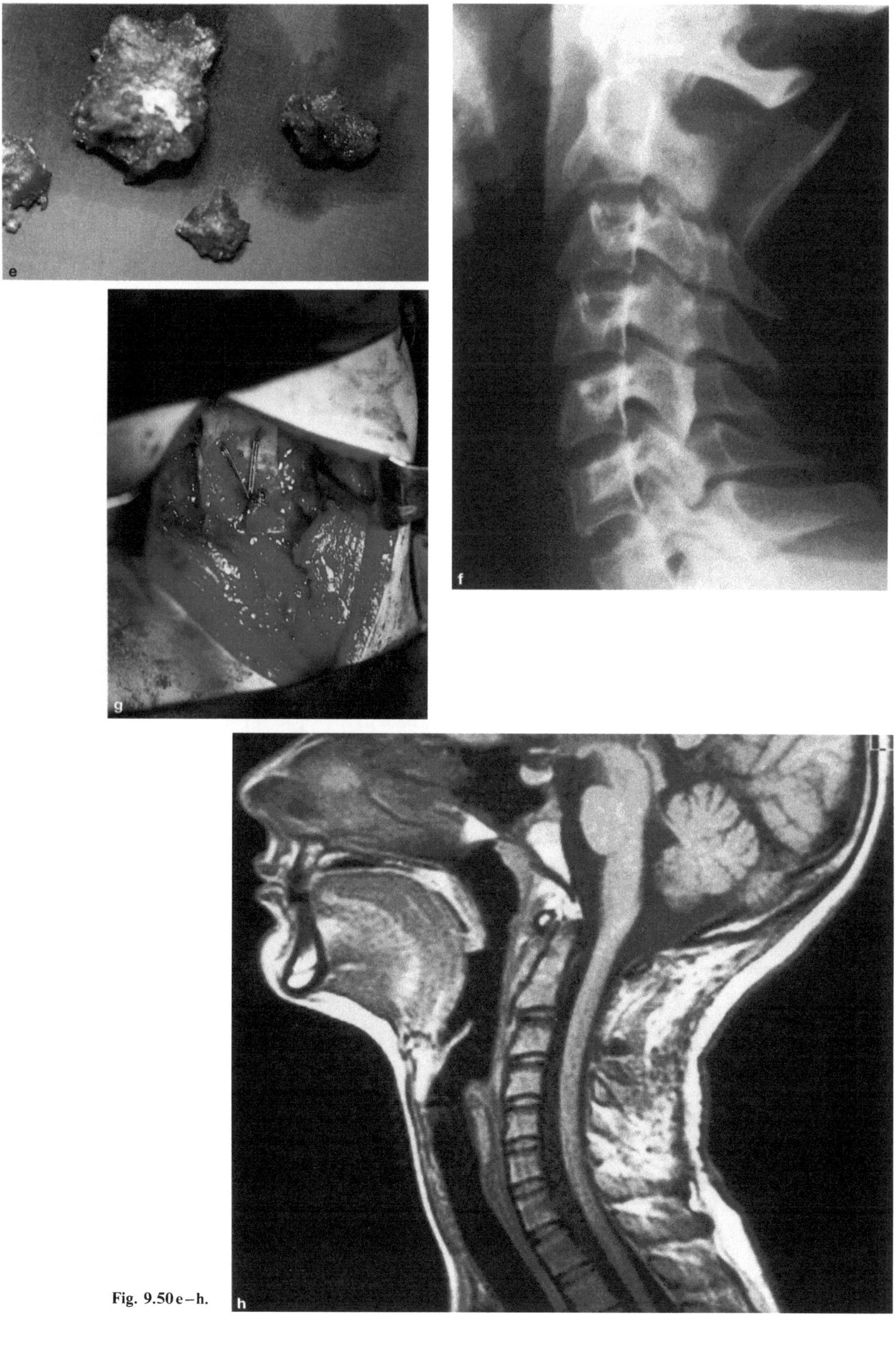

Fig. 9.50 e–h.

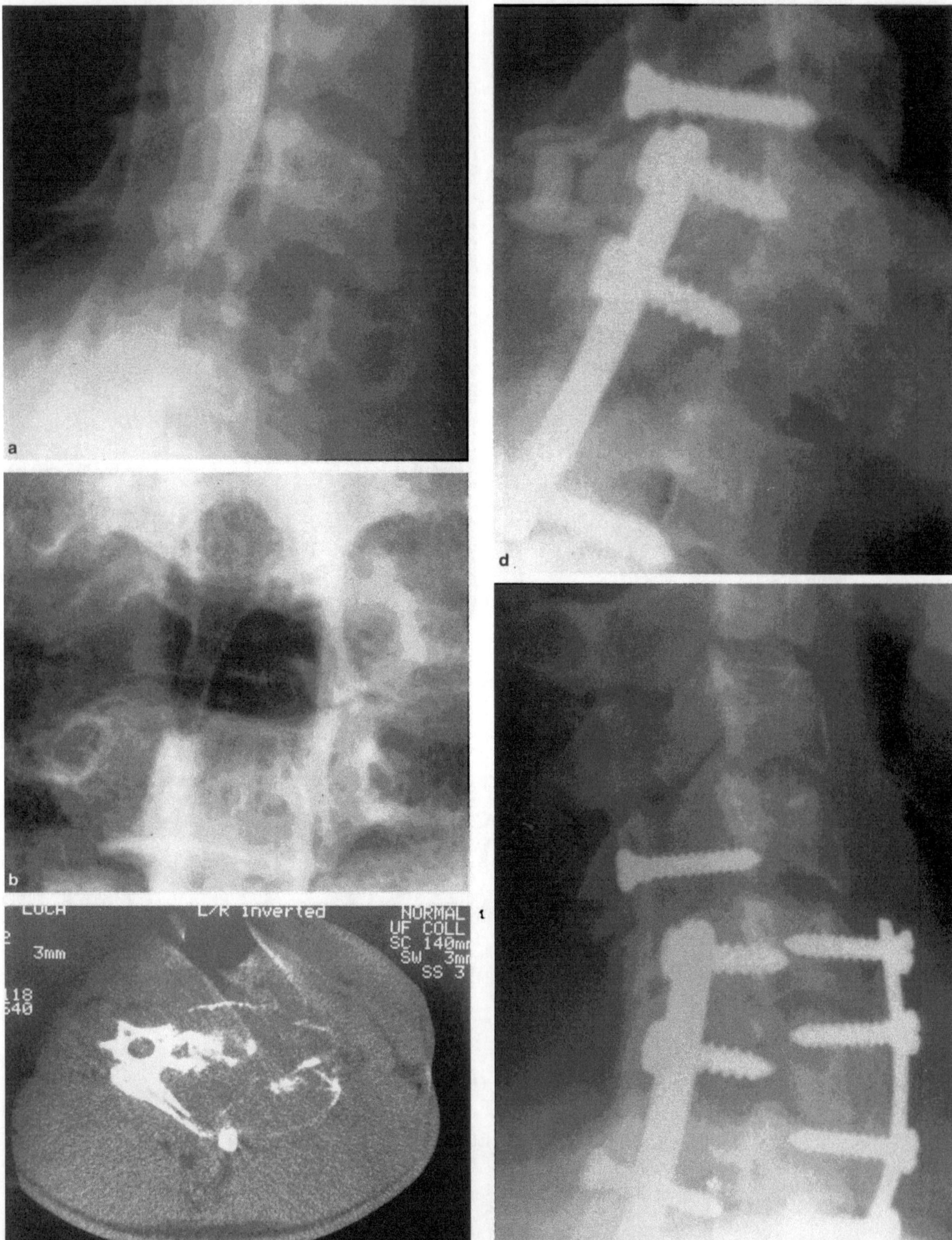
a
b
L/R inverted
NORMAL
UF COLL
3mm
SS 3
c
d
e

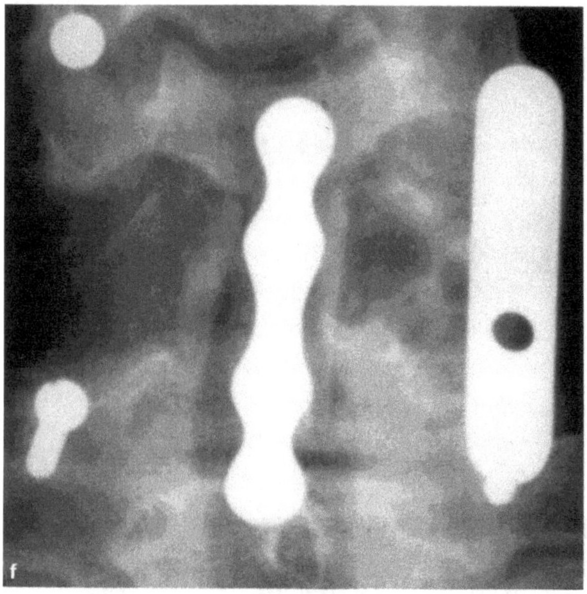

◀ **Fig. 9.51 a–f.** Radiological imaging in a 16-year-old male patient. This patient had an osteosarcoma at C6. The myelograms in both anteroposterior (**b**) and lateral (**a**) projection show compression of the cord. **c** The computed tomograph shows complete destruction of the vertebral body with invasion into the vertebral canal. Of particular interest is the complete destruction of the right side of the vertebra including the body, the laminae, and the lateral masses with their joints. **d** At surgery, posterior fusion was achieved on the intact side with one Roy-Camille plate. The tumor was taken out posteriorly, and fusion was obtained on the opposite side with an osseous bar screwed onto the lateral articular masses. **e, f** Postoperative radiographs were taken after the tumor had been removed through the anterior approach. After wide resection, the body was reconstructed anteriorly with autograft and plates anchored with screws

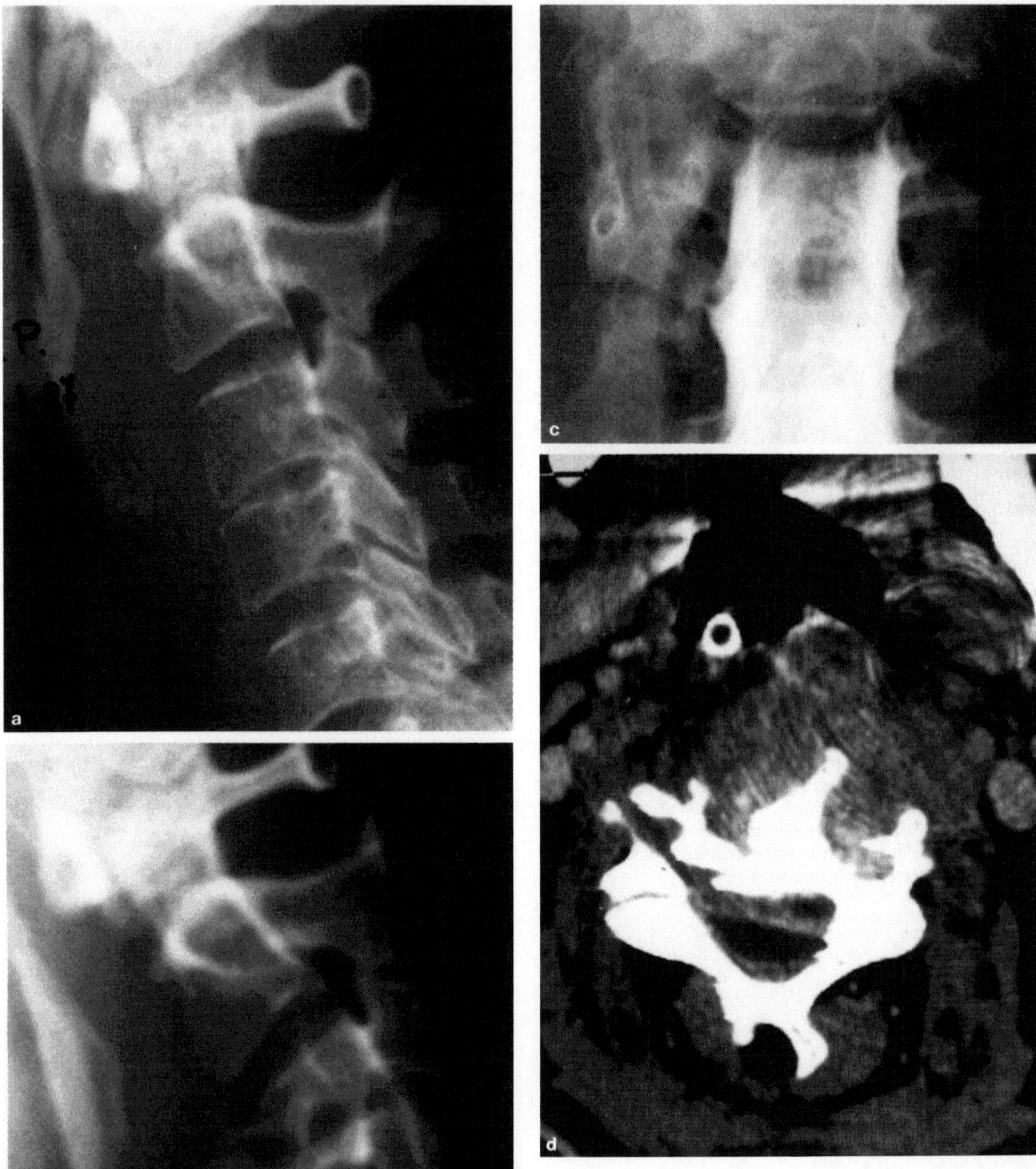

Fig. 9.52 a–d.

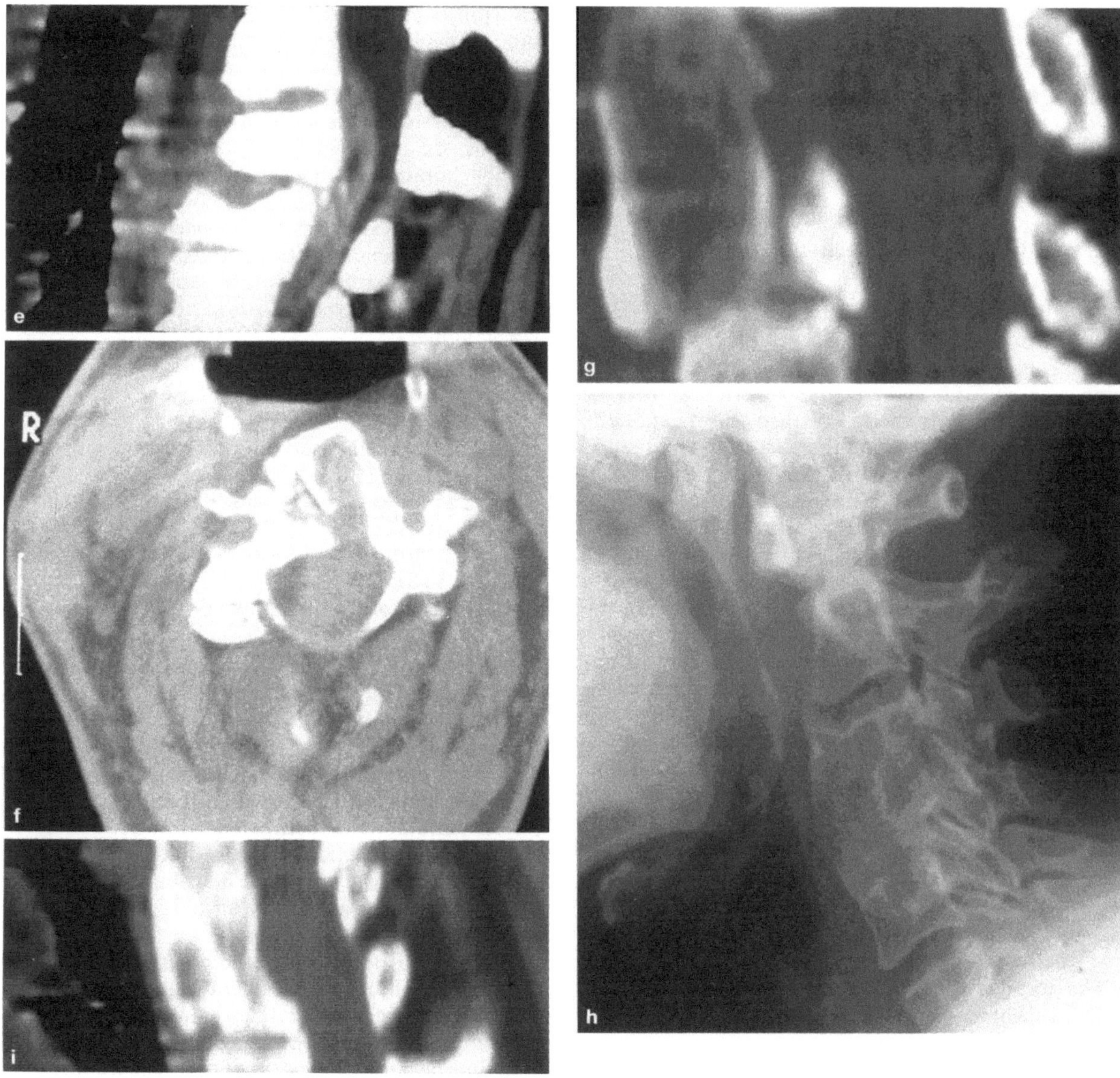

Fig. 9.52e–i. Radiological imaging in a 47-year-old male patient with tuberculous spondylitis. This patient had severe pain in the neck, which was diagnosed elsewhere as a discopathy and was treated with analgesics and cortisone. **a, b** Plain radiographs show destruction of the vertabral bodies of C3 and C4, this was associated with a severe tetraparesis. **c** Myelogram shows complete block of the radiopaque contrast medium, indicating that the lesion is not only protruding into the vertebral canal, but is also compressing the cord. **d** Horizontal computed tomograph cuts, with longitudinal reconstruction (**e**), clearly indicate the extent of the destruction of the vertebral body as well as the extent of the lesion into the canal. Needle biopsy carried out transorally confirmed the diagnosis of tuberculous spondylitis. **f** Horizontal computed tomograph cut and longitudinal reconstruction (**g**) taken after the evacuation of the lesion, with reconstruction using a tricortical bone graft to achieve longitudinal stabilization. **h** The radiograph taken 6 months after surgery shows that the bone has been reconstructed, the graft has been incorporated, and healing is occurring. **i** Computed tomograph with longitudinal reconstruction showing follow-up 6 months after surgery

Anterolateral and Anteromedial Combined Approaches in the Surgical Management of Cervical Osteoarthrosis

P. H. Kehr

Introduction and Pathogenesis

It is well known that cervical arthrosis (also called osteoarthritis) may develop in several locations and in overlapping structures of and close to the cervical spine such as cord, nerve roots, or vertebral arteries. By cervical arthrosis uncodiskarthrosis is meant here, since the uncus and disk are the parts most frequently affected, at least as far as the lower cervical spine is concerned. One of the characteristics of the cervical spine is the presence of the vertebral artery on each side of it; the V2 segment of this artery passes through the transverse foramina between C6 and C2, and is named the transverse segment for this reason. Another peculiarity is the existence in the lateral side of each intervertebral disk of an uncovertebral split, along which it will be possible for uncovertebral arthrosis, still called uncarthrosis, to develop. The origin of this uncovertebral split has been the subject of much discussion. It plays a part in real articulation for some, but is only considered to be a mere horizontal degenerative fissuring of the cervical intervertebral disk, which appears with physiological aging, for others. This last hypothesis seems to be the more plausible, and there is no lack of arguments in its favor. These include:

- The absence of the uncovertebral split in the child
- The appearance and development of the uncovertebral split in the young adult
- The continuity between the horizontal diskal split and the uncovertebral split visible on anatomical and histological section
- The lack of synovia (disputed by certain authors, but the synovia they found might, in reality, only be a metaplasia of the peridiskal connective tissue)
- Preoperative observations such as the constant presence of the diskal material in the uncovertebral split, or even the existence of extruded soft hernias through the uncovertebral split

This uncovertebral split might therefore be the result of a rachidian adaptation linked to natural aging and to the biped stance of higher primates such as man as a result of biological evolution. This theory provides an explanation for the increasingly important development of these splits in the inferior part of the cervical spine, from C4 to C7, the part most liable to microtrauma in everyday life. Why is this uncovertebral split complicated with an exuberant arthrosis in some patients and not in others, and why is this arthrosis clinically manifest in some and silent in many others? It is difficult to answer these questions, but the answer seems to lie in the intensity of microtraumas, the age at which they occur, and, finally, the possible addition of macrotraumas, which condition the clinical expression of the uncodiskarthrosis.

The uncodiskarthrosis (uncovertebral arthrosis) is very often associated with an anterior and posterior osteophytosis existing in other rachidian segments. One or the other of the following situations may thus be encountered:

- Cervical diskarthrosis with anterior osteophytosis (Fig. 9.53 a)
- Cervical diskarthrosis with posterior osteophytosis (Fig. 9.53 b)
- Cervical diskarthrosis with lateral uncarthrosis (Fig. 9.54 a)
- Cervical diskarthrosis with posterior uncarthrosis (Fig. 9.54 b)
- A combination of the above

The combination of cervical diskarthrosis with posterior osteophytosis and posterior uncarthrosis (Fig. 9.55 a) and cervical diskarthrosis with posterior osteophytosis and lateral and posterior uncarthrosis (Fig. 9.55 b) are particularly frequent. The affected levels are, in decreasing order of frequency, C5–C6, C6–C7, and C4–C5. The osteoarthritis which develops in posterior articulations is much less common and most readily affects the C3–C4 and C4–C5 levels. It may sometimes follow an old ignored fracture of an articular pillar.

The surgical treatments recommended here result from these pathogenic considerations. Priority is given to freeing operations rather than to simple segmentary immobilizations, which were advocated for a long time because of their simplicity. The frequency of arthritic associations led us to favor combined operations, too, in order to be able to work at the same time on different sites and decompress in one single sequence the vertebral artery, the nerve root, and the medulla. These operations are based, of course, on precise clinical indications, supported by good quality imaging.

Clinical Studies and Imaging

Here, the different clinical syndromes encountered and their surgical indications will be considered in turn. For each of them a brief clinical description and list of the complementary examinations necessary or desirable in order to speed up the diagnosis and prove the pathogenicity of arthritic lesions will be provided.

One must always remember that cervical arthrosis is more a state than a pathology, and that many arthritic lesions are tolerated very well and remain clinically silent. The discovery of a cervical arthrosis on standard X-rays does not mean ipso facto that this arthrosis is responsible for the patient's symptoms. It is important to remember from the outset that only those patients will be proposed for a surgical operation who have not been filtered out by the aforementioned complementary examinations, and in whom a variety of medical treatments and physiotherapy have been unsuccessful. We are also in the habit of asking for preoperative psychiatric advice, especially when an accident liable to compensation is supposed to be the origin of the symptoms. These notions will not be referred to again, but will be assumed to have been discussed in each of the following segments.

The Local Cervical Syndrome

Definition

In the local cervical syndrome, neck pain is always present, but quite often intermittent, and is localized either in the lower part of the nape or in the lateral side of the neck.

Typical Description

1. The neck pain corresponds to the cutaneous and musculoligamentary projection of painful osteoarticular zones and may well have varied expressions:
- Neck pain itself, the seat of which must be precisely determined by palpation, i.e., whether its origin is interspinous or facing the posterior articulations.
- Anterior cervicalgia which may be localized with palpation on one or several anterior transverse tubercles, most often that of C6 (tuberculum caroticum) and that of C5.
- Pain projected in the shoulder, along the trapezius muscle.
- Pain projected in the territory of the posterior branch of one or several rachidian cervical nerves, along the spinal edge of the scapula; it is known that the painful sites are tiered in structure, depending on the metameres involved.

2. The particularity of this neck pain is that it is precipitated and/or worsened by head and neck movements, in particular contralateral rotation and extension.

3. Most of the time this pain takes the form of attacks, but in the typical uncodiskarthrosis, it exists almost always as a continous aching background with occasional paroxysms, which are triggered off either by uncomfortable prolonged positions, meteorological conditions, or rest. In the latter case, it leads to a venous stasis, of which the classical early morning pain is the best example.

Imaging

Standard X-rays are of course essential and should consist of at least four views: front view, side view, and two oblique views (three-quarter views). These will show up one or several diskarthroses or diskopathies, possibly as a shift on the front view or side view of the usual marks. Views centered on C1–C2 must be added whenever there are superior cervical symptoms. Since cervical arthrosis is often post-traumatic, X-rays must always be read carefully, as it is not uncommon to find missed fracture lines or posterior osteoarthritic changes, which are often only retrospectively diagnosed.

Dynamic X-rays are a valuable asset in functionally assessing the cervical spine, and are, in our opinion, as necessary as standard X-rays. Only here can dynamic instabilities due to post-traumatic ligamentary strains which are not evident in a neutral position on a standard X-ray be recognized. Side-view dynamic X-rays provide the most information. In flexion, anterior diskal compression, interspinous diastasis, or even articular uncovering must be looked for in particular; in extension, anterior diskal gaping or the persistency of an interspinous diastasis may be noticed.

Centered X-rays and Tomographies may indicate the precise location of an osteophytic protrusion on the posterior side of the disk or the vertebral body or of the origin of an uncarthrosis, when compared with and superimposed on standard X-rays, but they are under increasing competition from and being replaced by scanography, which is more anatomical and offers the third plane, the axial plane.

Scanography (CT) is the key examination because, as mentioned above, it provides not only the third plane, the axial plane, but also allows density measurement and, above all, secondary processing of the image, without the necessity of the patient's presence. It is indicated, nevertheless, more frequently in diffuse syndromes than in the isolated local syndrome, even though sequelae of missed fractures may be responsible for the latter and may only be diagnosed using scanographical sections.

Diagnosis

A *positive diagnosis* is one of an arthritic or prearthritic origin of disease, e.g., a diskopathy or a traumatic ligamentary or even osseous lesion such as an missed unilateral fracture of a posterior arch which has led to the development of a post-traumatic arthrosis. This diagnosis will, as already mentioned, be established according to a network of clinically subjective, objective, and radiological evidence. Considering the great frequency with which degenerative signs in the cervical spine occur in patients over the age of 40, it is important to be able to prove the pathogenicity of a lesion diagnosed radiologically as uncarthrosis. This is possible using the therapeutic Xylocaine infiltration test. After the test has been carried out, the pain often surprisingly disappear totally for 1 or 2 hours, proving that the lesion really is responsible for the pain.

The *differential diagnosis* is very informative and space is lacking here to talk about it in detail. One must emphasize the frequency of neck pain of neurovegetative origin which must be particularly considered among women in the menopause.

The Cervicocephalic or Cervicocranial Syndrome

Definition

The cervicocephalic syndrome (CCS) is a vertebrobasilar insufficiency induced by a compression or an extrinsic irritation acting on the adventitia of either one or both vertebral arteries. The vertebrobasilar insufficiency of interest here is that induced by uncovertebral arthrosis, i.e., between C7 and C2 in the V2 segment of the vertebral artery.

Typical Presentation

Apart from neck pain due to the local syndrome, the patient complains about one, several, or even all of the following symptoms:

- Headaches situated in the occcipital or cervico-occipital regions and radiating often toward parietofrontal regions; they are unilateral (migraine) or bilateral.
- Cochlear signs such as tinnitus or hypoacousis.
- Vestibular signs such as episodes of vertigo or falso vertigo (vertiginous feeling), a sensation of intoxication, and feelings of insecurity.
- Drop attacks or sudden collapse of the legs through a loss of coordination force and linked to a sudden ischemia of the medulla oblongata.
- Eye trouble such as eye tiredness, a reduction of the field of vision, a feeling of having a foreign body in the eye (sensation of sand in the eye), or a conjunctival burning sensation.
- Psychic trouble. Psychasthenia, depression, and memory losses are the symptoms most often presented by patients and which lead to their being considered neurotic, hypochondriac, or pension neurotic.

The characteristic feature of this syndrome lies in the appearance or worsening of symptoms during rotation and/or extension movements of the cervical spine.

Involvement of the vertebral artery can be proved anatomically, arteriographically, hemodynamically, and therapeutically.

Anatomical evidence of involvement is that the respective dimensions of the transverse foramina and the vertebral arteries are very similar. A histological study on classified sections shows that the adventitia of the vertebral artery normally adheres in places to the periosteum of the transverse foramen and that of the uncus.

Arteriographic evidence of involvement is the existence of a narrowing (stricture) of the vertebral artery opposite an uncarthrotic prominence or inside a transverse foramen. This narrowing may be isolated or combined with a displacement. The displacement alone is not really significant, but the narrowing is, even when moderate.

Hemodynamic evidence of involvement is the total similarity between the CCS caused by unarthrosis and the vertebrobasilar insufficiency of an intrinsic origin, i.e., atherosclerotic stenosis or subclavian steal syndrome.

Therapeutic evidence of involvement is the regularity with which positive effects occur after surgical intervention to free the vertebral artery from compression. Any surgeon who has witnessed the change in a patient after the operation – he smiles again and has become happy to live – can only be convinced that this compression was the decisive factor. This conviction is strong enough for the surgeon to consider this operation when a simple immobilization with intervertebral fusion would otherwise have been his first decision!

Imaging

Vertebral arteriography is the only possible way of giving the proof of the pathogenic role of the vertebral artery, since all the other methods, such as Doppler sonography or cochleovestibular examinations, even if improved by electronystagmography, bring only suspicions. We prefer to use selective arteriography through the aortic approach (puncture of the femoral artery and Seldinger catheterization), as realized by our neuroradiologist colleagues, A. Wackenheim and his team. One may also use the retrograde humeral approach, but this requires greater dexterity and more cooperation from the patient, and it is unlikely that the surgeon would visualize a vertebral artery of low origin on the subclavian when using this method.

Digitalized or numerized arteriography has appeared more recently; it is less aggressive, not so much because the amount injected is lower, but rather because it can be performed intravenously and thus may be conducted on an outpatient basis. We consider it an excellent screening examination, classical arteriography becoming, thanks to it, an examination of secondary importance, which is required only if an abnormality is suspected. In some cases, on the other hand (Fig. 9.59), it allows sufficient visualization, especially when the symptomatology is not solely arterial and the freeing of the vessel only part of an operation which has been planned anyway.

Differential Diagnosis

To arrive at a differential diagnosis, vertebral arteriography is very useful. This may indicate an intrinsic lesion such as ostial atherosclerotic stenosis. If arteriography shows no abnormalities, a menopausal neurovegetative syndrome may be diagnosed; if other symptoms can then be additionally induced, particularly during cervical spine rotation, this will signal the presence of the organic cause rather than the neurovegetative syndrome, which is more vague and difficult to define. An important problem in differential diagnosis may arise in the case of post-traumatic uncarthrosis; on the one hand there is pension neurosis, in which case it is again the induced symptoms which indicate the presence of the syndrome and arteriography which removes any remaining doubts. On the other hand there is the postconcussional syndrome in patients with cranial trauma. Here again the cervical origin will be recognizable if local aching points exist and from the way troubles started; if a true postconcussional syndrome is present, there will be electroencephalographical signs and, of course, the notion of cranial trauma.

The Radicular or Cervicobrachialgic Syndrome

Definition

The radicular or cervicobrachialgic syndrome is characterized by a radicular pain, possibly with either clinical or merely electromyographical signs of motor deficit. These signs may be induced either by stenosis in the intervertebral foramen because of uncarthrosis or by stenosis. Of the spinal canal because of posterior diskal osteophytosis. Furthermore, both arthritic processes may often be combined in the syndrome. The existence of a constitutional stenosis in the spinal canal may coexist and, if it does, the clinical expression will be more severe even if the osteophytes are less developed.

Typical Description

The radicular pain radiates in the metameric territory, most often C6 (thumb) or C7 (index finger), and is exacerbated or induced by neck movements, in particular by contralateral rotation.

Clinical Forms

The most interesting clinical form is the one associated with a vertebrobasilar syndrome, as this is as frequently encountered as uncarthrosis. Nevertheless, it must often be sought carefully, since the patient does not spontaneously remember to mention attacks of vertigo and headaches when consulting about cervicobrachialgia.

Imaging

Imaging constitutes the key to a positive diagnosis as well as to a diagnosis of pathogenicity, and, consequently, to possible indications for surgical treatment.

Noncontrasted X-rays remain interesting despite the recent progress of medical imaging. They permit initial filtering and, with detailed reading, often even allow a very precise diagnosis. Of course, oblique views foramen and possible show the intervertebral foramen and possible narrowing of it best.

Myelography was an essential examination for a long time, but it is an aggressive, invasive technique, which will become rarer and eventually disappear in future as an isolated examination. It is still indicated, however, particularly when delays in appointments for scanography or MRI are too long! Root amputation and canalar stenoses with premedullary narrowing are well-known findings.

Computed tomography (CT) used together with intravenous injection of an iodized product to visualize epidural venous circulation, or, in former times, used together with myelography and Amipaque or tomodensitometry to give the axial view permits precise measurements of distance and densities. The pathogenicity of lesions seen on standard X-rays can thus be affirmed or invalidated.

Magnetic resonance imaging is an excellent technique for examining the spinal cord, but does not give enough details of the osseous structures. However, modern MRI techniques allow visualization of the vertebral arteries without the injection of contrast medium and represent true progress. We do not have any personal experience of this type of angiography at present.

Electromyography is as necessary to detect clinically silent motor deficits as it is to distinguish between medullary and radicular attacks. It should be employed systematically when any cervicobrachial suffering is present.

Differential Diagnosis

Radiculalgia of Other Origin. Soft diskal hernia also induces radiculalgia, but there the motor deficit predominates and soon becomes more important. The presence of trauma, effort, an initially isolated torticollis which is then followed by the appearance of the aching syndrome and then of the motor deficit, or the absence of arthrosis but the existence of signs of diskal involvement (static or dynamic compressions or functional blocks) make the diagnosis possible. The radiculalgia may also result from minimal traumatic lesions which lead to closed radicular compression and may be recognized by using imaging.

Nonradicular Neuralgia. There may be nonradicular neuralgia of medullary origin. With electromyography, acute medullary ischemia will be recognized. It is clinically expressed as a violent radiculalgia accompanied by motor deficits and electromyography shows an incomplete multiradicular attack. Peripheral nonradicular neuralgia may also be present. The thoracic outlet syndrome and the other various canalar syndromes all have their own clinical and electromyographical signs.

Combined Syndromes

The Cervicocephalobrachialgic Syndrome

The cervicocephalobrachialgic syndrome is due to the simultaneous compression of the root by the uncarthrosis narrowing the intervertebral foramen and of the vertebral artery by the lateral part of this some uncarthrosis. Of course, the presence of a radiologically diagnosed narrowing does not necessarily mean that there is a neuralgia, and the radiologically visible lateral development of an uncarthrosis does not automatically correspond to a syndrome of compression of a vertebral artery. Tolerance must be allowed for the soft tissues and the relations between the structures. There are some intervertebral foramina which are wide and welcoming, where the root may coexist for a long time with the exostosis, and there are some where the opposite is true!

The Cervicocephalomedullary Syndrome

It is interesting to know about the cervicocephalomedullary syndrome, since this combination is the subject of diagnostic and therapeutic discussion. It is not a true cervical myelopathy. It either means the coexistence of an uncarthrosis and a posterior median diskal osteophytosis, each leading to compression, or the presence of just one uncarthrosis, which, however, compresses not only the vertebral artery and the nerve root, but also acts on the medulla by compressing a nutrient artery originating from the vertebral artery. The clinical expression of the medullary syndrome may range from simple intermittent and reversible medullary irritation to paraplegia or paraparesis.

Imaging. Imaging is indicated most illustratively here, be it CT or MRI combined with myelography and Amipaque, which allows visualization of the vertebral arteries.

Surgical Management

Methods

Anterolateral Freeing Approaches

The anterolateral freeing approaches were first described by Jung in Strasbourg in 1963. I and my colleagues have used them ever since, together with Jung until 1974 and then on our own as his students thereafter. These approaches are defined as surgery of the uncodiskalradicular carrefour and consist of three successive steps, each of which may constitute an operation. The three steps are transversectomy, uncusectomy, and uncoforaminectomy:

The *transversectomy* consists in opening one or more transverse foramina. It thus frees the vertebral artery by removing the stenosis which may be compressing it in the foramen and is the only step which needs to be taken if there is no uncarthrosis. It is insufficient, however, if an uncarthrosis overlaps a vertebral artery in the region of the uncoarterioradicular junction.

The *uncusectomy* frees the anterior part of the junction by removing the anterolateral part of the uncovertebral exostosis which is compressing the vertebral artery.

The *uncoforaminectomy* frees the posterior part of the junction by removing the posterolateral portion of the uncal spur which is narrowing the intervertebral foramen and compressing the nerve root. The vertebral artery may be freed at one or two levels during the same surgical procedure, but we have never operated on both sides during the same procedure and consider this to be excessive.

Principles and Common Steps. The incision is made along the anterior edge of the sternocleidomastoid muscle and provides access to the levels C3–C7. Whenever the vertebral nerve is encountered, it is severed. The site of the uncarthrosis is usually at C5–C6, but may also be found at C4–C5 or at C6–C7.

The patient should be placed in a half-sitting position with the head in moderate extension and slightly turned away from the surgeon, a hard roll is placed under the neck. General anesthesia with endotracheal intubation is necessary.

After the incision has been made, the same approach is used for all three steps, i.e., between the visceral and vascular sheats. The lamina pretrachialis fasciae cervicalis is incised and the omohyoid muscle severed. The thyroid gland and the esophagus are retracted medially, the carotid and jugular vessels laterally. The dissection has now reached the prevertebral level.

By scraping the long muscles of the neck and head away, the anterior tubercles of the involved transverse processes can be freed. In all cases, it is advisable to start by freeing the anterior tubercle of C6 (tuberculum caroticum), since this is the most prominent and since the vertebral artery usually enters the transverse foramen of C6.

After completion of the surgical procedure, in all cases a suction drain is used and closure is achieved by reconstituting the omohyoid muscle and suturing the platysma.

Transversectomy. The first step of the transversectomy is to identify the vertebral artery upstream from where it enters the transverse foramen of C6. The vessel and the veins around it are then freed from the periosteum of the transverse foramen, to which they adhere in all cases. The same procedure is repeated in as many of the foramina above this level as necessary for the operation intended. At this stage, the transverse foramen (or foramina) may be opened progressively using a gouge-forceps, or a punch and taking care never to tear bony fragments off briskly, since this may provoke venous bleeding, which although never serious will delay the operation.

Uncusectomy. The form of uncusectomy recommended here may only be performed after transversectomy at least above and preferably also below the involved level. During this operation, the vertebral artery must be protected with a blunt dissector or small retractor. If the vertebral artery adheres to the periosteum of the uncus, it must first be removed by cutting into and scraping the periosteum, thereby separating the artery from the subperiosteal bone. A groove can then be made with a chisel or, if preferred, with an air drill in the lateral part of the vertebral bodies carrying the uncal spur. The uncovertebral exostosis should then be levered out so that the last part breaks and is removed using the punch or forceps, taking care not to tear the bone off.

Uncoforaminectomy. According to the procedure first described by Jung (1963), uncoforaminectomy must follow transversectomy and uncusectomy, and consists in removing the posterior portion of the uncarthrosis. The chisel should be directed obliquely backwards at an angle of 45° in front of the vertebral artery (and not behind it, as the nerve root passes here). In order to direct the chisel, a spinal needle may first be inserted into the transverse foramen. We have given up using the technique as it was first described because we think that whenever an anterolateral foraminotomy (or uncoforaminectomy) is indicated, there is also an indication for transdiskal osteophytectomy. It is then easier to carry out the uncoforaminectomy by approaching simultaneously medially and laterally.

Anteromedial Freeing Approaches

When the vertebral artery is not involved in the arthritic process, we use the transdiskal osteophytectomies according to Cloward or Robinson (cf. Cervical Spine Research Society 1983). For a description of these, the reader is referred to the transdiskal step described below for combined operations.

Combined Anterolateral and Anteromedial Approaches

Combined Disk and Vertebral Artery Approach (Kehr 1984, 1987; Kehr and Jung 1985). This operation consists of a combination of decompression of the vertebral artery by transversectomy or uncusectomy on the one hand, and transdiskal osteophytectomy with arthrodesis according to Robinson on the other hand (Fig. 9.56). The approach used is the same as that used in the anterolateral approaches. This combined operation offers only advantages, in particular the fact that the vertebral artery is permanently under control, thus avoiding the risk of injury, stretching, or compression during intervertebral distraction.

Combined Disk and Uncoarterioradicular Junction Approach (Kehr 1984; Kehr and Jung 1985). This operation consists of a combination of an uncoforaminectomy and a transdiskal osteophytectomy followed by intervertebral fusion according to Robinson (Fig. 9.57). There are only advantages to be gained from this operation, in particular the double approach – medial and anterolateral – to the transverse foramen permitting the complete removal of the uncal spurs. It is essential to cut down the first fragment of the posterior osteophyte very gently, starting from the vertebral plate and with the instrument angled 30° upwards or downwards, depending on whether the osteophyte to be removed is on the vertebra above or below this level. Only light taps with the mallet followed by lever movements are necessary to fracture the posterior cortex. Since 1988, we have preferred to use a curette to perforate the posterior cortex; this method provides more security but can only be used in older patients with softer, arthrotic bone. It is then possible to remove a piece of the osteophyte, to introduce a punch gouge into the hole thus formed, and to progressively scrape out the last remnants of the osteophytic spur. This is facilitated when there is an old exteriorized diskal hernia, since in this case the hole is already present and fibrous diskal tissue is often found around the spur.

Indications

The Local Syndrome

In the case of the localized syndrome, management of an instability is indicated. This means stabilization with intervertebral fusion, for which we prefer the Robinson technique, possibly combined with an osteosynthesis with insertion of a screwed plate whenever two-level fusion is involved or where there is post-traumatic instability.

The Cervicocephalic Syndrome

Vertebral artery freeing is indicated for the cervicocephalic syndrome. This may be achieved either with transversectomy alone, if the narrowing occurs in only one transverse foramen, or, most often, by transversectomy followed by uncusectomy.

The Radicular Syndrome

In the case of the radicular syndrome, root decompression is indicated through the medial transdiskal approach whenever the vertebral artery is not involved.

The Combined Syndromes

Complete decompression is indicated if combined syndromes are present. In our opinion, the existence of a combined syndrome justifies a combined operation, which allows the vertebral artery, nerve root, and the anterior side of the cord to be decompressed in a single surgical procedure. This is justified on condition that the pathogenecity of the bony spurs is authenticated by undisputed neuroradiological examinations and that conservative treatments have proved their inefficiency (Figs. 9.58–9.60).

Results and Conclusions

Between 1962 and June 1989, we performed 508 operations using an anterior cervical approach, 365 of which could be followed up. The operations most frequently performed were uncusectomies (117 cases), followed in frequency by transdiskal osteophytectomies (112 cases), simple grafts according to Robinson (73 cases, of which 46 were simple grafts and 27 osteosynthesis grafts), combined transdiskal osteophytectomy and uncoforaminectomy (Kehr operation; 46 cases), simple transversectomies (46 cases), uncoforaminectomies according to Jung (39 cases), freeing of vertebral arteries with graft (26 cases). The 32 corporectomies, the 11 Cloward operations, and the 6 anterior exostosectomies (because of Forestier disease) were not reviewed for this study.

Not all of these operations are performed regularly anymore. The uncoforaminectomy described by Jung, for example, was not performed as an isolated procedure after 1979. Similarly, freeing the vertebral artery with a graft was last performed in 1982.

Of the 365 patients treated, 223 were men and 141 were women; this male preponderance is typical. The 365 operations may be classified into four groups:

Group I	Anterolateral approaches, i.e., approach to the uncoarterioradicular junction (164 cases)
Group II	Medial anterior approaches using pure graft according to Robinson, with or without osteosynthesis (50 cases)
Group III	Medial anterior approaches with transdiskal osteophytectomy, i.e., decompression and graft with osteosynthesis (88 cases)
Group IV	Combined operations with medial anterior and anterolateral approaches (63 cases)

The results were classified into the categories excellent (complete disappearance of the symptoms), good (persistence of one clinical sign, disappearance of the others), fairly good (reduction but not disappearance of the symptoms), nil, bad, and, even in a a few cases, worsening. The number of excellent, good, and fairly good results were added together to represent the number of successes. The categories nil and below were added together to represent failures.

The results of these four groups are varied (Figs. 9.62, 9.63). The 88 transdiskal osteophytectomies achieve the best score with 90% successes, while the 164 anterolateral approaches have an overall success rate of 80%. Of course, the decision to perform these operations is made for a variety of comparable but different clinical pictures. It must be remembered that patients are included here in whom the possibilities of conservative treatment have been exhausted; with this in mind, an 80% chance of cure or improvement is really good! If we study the results for each type of operation (Fig. 9.64), more significant differences appear.

Transdiskal osteophytectomy, transversectomy, combined operation of Kehr, pure graft Robinson operation, and uncusectomy all have a rate of success between 83% and 90%, whereas freeing the vertebral artery with graft and uncoforaminectomy have a success rate of only 71% and 66%, respectively. This is an argument for abandoning the use of these two methods as isolated surgical procedures. If a nerve root needs to be freed, we now recommend that it be performed medially through the transdiskal approach without freeing the vertebral artery. If a vertebral artery is to be freed where the nerve root and medulla are not involved, it is merely necessary to free the vertebral artery concerned by transversectomy or uncusectomy; association of a graft should then be avoided. If, on the other hand, vertebral artery, nerve, and medulla are all involved, the combined transdiskal osteophytectomy with uncoforaminectomy and graft (Kehr operation) is indicated, the value of which is shown by its success rate.

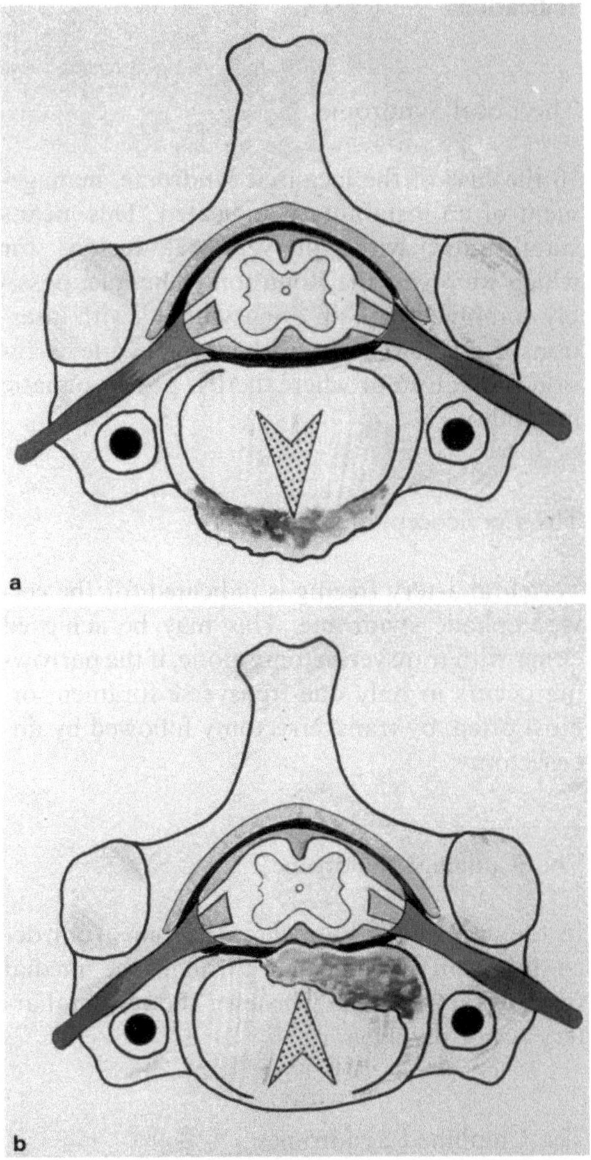

Fig. 9.53 a, b. Cervical diskal osteophytosis. **a** Development of diskarthrosis (*arrow*) limited to anterior of vertebral body in a clinically silent zone. Only if the prominence is very big (Forestier's disease) will esophageal function be hampered. **b** Development of diskarthrosis limited to posterior of vertebral body (*arrow*) in a clinically significant zone with circulatory symptoms or intermittent compression of the medulla itself

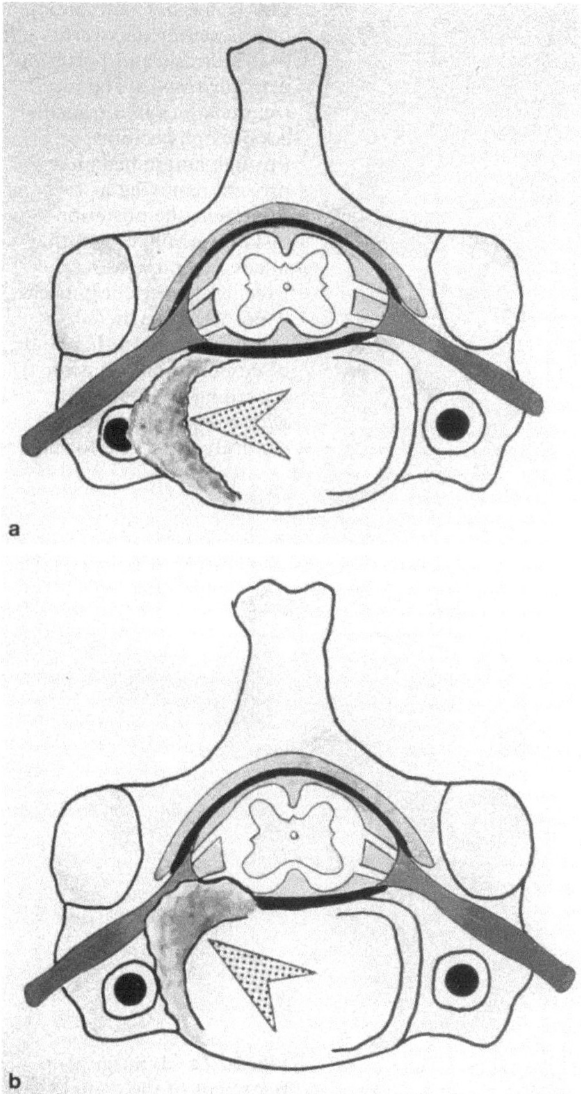

Fig. 9.54 a, b. Cervical uncodiskarthrosis. **a** Development limited to lateral uncovertebral exostosis (*arrow*), which comes in close contact with the vertebral artery at the uncoarterioradiculary crossroads. A cervicocephalic syndrome or syndrome of the vertebral artery may result from it. **b** Development limited to posterior uncovertebral exostosis (*arrow*) coming close to the root in the intervertebral foramen. Radiculalgia may result from it

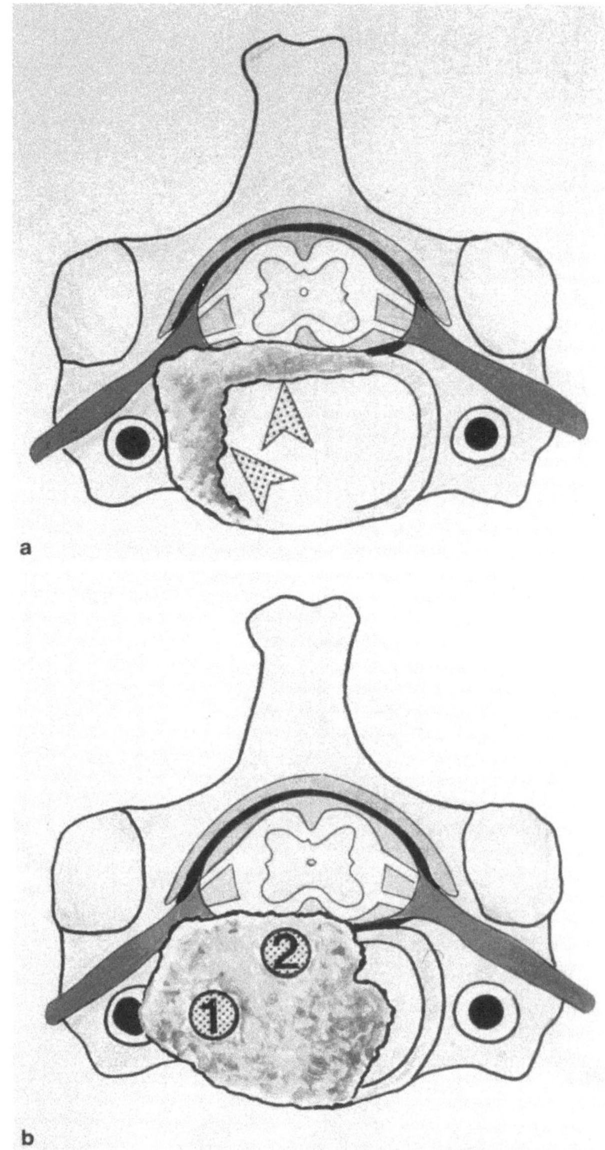

Fig. 9.55 a, b. Combined uncodiskarthrosis. **a** Combination of a posterior uncovertebral arthrosis (*lower arrow*) with a posterior diskal osteophytosis (*upper arrow*); the clinical expression may be only radicular or radiculomedullary. **b** Total uncodiskarthrosis with lateral as well as posterior (*1*) uncarthrosis and posterior osteophytosis (*2*); the clinical expression may be either cervicocephaloradicular or cervicoradiculomedullary

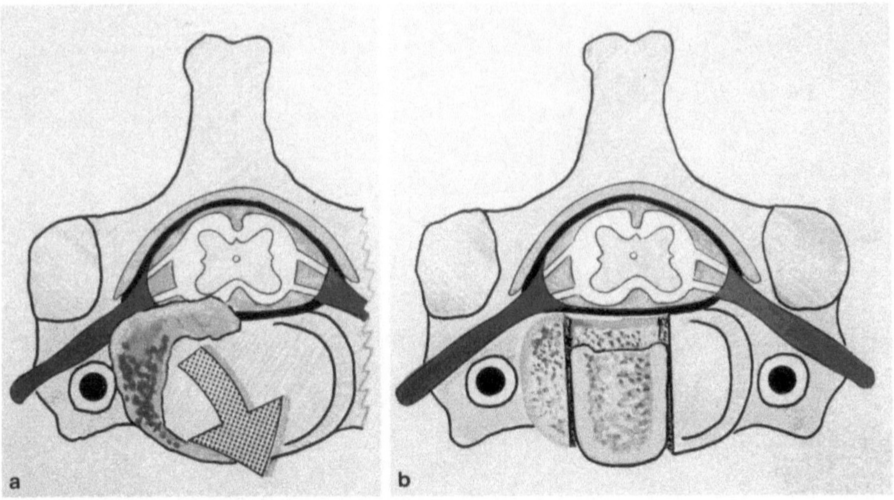

Fig. 9.56 a, b. Combination of a posterior uncovertebral arthrosis and posterior osteophytosis. **a** The ideal treatment lies in a transdiscal osteophytectomy through anteromedian approach, removing at the same time the posterior diskal osteophyte and the uncovertebral exostosis. Freeing the vertebral artery is not necessary here as it is not involved in this kind of combination. **b** fusion according to Robinson with a sole iliacal tricortical graft is then performed

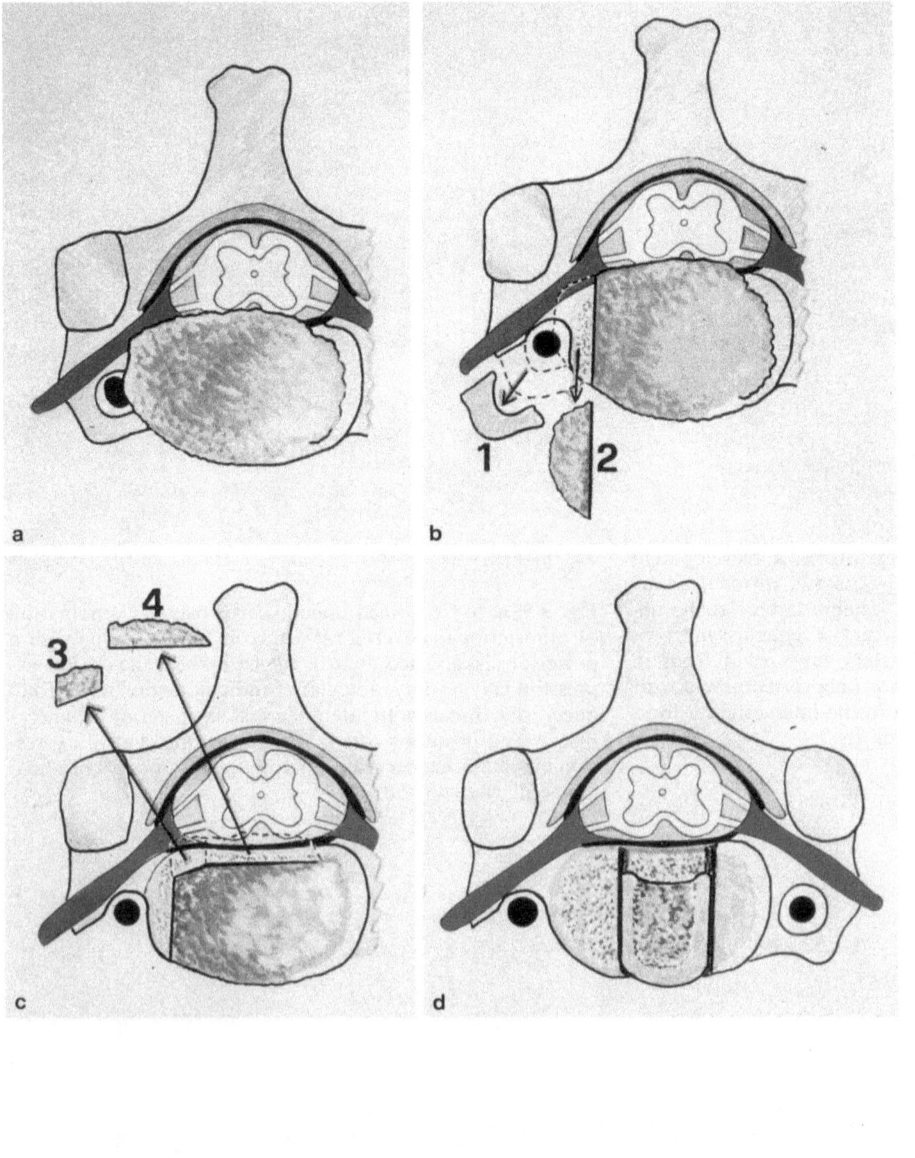

Fig. 9.57 a–d. Surgical treatment of the complete combined uncodiskarthrosis. **a** Preoperative stage with a both uncovertebral and posterior diskal osteophytic arthrosis; vertebral artery, root nerve, and medulla are pressed together. **b** Initial freeing of the vertebral artery by transversectomy (*1*) then uncusectomy (*2*). **c** Uncoforaminotomy (*3*) by resecting the posterior part of the uncovertebral exostosis and transdiskal osteophytectomy (*4*). **d** Interbody fusion according to Robinson with a sole iliacal tricortical graft

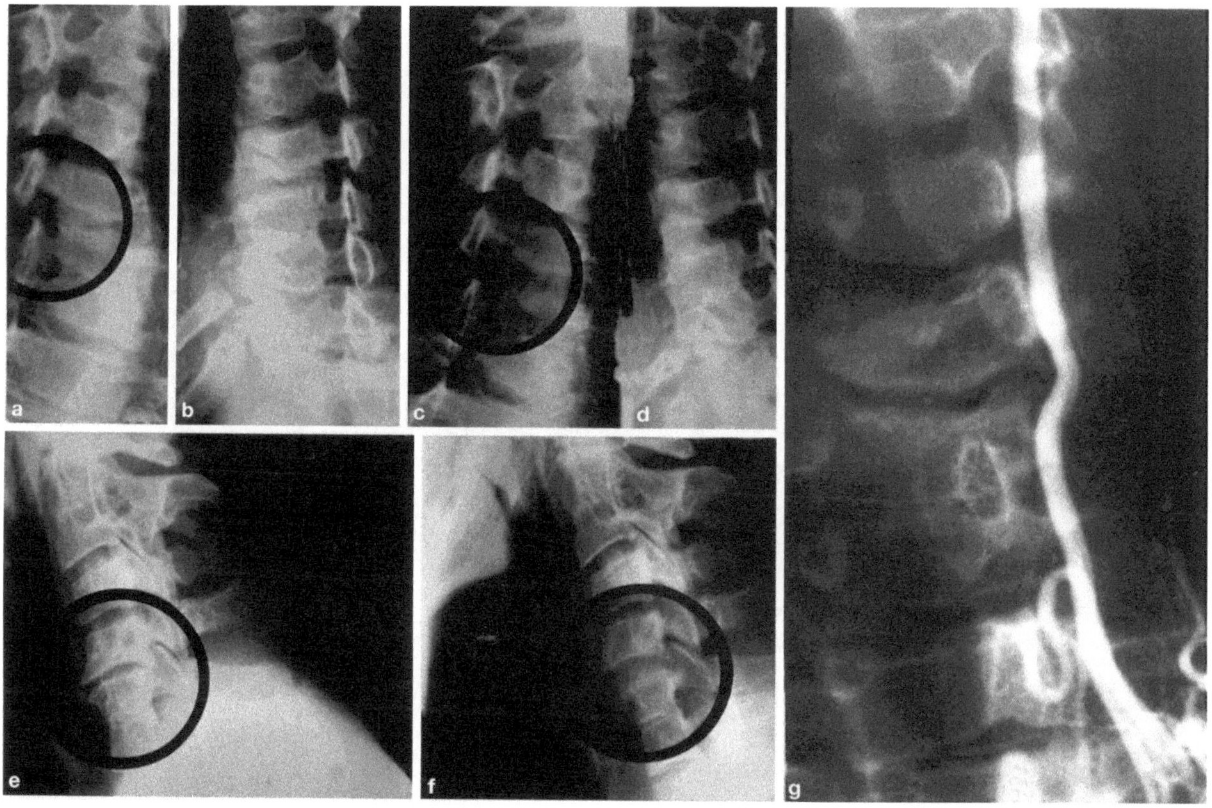

Fig. 9.58 a–g. Example of a combined syndrome, cervicobrachialgic, cervicomedullary, and cervicocephalic in a man aged 37 presenting an early C4–C5 uncodiskarthrosis, lying above a congenital C5–C6 block. The symptoms consisted of constant nuchal pain, headaches, vertigo fits related to head rotation, movements to the right, drop attacks (a dozen), fasciculations, and a Lhermitte's sign induced by flexion of the neck. **a, c** Left C4–C5 intervertebral foramina before (**a**) and after (**c**) the operation which consisted of a transdiskal osteophytectomy associated with a left C4–C5 uncoforaminectomy. **b, d** Right intervertebral foramina. **e** Dense diskarthrosis with preoperative canalar stenosis. **f** Postoperative state. **g** shows clearly the stenosis and the displacement of the left vertebral artery facing the C4–C5 uncarthrosis. The result of the operation was exellent, with disappearance of all the symptoms and complete work resumption; operation on November 16, 1977, latest last follow-up December 1985

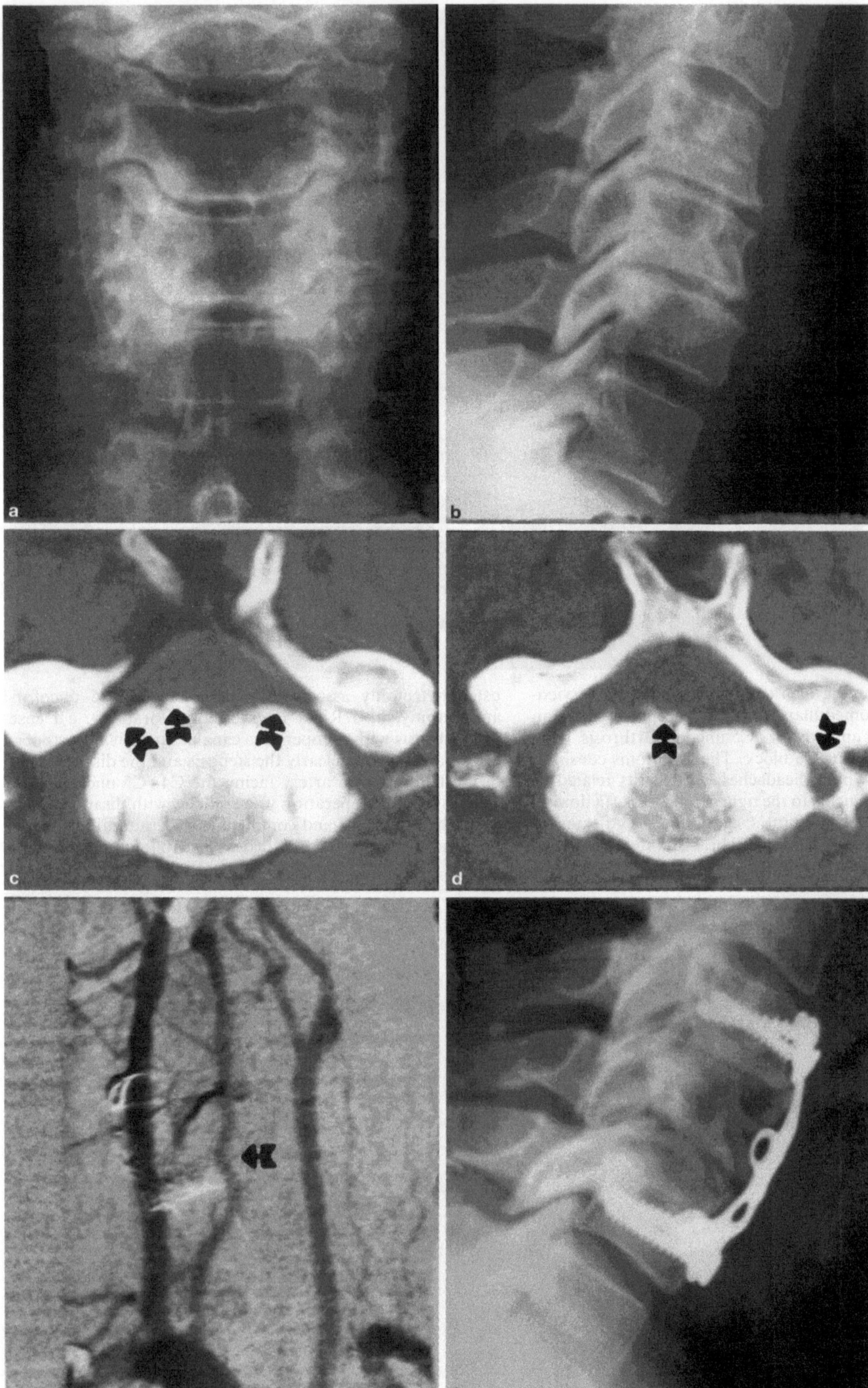
a
b
c
d
e
f

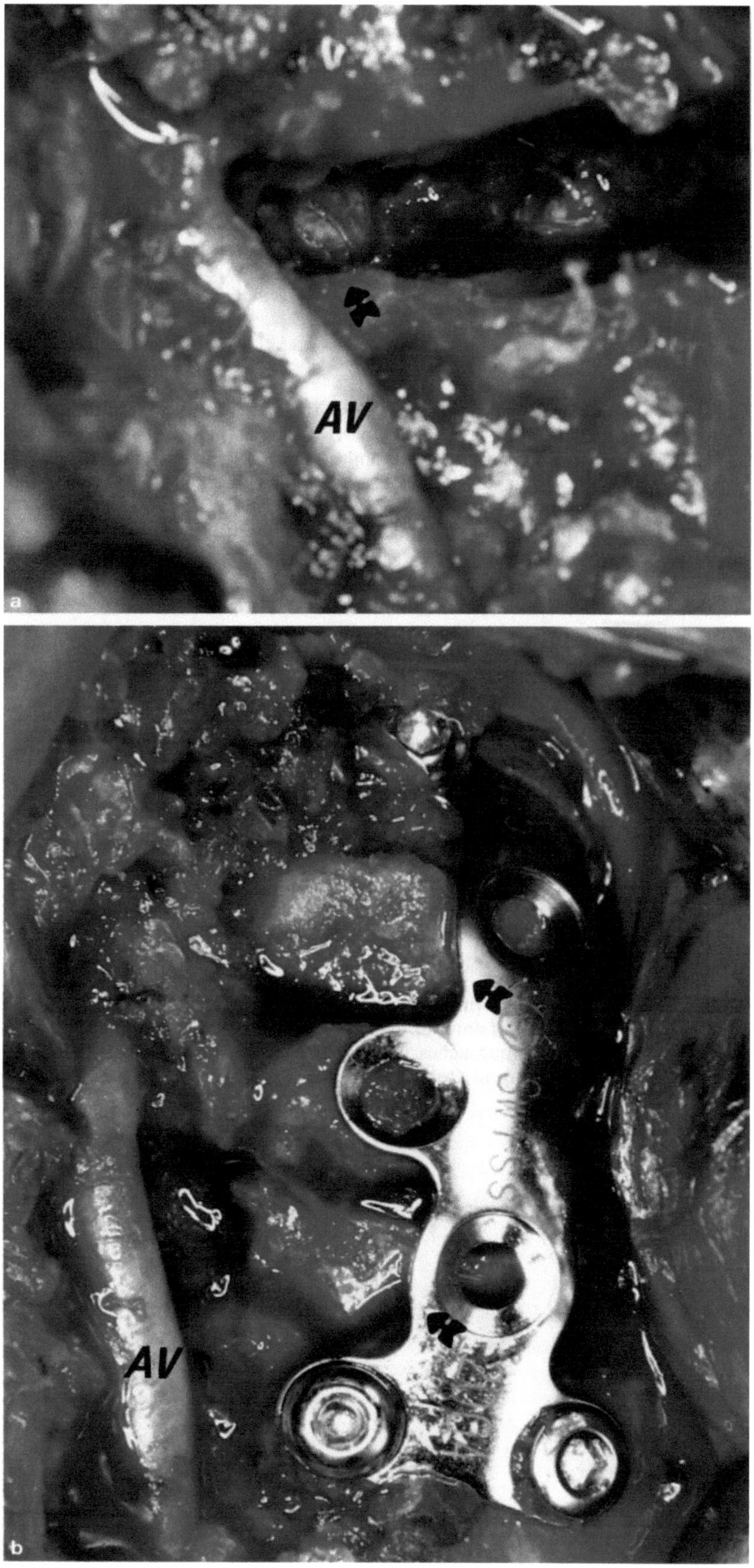

Fig. 9.60 a, b. Preoperative photographs of same patient as in Fig. 9.59. **a** The right vertebral artery is freed through C6, C5, and C4 transversectomy (*AV*); the dura mater is visible thanks to the transdiskal osteophytectomy which freed dura mater and medulla as well as the roots laterally (*arrows*). **b** The osteosynthesis plate is set in; the right vertebral artery is again recognizable (*AV*) with the grafts (*arrows*)

◀ **Fig. 9.59 a–f.** Example of a combined cervicobrachialgic and cervicocephalic syndrome which developed over many years in a man aged 54. Casualty at the age of 32 of a very serious road accident, suffering from a indirect craniocervical trauma, but with contact and fracture of the cheek bone. Symptoms arose step by step as the C4–C5 (**a**) and C5–C6 (**b**) uncodiskarthroses developed. Scanographical sections (**c, d**) clearly indicated the canalar stenosis (*arrows*) due to the posterior osteophytosis, the stricture of the intervertebral foramina because of the posterior development of the uncarthrosis, and even the stenosis of the C6 transverse foramen by lateral overlapping of the uncarthrosis. **e** Digitalized arteriography showing a displacement of the right C5–C6 vertebral artery and a stenosis in the transverse foramen of C6. **f** lateral view radiography after the operation. The posterior osteophytes have been resected through a transdiskal approach, grafts have been set in and, two levels have been operated on, with osteosynthesis using an AO plate has been realized (see also Fig. 9.60). Operated in October 1985 with very good results a follow-up at six month

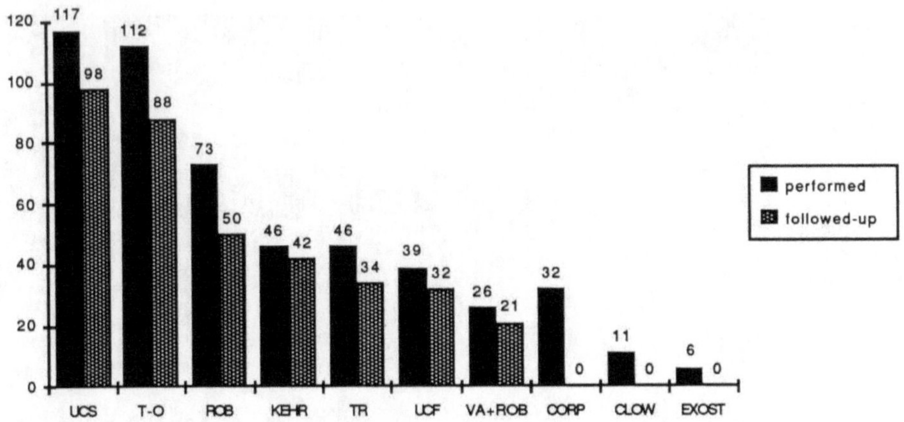

Fig. 9.61. Comparative histogram showing the 508 cervical approaches realized and their follow-up: 117 uncusectomies (*UCS*), 112 transdiskal osteophytectomies (*T-O*), 73 interbody fusions according to Robinson (*ROB*), 46 combined approaches according to Kehr (*KEHR*), 46 transversectomies (*TR*), 39 uncoforaminectomies (*UCF*), without bone grafting, 26 freeings of the vertebral artery and bone grafting according to Robinson (*VA + ROB*), 32 corpectomies (*CORP*), 11 interbody fusions according to Cloward (*CLOW*), 6 anterior exostosectomies (Forestier disease) (*EXOST*)

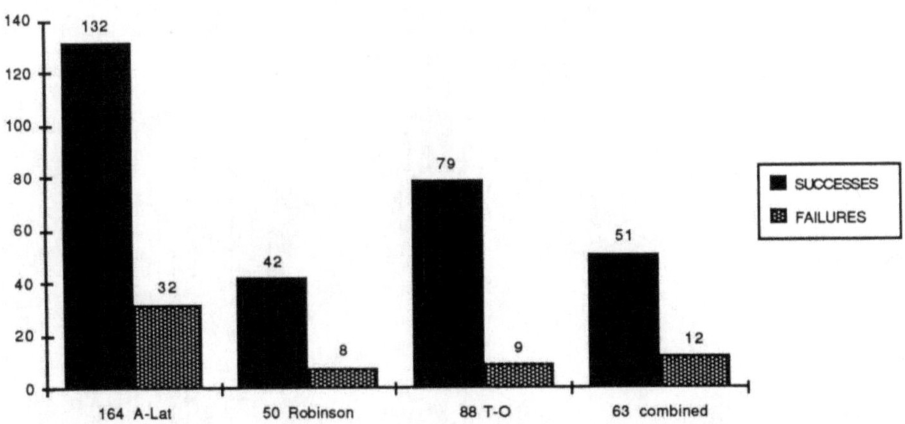

Fig. 9.62. Histogram showing the rate of successes and failures in the four groups of anterior approaches to the cervical spine. Anterolateral approaches (*A-Lat*; 164 cases), interbody fusions according to Robinson (*Robinson*; 50 cases), transdiskal osteophytectomies (*T-O*; 88 cases), and combined approaches according to Kehr (*combined*; 63 cases). The best rate of success was obtained in the transdiskal osteophytectomies

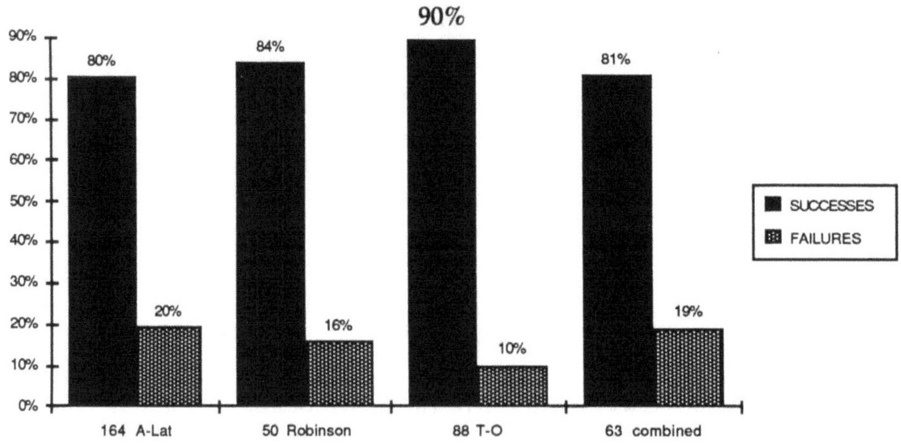

Fig. 9.63. Same data as in Fig. 9.62 presented in the form of comparative percentages. The best rate of success was obtained in the transdiskal osteophytectomies

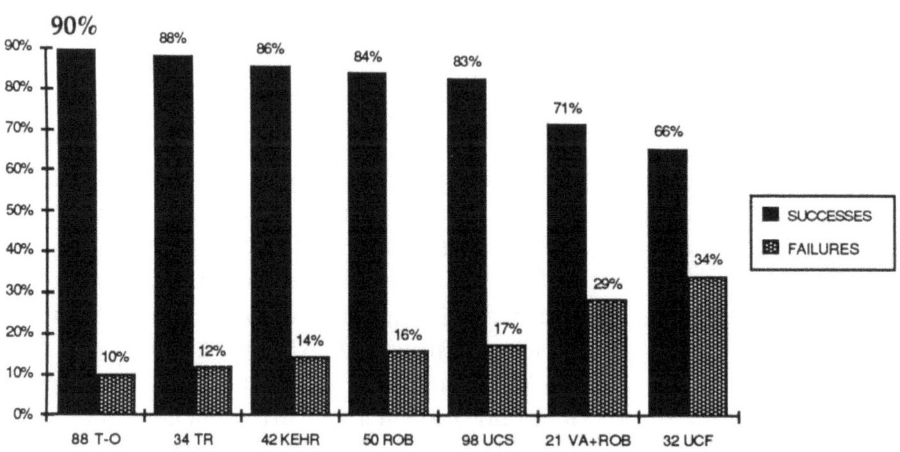

Fig. 9.64. Comparative histogram showing in percentages the rates of success and failure in all operations. The 10 % failure rate of transdiskal osteophytectomies contrasts with the 34 % failure rate of the old uncoforaminectomies without bone grafting

Posterior Decompression

From the discussion it is apparent that the surgical indications and the surgical procedure selected will depend on the cause of the stenosis. In some patients the stenosis is the result of specific posterior abnormalities such as hypertrophy of the ligamentum flavum, anomalies of the laminae and of the pedicles, hypertrophy or arthrotic changes involving the posterior facet joints, and uniform concentric narrowing of the canal, either on a congenital basis resulting from diseases of the posterior longitudinal ligament. When these are not associated with detectable anterior abnormalities, they can be dealt with successfully using surgical procedures that widen the spinal canal from the back. The most common surgical procedures will be discussed here. These include partial or complete hemilaminectomy, the type of hemilaminectomy described by Frykolm in 1951, wide laminectomy, and procedures such as expansive laminoplasty, which involves the spinal canal without removing the laminae or spinal processes.

Hemilaminectomy

Hemilaminectomy, with or without arthrectomy is useful in segmental stenotic pathology associated with posterolateral compression. It permits exploration of the nerve roots, the posterior wall, the root canal, the facet joints, the posterolateral wall, the vertebral canal, and the disk (e.g., soft hernia produced in the posterolateral wall or tumor protrusions).

Technique

Following the posterior approach described in Chap. 8 the spine is reached. Before proceeding, the operative level must be confirmed with appropriate intraoperative radiographs. The distance between the laminae in the cervical spine is very short, particularly in comparison with that in the lumbar region. Even with the anterior flexion of the head that tends to separate the laminae, the amount of space remains limited.

The ligamentum flavum is detached from the lamina above and below the operative level using a small 45° curet (Fig. 9.65). If the necessity for a much wider exposure is anticipated, then it may be necessary to remove the spinal apophysis and the interspinal ligaments. In addition to providing a wider field of view, this will facilitate detachment of the ligamentum flavum.

Having detached the ligamentum flavum from the margins of the laminae, one can then introduce a small Kerrison forceps with a large case of up to 4 or 5 mm (Fig. 9.66). One then begins to remove the edges of the laminae above and below. The exposure is gradually enlarged and the removal of approximately one half of the lamina should be planned. The ligamentum flavum while in place protects the dura mater and cord from the instruments. Once it is exposed, however, it may be easily removed from the remaining points of attachment with curets or with a Kerrison punch.

Often, however, this limited hemilaminectomy is not sufficient to provide adequate exposure of the root canal for inspection of the nerve root. In this case, therefore, the removal of one half to two thirds of the lateral mass with the facet joints (hemilaminectomy and arthrectomy) must be removed. At this point, curved curets should be used, or, if available, a high-speed diamond burr on an air drill which is very useful in advancing the dissection (Fig. 9.67). Placing a flat blunted spatula behind the facet joint below the level to be enterd, the dissection may be quickly extended into the periarticular lateral masses. It must be ensured that the neuromeningeal and cord structures are well protected as described. Drilling continues until the anterior cortical wall of the inferior articular apophysis is reached. The remaining wall and the remnants of the lateral aspect of the ligamentum flavum that form the posterior wall of the root canal can then be removed with small curved curets (Fig. 9.68). This exposure permits access to the lateral course of the dural sac along with the related nerve root. The nerve root may be mobilized by pushing it up or down, while the dural sac will move more easily laterally. This allows a full view of the root canal, the posterolateral margin, the intervertebral disk, and the adjacent vertebral body (Fig. 9.69).

In cases where there are specific abnormalities of the lamina, such as in congenital deformities or tumor, greater exposure of the bodies may be obtained by completing the hemilaminectomy at one or more levels. The surgical steps are identical to those that have been already described. In the literature, removal of the soft disk hernia or posterior and posterolateral vertebral osteophytes has been described using this approach (Fineschi 1962; Epstein 1963).

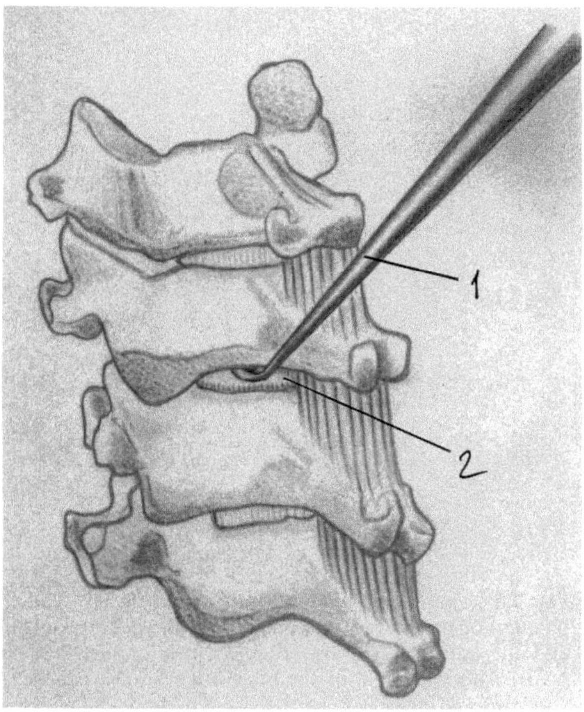

Fig. 9.65. The curet (*1*) is used to detach the ligamentum flavum (*2*) from the interlaminar space, which will be the operative site

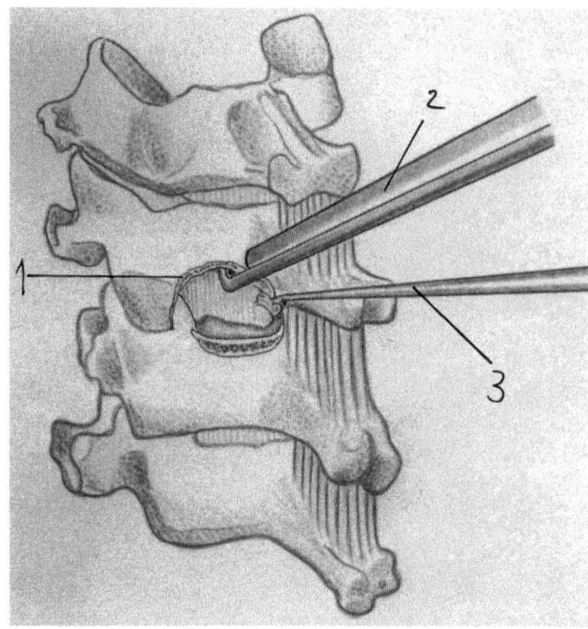

Fig. 9.66.

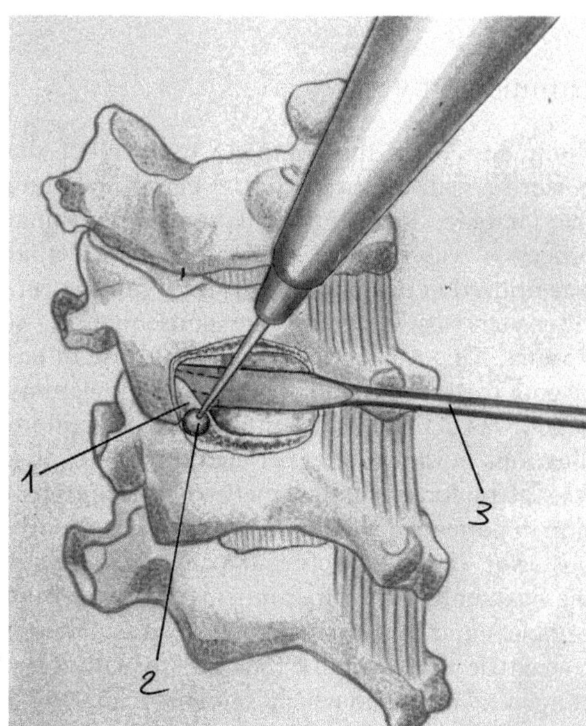

Fig. 9.66. Following the removal of the ligamentum flavum, a conservative or limited hemilaminectomy (*1*) is carried out using Kerrison forceps (*2*). The removal of the ligamentum flavum is completed using curved curets (*3*)

Fig. 9.67. The decompression is extended along the apophyseal masses (*1*) towards the nerve root canal using different-sized drill bits of different sizes (*2*). The underlying nerve and cord are protected with a thin spatula (*3*) ▶

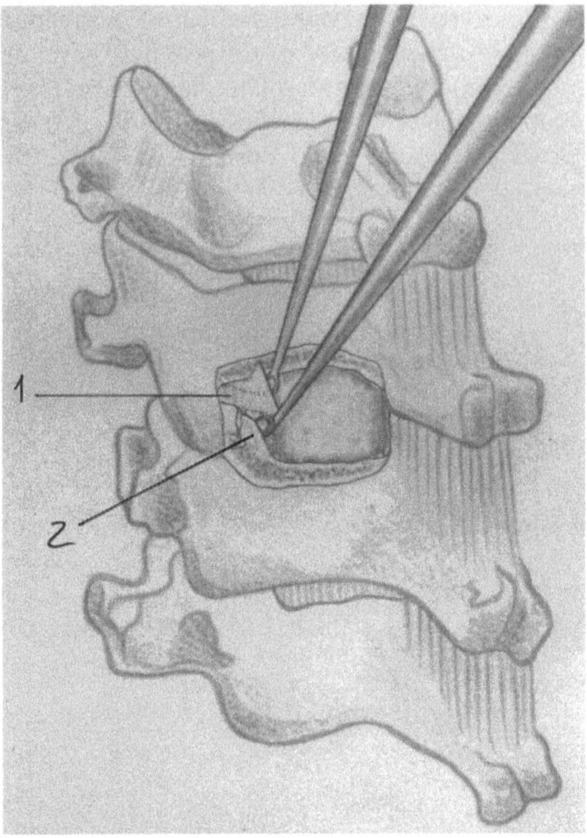

Fig. 9.68. Removal of the lateral masses exposes more ligamentum flavum (*1*) which must be removed. The anterior surface of the inferior facet (*2*) is removed with curved curets

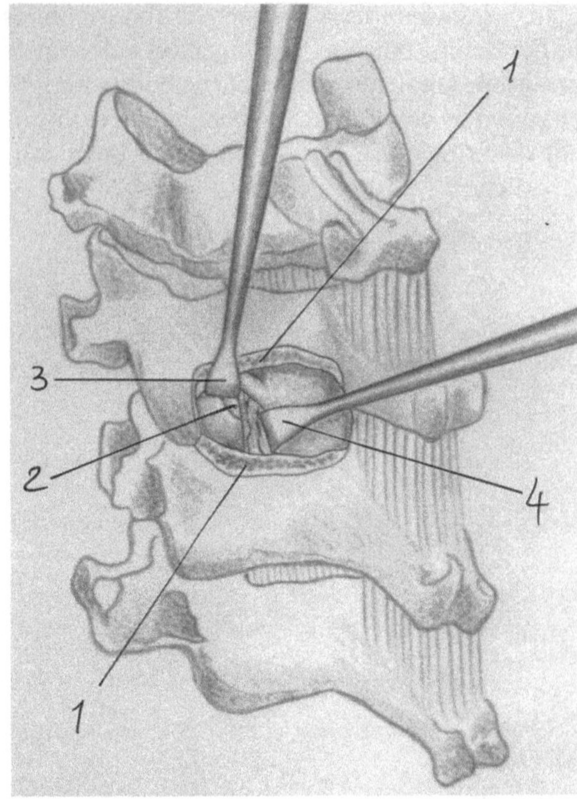

Fig. 9.69. Completed limited hemilaminectomy (*1*) and the opening of the nerve root canal (*2*). If the neural roots (*3*) and the dural sac (*4*) are retracted, the foramen and the posterolateral margin of the intervertebral disk can be inspected

Laminectomy

For many years the complete removal of the posterior wall of the vertebral canal including the laminae, ligamentum flavum, and spinal processes was the one surgical procedure that was utilized in dealing with diseases causing cervical stenosis, including the consequences of trauma. This was done with the purpose of enlarging the spinal canal. This wide laminectomy which was defined as decompressive has real indications in the relief of cervical spinal stenosis. It is the preferred surgical method of decompression in patients in whom the stenosis is primarily posterior (laminar deformity, hypertrophy of the ligamentum flavum, and enlargement of the pedicles) and in cases where there is a uniform concentric narrowing of the canal usually on a congenital basis and which is not associated with localized compression of the cord. It is also useful as a method of treatment for cases associated with calcification of the posterior longitudinal ligament.

Technique

Obviously, the approach to the spine will be through the posterior approach described in Chap. 8. The patient is placed in the anti-Trendelenburg position. Intraoperative X-rays are used to check and confirm the levels of the spine in preparation for the surgery. Usually, the approach is undertaken at a level above and a level below the level which is to be decompressed. The first step is the removal of the spinal apophysis. The interspinous ligament is cut with a scalpel in the space below, and the spinous processes of the laminae to be removed can be cut with a Luer forceps (Fig. 9.70). It is best to check visually the level of the transection of the spinous apophyses because there is a risk that it may be too low. If it is too low, the surgeon might enter the vertebral canal at a point corresponding to the interface between the laminae and the spinous processes themselves.

Having removed the spinous processes, dissection of the ligamentum flavum away from the distal laminae is begun with a curved curet. The detachment of the ligamentum flavum is carried out with blunt dissection extending laterally as far as the facet joint (Fig. 9.71). Once the first lamina has been freed, the actual laminectomy can begin using Kerrison punches or rongeurs (Fig. 9.72). The ligamentum flavum should be left in place during this part of the procedure since it will act as a buffer between the instrument and the subjacent nerve structures. As the laminectomy proceeds, the surgeon can contemporaneously begin to remove the ligamentum flavum. Once this has been done, the peridural fat appears indicating that the dura mater has been reached. This procedure is repeated at each level as required to achieve the needed decompression. Throughout the dissection bleeding must be carefully controlled using coagulation and bone wax. In some cases, particularly those with a severe stenosis of the canal, the surgeon must proceed with extreme caution throughout the procedure because the deformity will be such as to exclude any amount of peridural fat. The dura mater is therefore immediately behind the level of the section and runs the risk of being injured by the instruments. The peridural venous plexus will also produce extensive bleeding. This must be controlled with electrocoagulation, Surgicel, or Spongostan impregnated with coagulants.

Should it be necessary to expose the root canal in order to free the nerve root posteriorly, the laminectomy must be extended as far as the facet joints, removing one third to one half of the surface according to the individual case. Particularly in cases where the bone is osteopenic, all this can be achieved with curved curets. In most cases, however, as indicated above, all of this can be more easily achieved with an air drill (Fig. 9.73). Great care must be taken not to remove the entire articular facets. If this were to be done, it would result in significant segmental instability. A modification of this technique is to remove the entire posterior wall including spinous processes, laminae, and ligamentum flavum with the use of a high-speed air drill (as is usually done in a laminoplasty) or a small Kerrison punch. The procedure in these cases is to use the tip of the drill to cut the most lateral portion of the lamina at a point where it joins the apophyseal masses (Fig. 9.74). The drill will easily cut the external cortex and drilling can be extended to the internal cortex. Bleeding is controlled with bone wax. The cut is placed at each end of the laminae at every level at which they are to be removed. The insertions of the ligamentum flavum are then detached with a fine curved curet. A small spatula is pushed under the edge of the lamina above the ligamentum flavum. The drill can now safely transect the internal (deep) cortex of the lamina to complete the transection. After this first breach of the lamina, the separation is completed with the drill or with a very small Kerrison punch that we have had designed. It has a very narrow cutting surface and will easily complete the transection of the lamina as required (Fig. 9.75). The dissection may be completed at the various levels and from side to side. Once the laminae have been cut at both ends then they can be removed en bloc. Even when the laminae have been completely removed, there will be remnants of the ligamentum flavum both proximally and distally to the first and last lamina. When these have been freed, then mobilization and eventually removal of the complete posterior wall of the canal can begin. When adhesions within the peridural fat are encountered, they must be very carefully released in order to permit the removal of the laminae. Because the peridural venous plexus will be the source of extensive bleeding, particularly in the lateral regions of the dura mater, coagulation and packing with Surgicel, Spongostan, and coagulants will be needed for control. The subsequent steps leading to the exposure of the root canal (by way of arthrectomy) are as described above (Fig. 9.73).

The laminectomy may be extended down as far as the first thoracic vertebral levels where the necessity for any additional steps is not anticipated and no specific problems are envisaged. Proximally, the resection may be extended to reach the first cervical levels, right up to exposure of the foramen magnum.

However, great care must be taken in the upper cervical region, particularly when removing the arch of the atlas. Here the dissection must be very careful and very deliberate. The first step is to strip the arch of the atlas, beginning at the posterior tubercle. A blunt periosteal elevator of the type that is often used for packing sponges is used to separate the muscle attachments on either side of the arch to within 15 mm of the posterior tubercle. This dissection is always the cause of heavy bleeding that must be controlled by packing small pieces of Surgicel into the plane of cleavage between the bone surface and the muscular tissue being raised from it (Fig. 9.76). Once this has been completed on both sides, the greater part of the posterior arch of C1 is exposed. Extending the dissection more laterally exposes the vertebral artery, which may be injured. If it is necessary to enter this area, then one must be careful to first fully identify the vertebral artery and mobilize it where it passes through the bone of the atlas.

The surgeon can now begin freeing the arch from the attachments of the atlanto-occipital membrane along its superior border and from the atlanto-axial membrane at its inferior border. The detachment of these ligaments is not difficult. It should be carried out at first with small curved curets and may be completed with the specially designed 90° curved periosteal elevator (Fig. 9.76). The transection of the bone should be carried out slowly with rongeurs. Proceeding laterally, then increasing care must be taken, for this is the area of the vertebral artery (Figs. 9.77, 9.78). Should the foramen magnum need to be widened, the procedure is a very delicate and difficult. If there is protrusion of the odontoid process or instability with compression that can be ascribed to the superior edge of the foramen pushing onto the cord, it then becomes necessary to widen the foramen on its superior side. The periosteum is removed from the surface of the occipital bone, beginning at the external occipital protuberance and extending for 10–11 mm on each side. If this is carried out exaclty along the surface of the bone, then there is no risk of injury to the greater occipital nerve. Small curved curets are used to detach the atlanto-occipital ligament. Although this part of the dissection is easy, it should nevertheless be carried out deliberately and with great care. The removal begins at the midportion of the foramen and extends for about 15 mm (Figs. 9.78, 9.79). The dissector must always be aware of the path of the nearby vertebral artery. If the lateral widening of the foramen is slow, careful, and well controlled, no difficulties should be encountered. Once the ligament has been completely detached using the small Kerrison punch (Fig. 9.78), widening of the foramen to a depth of up to 10 mm from its original edge can then begin. In cases of protrusion of the odontoid process or approximation of the atlas it is not unusual to find that the posterior stenosis with cord compression is not only due to the bony structures; once the bony structures have been removed and the foramen widened (Fig. 9.79), thickenings of the atlanto-occipital membrane may also be identified. These ubiquitous thickenings that follow the contour of the foramen may in fact be producing the compression of the underlying structures.

It is therefore important that after dissection of the osseous elements of the foramen, the structure be opened longitudinally. The adhesions between this level and the dural level may be very tight and may well necessitate opening the dura mater wide (Fig. 9.80). This requires a duraplasty with artificial dura mater or fascia lata and should always be followed by occipitocervical fusion (Figs. 9.81, 9.82). It is absolutely essential that all motion at this level be abolished since any movement, no matter how small, will cause instability and may even cause severe cord injury that may be fatal. Fusion therefore must be carried out. The arthrodesis may even cause severe cord injury that may be fatal. Fusion therefore must be carried out. The arthrodesis should be carried out with the patient's head and neck in the preoperative position. Any internal fixation that changes the relationship between the head and the cervical spine or any step that attempts to change this relationship must be categorically avoided. The established malalignment does not allow for changes of the preexisting fixed position; it has usually been there for a long time, often many years, and should not be changed. The fusion is therefore carried out with the patient's head immobilized in a halo, and the arthrodesis is achieved with dowel grafts from the iliac wing (Fig. 9.120). The external curve of the iliac wing on its outer posterior surface fits well with the occipitocervical curve. The graft is fixed in position with screws into the head and distally into the lateral masses (Fig. 9.82).

Closure

Once the posterior dural sac and the roots have been freed posteriorly and all of the surgical steps required for the procedure have been carried out with complete removal of the causes of the stenosis, the muscular and cutaneous layers are closed. It is not expected that any specific problems will arise associated with simple hemilaminectomy or combined hemilaminectomy and foraminotomy. The presence of an established plane at the level of the spinous apophysis provides a good support for the posterior muscles with the reconstruction of the tissue layers.

In complete laminectomy, however, the absence of the plane where the laminae have been removed along with the spinous apophysis leaves a gap in the tissue between the dura mater that envelops the cord and the muscles which have now lost their medial points of attachment.

Closure of the muscle layers must therefore be very careful. If any space is left under the muscles, this will favor the formation of blood pools (hematomata) which will resolve with great difficulties, even with time, and which act as an open invitation for a deep-seated infection. This risk can be minimized by closing the muscular levels in layers beginning with the deepest. One should close with at least three layers in the muscles. This step will avoid dead spaces or the necessity for deep suction drainage. Such deep suction drainage will obviously be deep enough to reach the dura mater. Particularly in cases where there may have been small dural tears, there is a risk of establishing iatrogenic CSF fistulas. Along the surface, it is wise to undertake careful closure, particularly in the approximation of the nuchal ligament. Careful and complete reconstruction of muscle in layers, particularly along the medial line, and the restoration of the nuchal ligament will have a very important bearing on postoperative stability. The postoperative immobilization will depend on the underlying pathology and will range from halo traction to a more simple collar such as the Somi brace (the latter in simple hemilaminectomy). If the surgery has been carried out accurately and skillfully, the vertebral column at the operative site will maintain its stability.

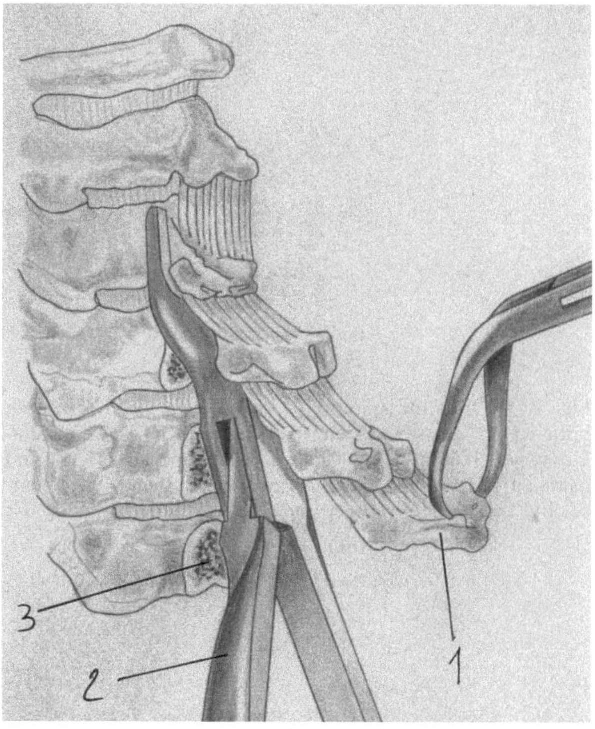

Fig. 9.70. First stage of laminectomy. The interspinal ligament is removed from the level of the first spinous process to be resected (*1*). Using a Luer forceps (*2*), the row of spinous processes is cut at the base at the point of confluence of the two laminae at each level (*3*)

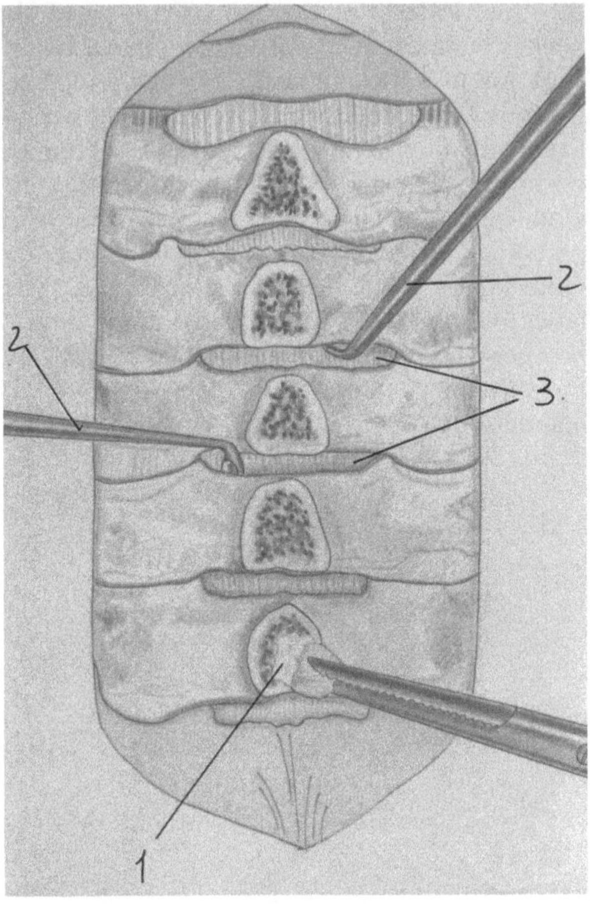

Fig. 9.71. Once the spinous processes have been removed, bone wax (*1*) is used to stem the hemorrhage from the spongiosa, which is now exposed. At each operative level and using curved curets (*2*), the ligamentum flavum (*3*) is elevated, but must remain intact and in place

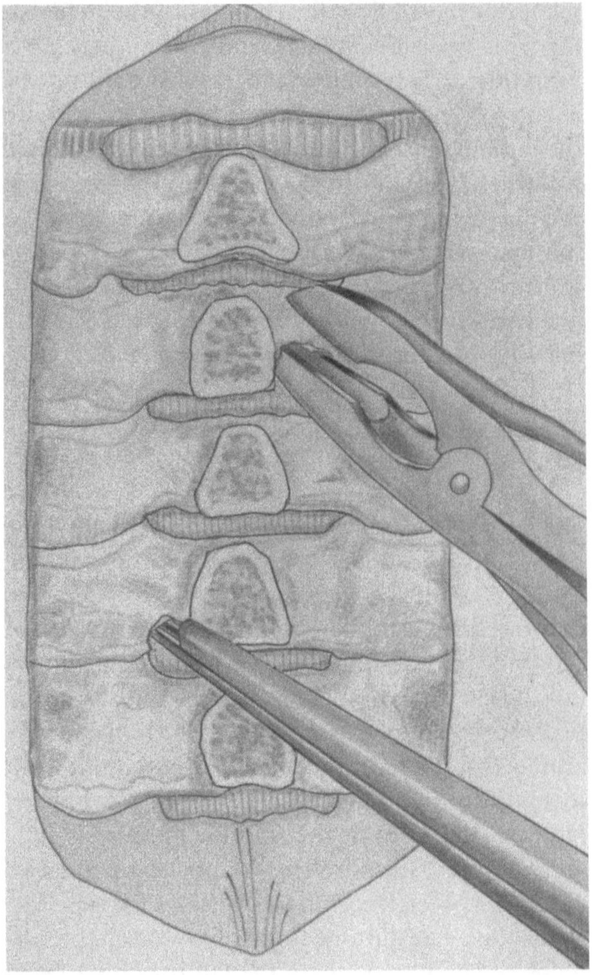

Fig. 9.72. The laminae are removed using selected sizes of either a Kerrison punch or rongeurs

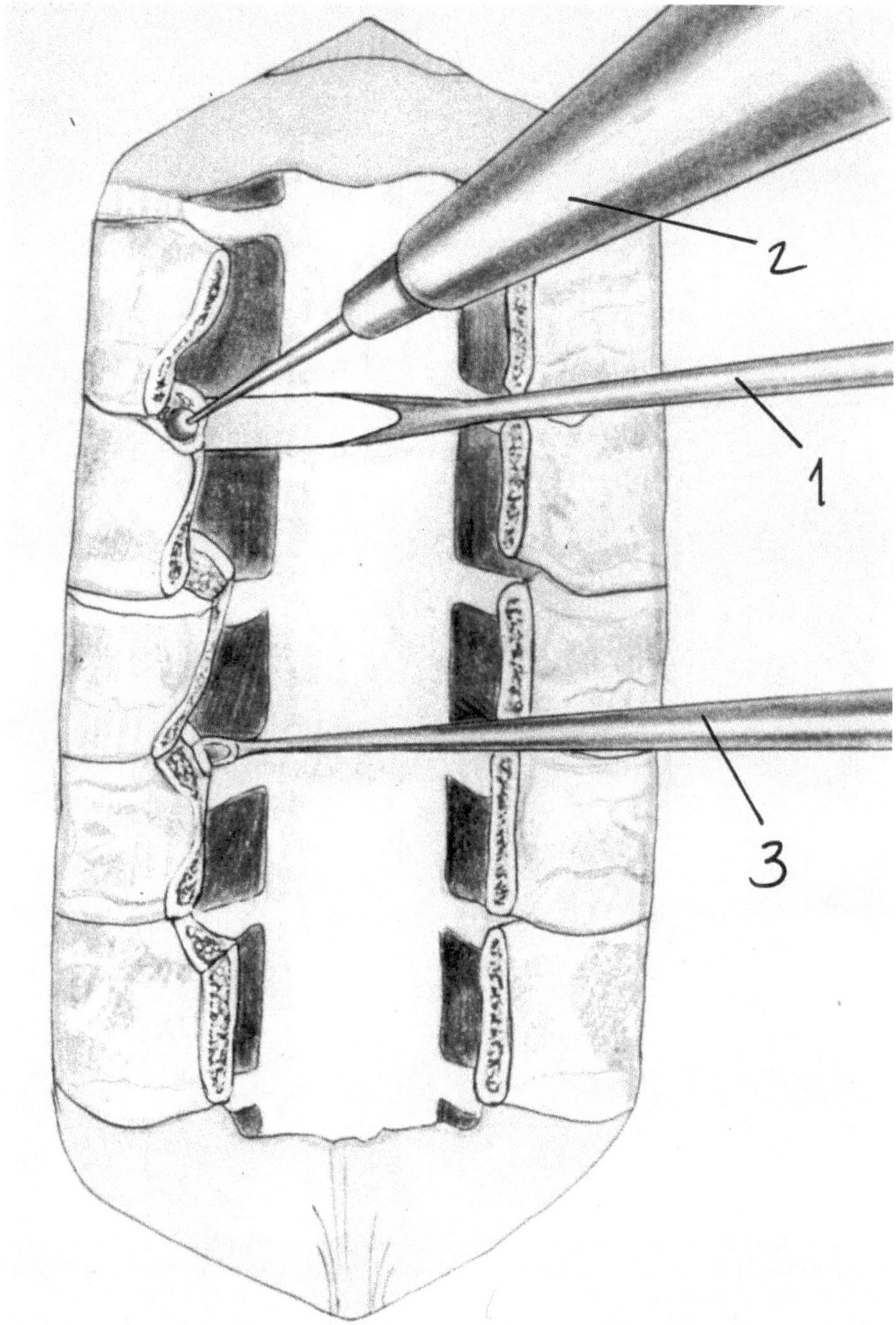

Fig. 9.73. After removal of the laminae and ligamentum flavum, the roots must be freed laterally to the level of the opening of the root canal. The roots must be protected during this procedure and this is achieved by placing a spatula (*1*) in front of the inferior facets and behind the nerve roots and the dural sac. Decompression is achieved with an air drill (*2*). Any remnants of ligamentum flavum or fragments of bone that remain on the wall at the inferior facet should be removed with curets (*3*)

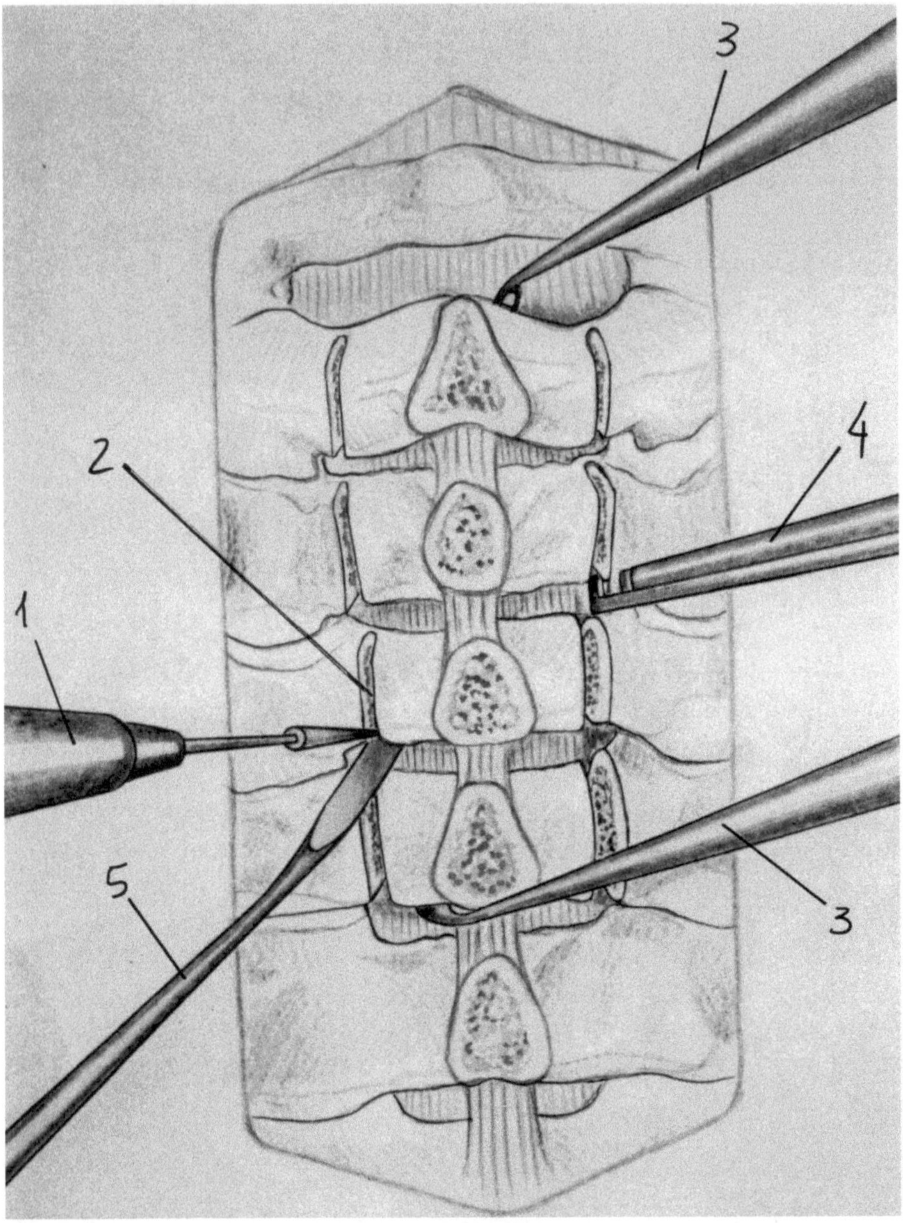

Fig. 9.74. Japanese authors have described a method for en bloc removal of the posterior wall of the canal including the laminae and the ligamentum flavum. They use a drill (*1*) to outline the limits of the lamina at the interface with the articular mass (*2*). The cut across the lamina is gradually deepened to reach the internal cortex. The ligamentum flavum is detached at its most proximal and most distal parts with curved curets (*3*). The anterior cortex of the lamina can then be removed with very fine Kerrison forceps (*4*) (which have a cutting edge), curets, or a very fine drill with a pointed bit. Great care must be taken to protect the underlying neural structures with a spatula (*5*)

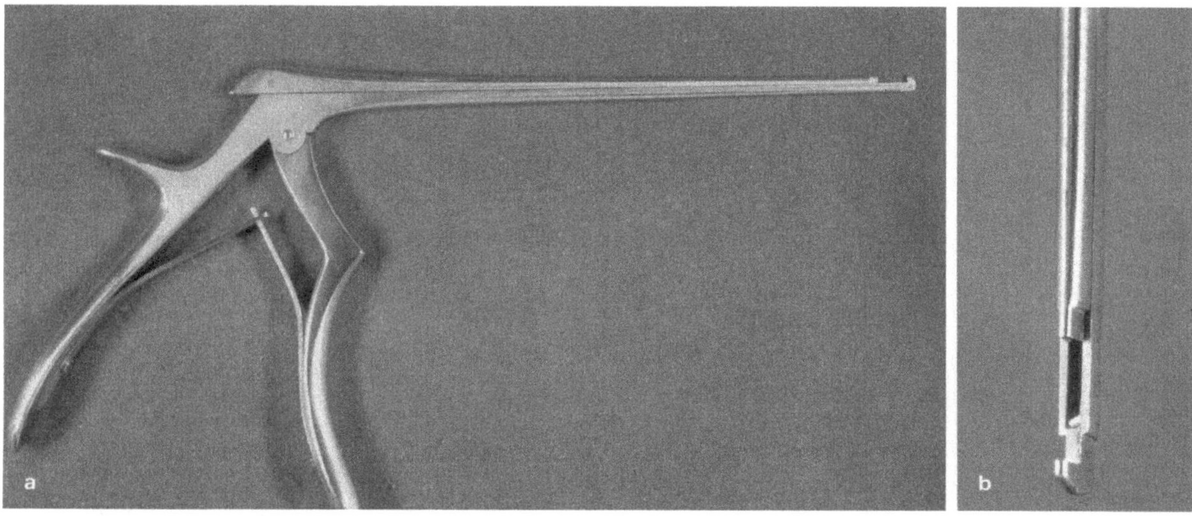

Fig. 9.75.a Full view and **b** detail of a very small Kerrison punch designed for lamina transsection

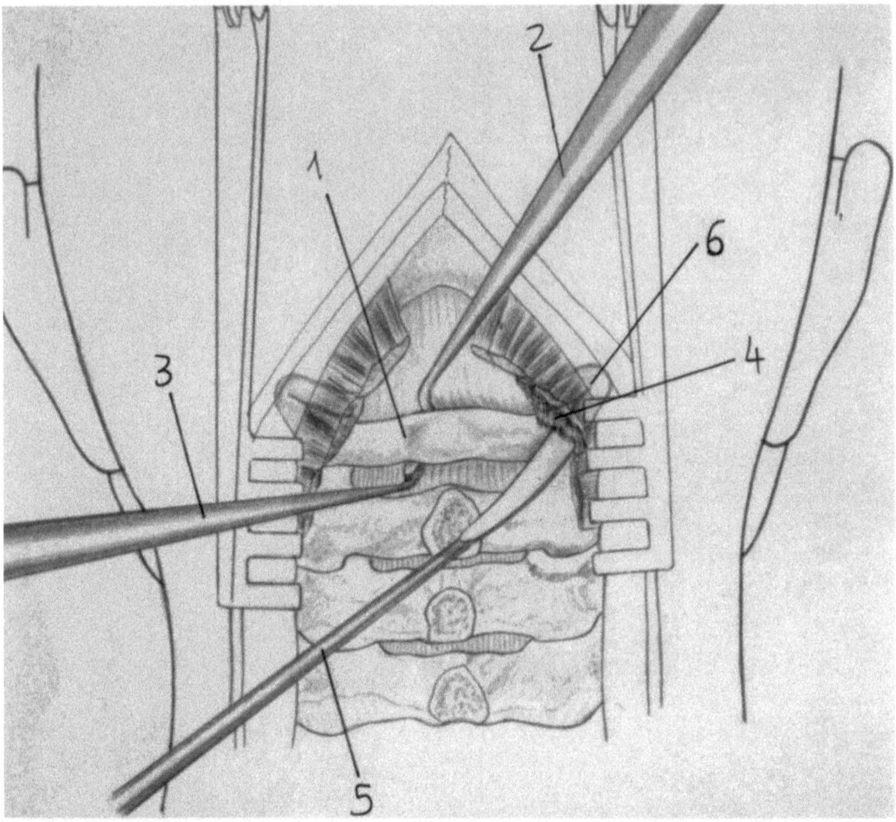

Fig. 9.76. In order to undertake laminectomy of the atlas (*1*), the atlanto-occipital (*2*) and the atlantoaxial (*3*) membrane must first be detached with curets. Great care must be taken in this dissection to assure that the posterior arch is elevated posteriorly during the dissection. Surgicel (*4*) is useful in providing protection during removal; it can be pushed laterally with a spatula (*5*), being careful to maintain visual contact with the vertebral artery (*6*). The osseous removal should not extend beyond 1.5 cm laterally from the posterior tubercle of the atlas

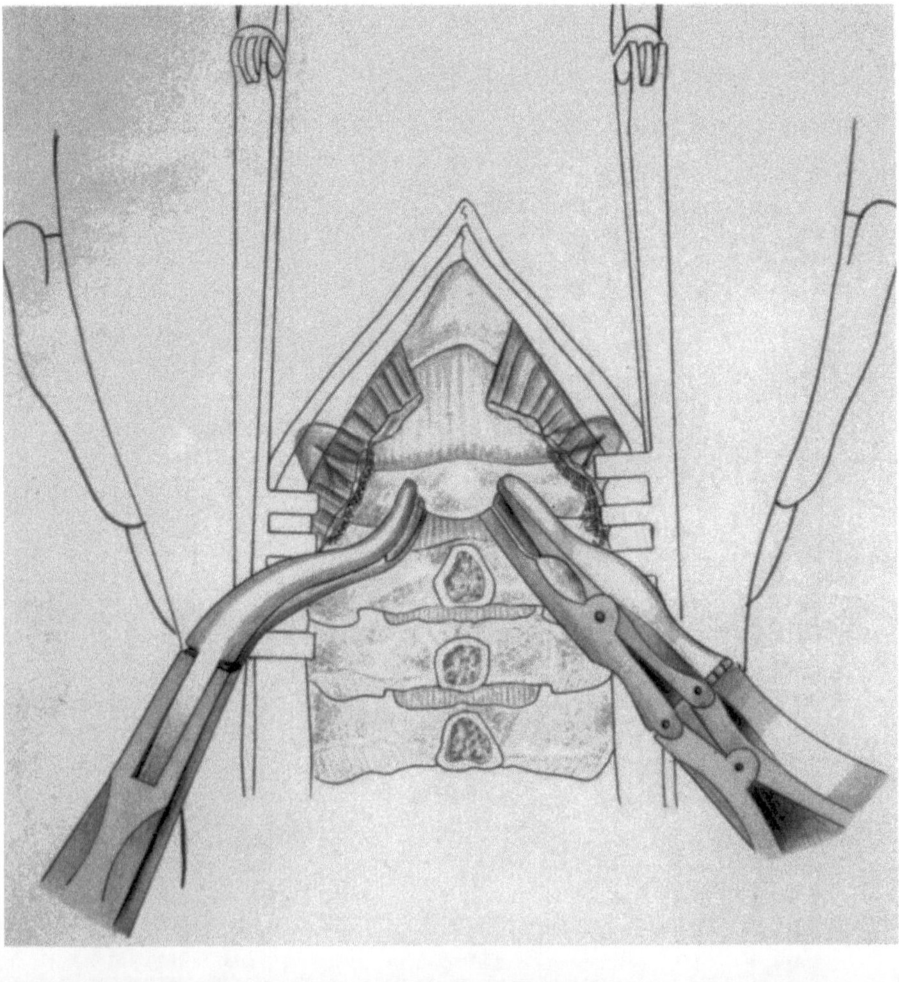

Fig. 9.77. The arch of the atlas may be removed. Using various sizes and configurations of the Kerrison punch

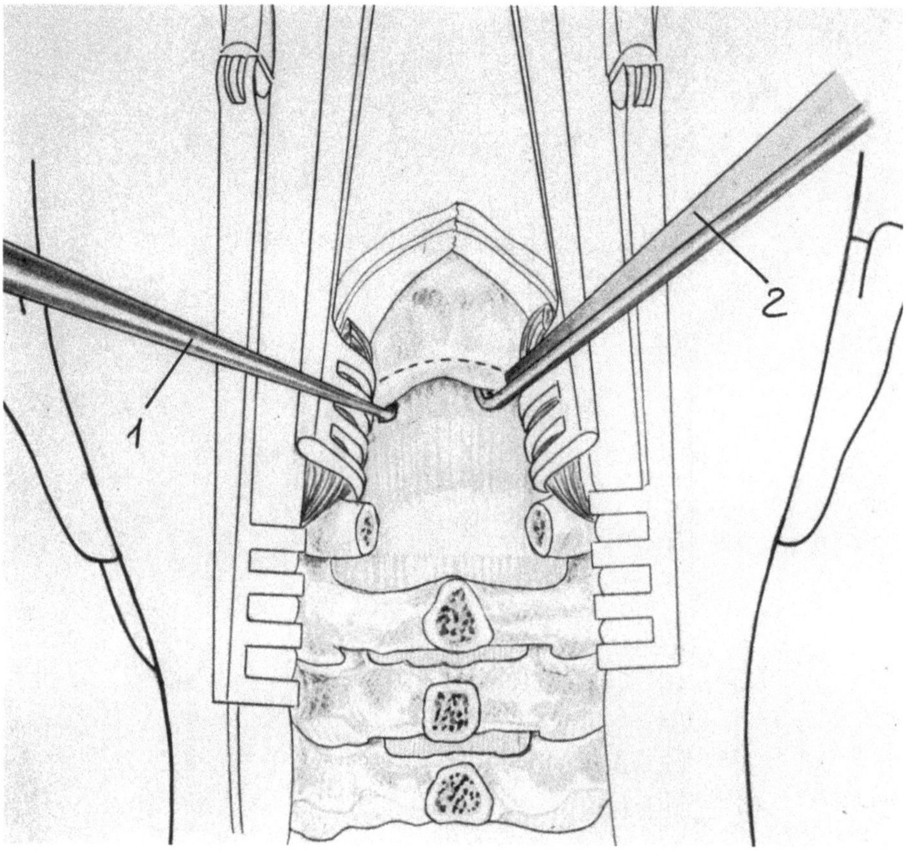

Fig. 9.78. If widening of the foramen magnum becomes necessary, the atlanto-occipital membrane must be detached with curets (*1*). The edge of the foramen can then be removed with a Kerrison punch (*2*)

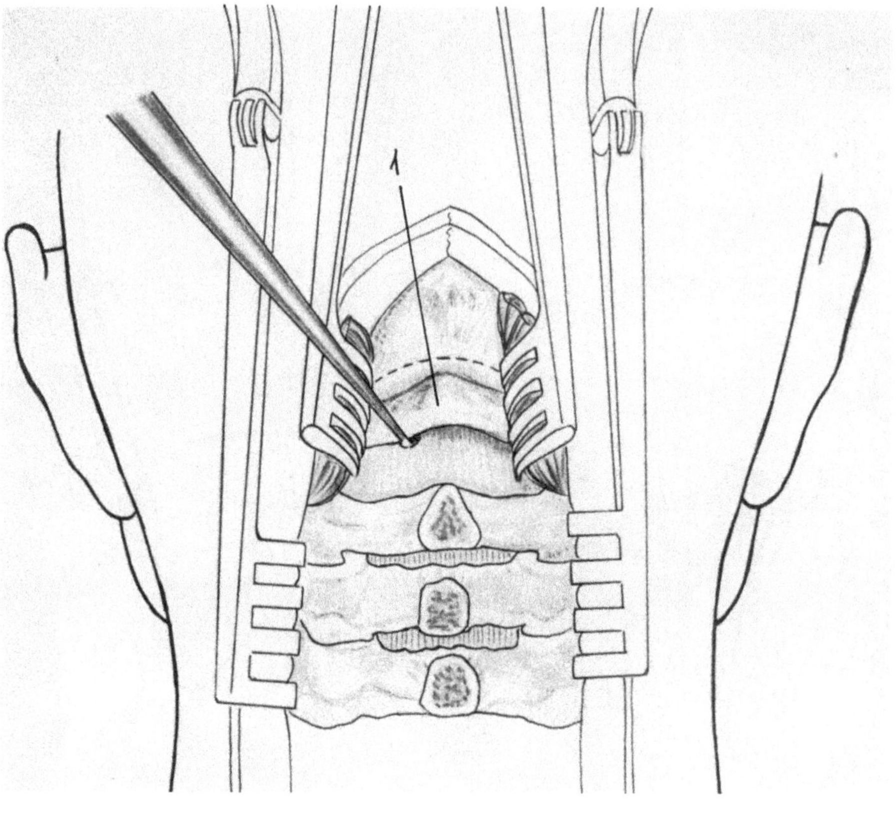

Fig. 9.79. The atlantoaxial membrane is released with blunted curets in cases of protrusion of the odontoid process or approximation of the atlas (*1*)

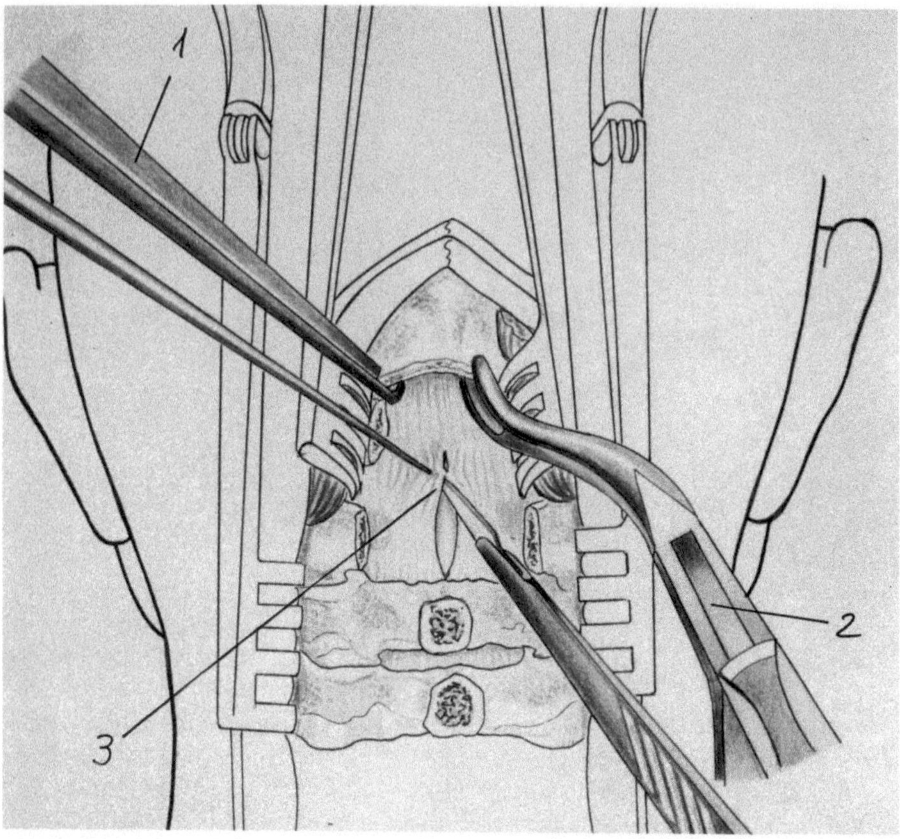

Fig. 9.80. The posterior arch is removed and the foramen magnum widened using a Kerrison punch (*1*) and rongeurs (*2*). The occipitoatlantoaxial membrane is opened and retracted to expose the dura mater (*3*)

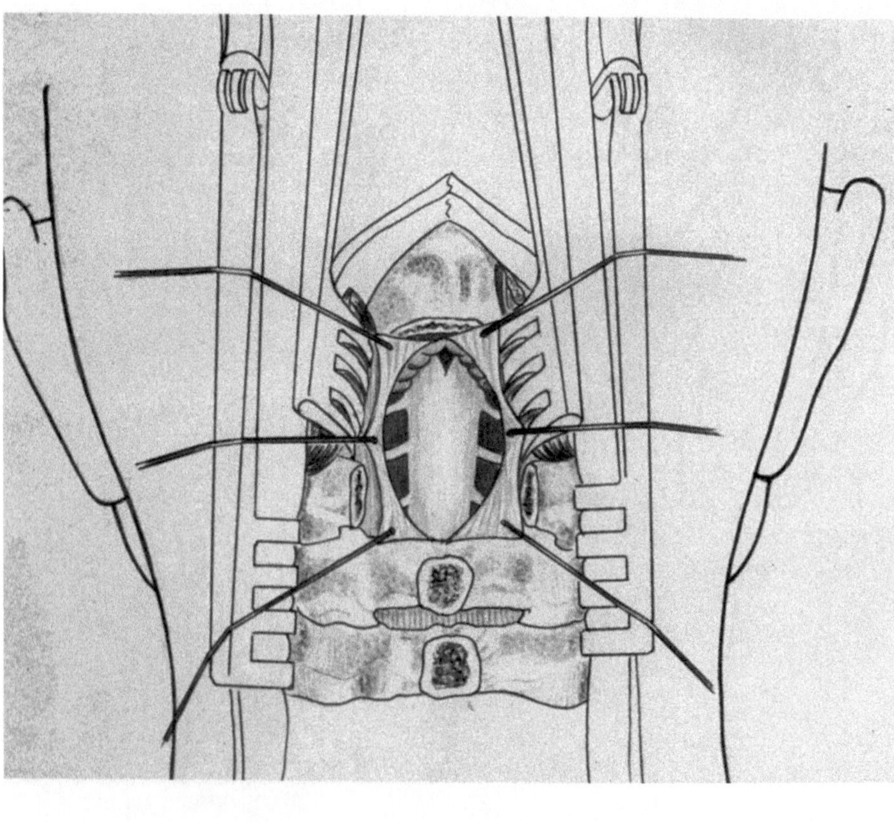

Fig. 9.81. The dura mater is opened

Technical Errors and Complications

In addition to the complication already described there are those complications that are strictly related to the approach. These include inappropriate positioning of the patient on the operative table or of the head in its supported position, lesions of the eye, poor anchoring of the endotracheal tube for anesthesia and inappropriate dissection leading to vascular or neurological damages. There are also complications specifically related to the definitive surgical procedure such as dural tears resulting from the careless use of curets or Kerrison forceps. As indicated above, in the first stages of the laminectomy, the ligamentum flavum should be detached but left in place to act as a buffer between the dura mater and the lamina during removal of the laminae. The use of curets or of Kerrison forceps must be careful and deliberate. As mentioned already, in cases of severe deforming malformation of the spine and in congenitally severely narrowed canals, there is very little peridural fat to protect the dura mater from the dissector. In these cases, the laminae and the ligamentum flavum lie immediately opposite the dura mater and often produce an imprint on the outline of the dural sac. In the act of removing the spinous apophyses, there is again the risk of injury to the dura mater. In cutting the bone, one may extend too deeply, particularly at the point of junction of the opposing laminae, and therefore enter the dural space. Dural tears must be sutured and the entire area of the tear must be covered with fatty tissue or fibrin glue. The consequence of neglect or underestimation of the significance of such tears include the establishment of CSF fistulas postoperatively and infection such as meningitis.

There may be injury to the cord or nerve roots from careless electrocoagulation. In the lateral region of the dural sag approaching the root canals, there is an abundant venous plexus that is quite superficial as well as a more important one situated more deeply in the canal along the posterior wall of the vertebral bodies. Whenever there is bleeding, these vessels must be coagulated and the bleeding stopped. When electrocoagulation is difficult, the area should be packed with Surgicel and Spongostan soaked in coagulant. If inappropriate coagulation is used, particularly with a very high voltage, it is possible to produce a greater degree of injury to the tissue since the heat penetrates deeply to affect the subjacent neurological tissues. Another complication may arise due to the fact that this procedure does not provide decompression of the roots in the lateral aspect of the root canals. If indeed there is segmental posterolateral stenosis, a simple laminectomy will provide no benefit in cases with such nerve root disease. It is also dangerous to remove too much or indeed all of the facet joints, since the stability of the segment or indeed of all the segments operated on is then undermined (a swan-neck deformity).

Techniques of Posterior Cervical Stabilization

Once the causes of the cervical spinal stenosis have been removed through a posterior approach, surgery must be completed with stabilization of the segments operated on. Removal of the cause of the stenosis results in enlargement of the canal, but this widening must be maintained by appropriate additional instrumentation. A selection of the techniques used by us most often and found most commonly in the literature are discussed here.

Occipitocervical Stabilization

Any procedure that removes movement at the occipitocervical joint will result in severe disability for the patient. By their very nature such procedures preclude any rotatory movement of the head on the neck. It is important therefore that very stringent criteria be used in identifying the indications in all cases. For the procedure to be justified, the type of stenosis present and the overall clinical situation must pose a significant threat to the patient. Often these are cases with advanced tumor, severe instability, and congenital malformations.

The most common techniques are:

Fusion with Bone Graft Only. Different methods may be used to achieve fusion with just a bone graft. It is important to realize that any such fusion will not produce immediate stability, unlike the methods that use internal fixation. The stability achieved will be potential and will only occur when the graft is fully incorporated. This predicates that external immobilization be applied in all these cases in order to produce the stability required for an appropriately long period of time, i.e. the time required for the incorporation of the graft. This can be achieved with halo casts, halo jackets, or an appropriately shaped minerva-type plaster jacket. Orthotic appliances or braces will not provide the required immobilization and will almost invariably expose the patient to the risk of the establishment of a nonunion or pseudoarthrosis.

The use of free bone graft presents problems here. Bars of bone graft are laid as a bridge between the occipital bone and the first cervical vertebrae. By this method, they are held in place only by the tension created by the closure of the overlying muscle and skin layers. This is not a very practical or reliable method of fusion. While the patient may well be fully immobilized in an appropriate halo, the graft, which is in loose juxtaposition to the bone, will be resorbed and fusion will seldom occur. This is therefore not a recommended procedure.

Fusion with Bone Graft Anchored by Screws. It is relatively easy to undertake fusion with bone graft and screws. The method is used in association with posterior decompression of the foramen magnum or the posterior arch of the atlas. Strips of bone harvested from the external surface of the iliac crest are commonly used, although a full thickness graft from the iliac crest that will cover the entire length of the fusion may also be used (Fig. 9.82). Since bilateral grafts must be used, the full thickness graft can be split in half. This provides a cortical and a trabecular surface. The cortical surfaces of the occipital and cervical vertebral bone are removed using a drill or a fine rongeur (Fig. 9.83). This exposes the trabecular bone of the host bone to the trabecular bone of the graft. Shaping the bed will also provide better seating for the graft and favor incorporation. The preparation of the seat for the graft should include the external surface of the occiput, the posterior arch of the atlas, and the lateral articular masses. Once the graft and the host site have been prepared, they are screwed into place, beginning at the occipital end. This should be within 15 mm laterally from the external occipital protuberance. The hole tapped to receive the screw should have a diameter approximately one half that of the screw. The thickness of the cranial cortex in the occipital region is less than elsewhere and the diploë is thinner (Fig. 9.82). Obviously, both cortical surfaces have to be penetrated and this should be done with great care. We prefer screws with a diameter of 3.6 or 4.5 mm and which barely reach the internal cortical plate in length. It is wise to use an appropriate depth gauge to assess the depth that can be drilled. The length of the screw must also take into account the thickness of the graft as well as that of the remaining internal plate of the occipital bone, remembering that the external plate of the occipital bone has been removed to create a seat for the graft (Fig. 9.84).

Laterally, the graft may extend along the apophyseal masses of C2, C3, or even C4. The screw is best placed exactly in the middle of the masses. This location can be determined by identifying the margins of the apophyseal masses and determining the center between these limits where there will be a slight elevation of the outline (Roy-Camille et al. 1987). This will also be the site of a small vascular foramen and the screw must be seated here. In order to ensure that the screw will not be directed toward the area of the vertebral artery but completely straight ahead (as described by Roy-Camille et al. 1987), experience has shown that a slight 15° inclination laterally is advisable (Figs. 9.84, 9.47).

The two bilateral grafts have a natural curvature that reflects the curvature of the iliac crest; this favors the accurate positioning of the fusion. Nevertheless, it cannot be ignored that the position of the head with regards to the neck may often be predicated by changes brought about by the disease process present. When there is protrusion of the odontoid process or malformation of the spine, the aim of the surgery with the fusion must be to maintain the same position that was present prior to the surgery. Any attempt to change the preoperative interrelationships between the bones and intervening structures may have serious consequences, possibly involving the cord right up to the bulbar level and which may well be irreversible.

Arthrodesis with a Single Rectangular Graft and Wires. A single rectangular graft may be placed along the external occipital surface and down the cervical spine to reach the desired level as low as C2–C3 or C4. The graft is placed like a dowel into its seat (Figs. 9.85, 9.86). In order to obtain a rectangular graft, the external or posterior external surface of the crest and wing of the ilium must be used. Once the graft has been harvested and prepared, it too will be fixed proximally on the external surface of the occiput, either with two screws, as described above, or with a metal wire that is passed through drill holes in the external occipital protuberance approximately 15 mm laterally on either side. The wire is introduced through the drill holes and brought back out through the occipital foramen. It will be brought externally through holes drilled in the graft. The wires are then tied to fix the graft in place on the external surface of the occiput. Distally, the graft is slotted into a seat above the spinal apophyses, and may be fixed with the use of two wires that run under the laminae and exit through the graft. Once tied, this will firmly anchor the distal aspect of the graft (Fig. 9.85).

A modification has been described that will permit the fixation of a large rectangular graft between the occiput and the laminae of the first vertebral bodies through a cerclage placed around the arch of the atlas through the central region of the large graft. When they are tied, they will force one end of the graft into the external theca of the occiput and the other end onto the laminae, thereby producing the fixation (Figs. 9.48 g, h, 9.86, 9.87).

Fusion Using Plates and Screws. A more immediate immobilization can be obtained if internal fixation is used with a combination of plates and screws. Our choice is the use of the plates designed by Roy-Camille. These are L-shaped plates and, once anchored onto the occiput and onto the apophyseal masses, they provide support and fixation (Figs. 9.49, 9.88, 9.89). These are available in various sizes, and their preshaped curvature maintains an angle of 105° between the occiput and the cervical spine. This predetermined angle will keep the head in a fixed position that permits the patient to retain a normal field of vision.

The plates are screwed into place approximately 15 mm on either side of the external occipital crest. Again, the selection of screws that we favor ranges between 3.6 and 4.5 mm. They are inserted after tapping a hole of far lesser diameter than the screws themselves. Before the screw holes are tapped, the plates must be tested in the desired position to assure that the proper alignment and fusion can be achieved. Special attention must be paid to the occipital placement before holes are drilled in the cranial bone. Once the use of the plates has been confirmed, as always, the surgeon must proceed cautiously in tapping the bone. This should be done slowly using a low-speed drill. A sudden maneuver due to over-enthusiastic drilling or because the relative thinness and fragility of the internal cortical plate of the occiput are not taken into account may result in a tear in the meninges. If this happens (as it did in two of our early cases) the CSF leak must be plugged with Spongostan and fibrin glue must be injected before proceeding to insert the screw. Our two cases with meningeal tears were treated as described and there were no postoperative or long-term consequences.

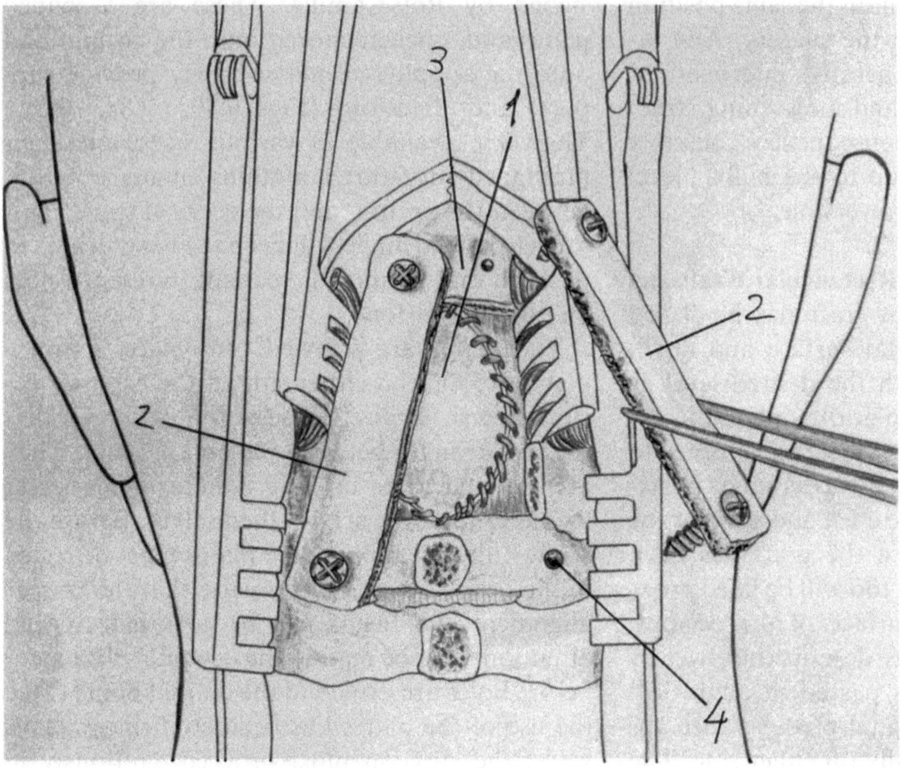

Fig. 9.82. The opening is closed using artificial dura mater or fascia lata (*1*). Fusion with shaped autografts and wires is carried out after decompression. The illustration shows an alternative method in which two bars of iliac crest graft (*2*) are used. They are fixed to the occiput (*3*) and to the lateral mass of C3 (*4*) with screws

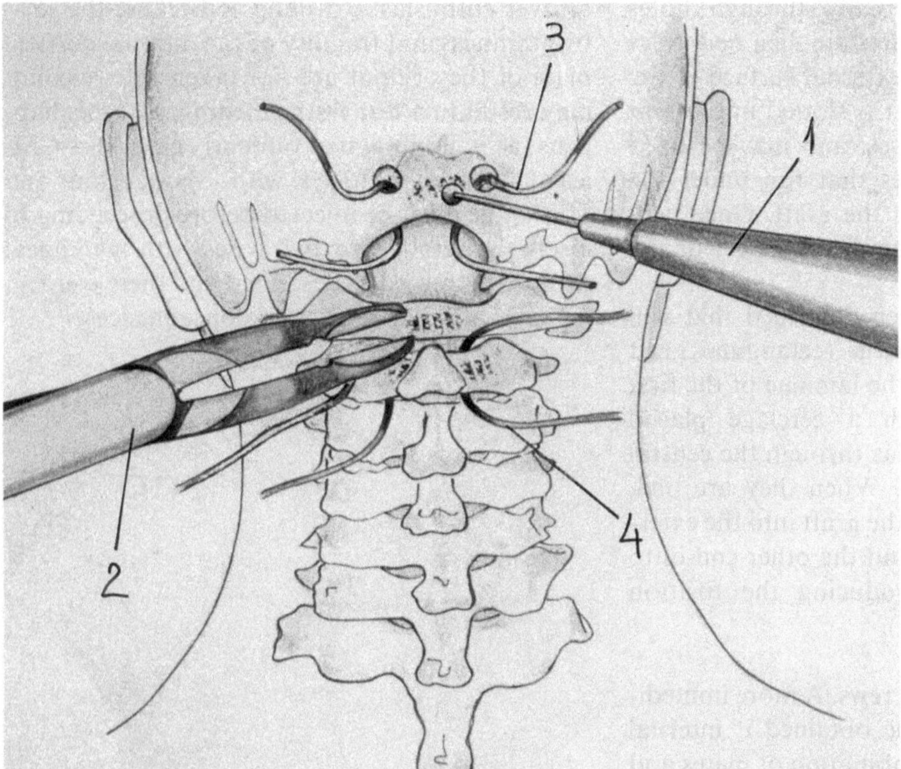

Fig. 9.83. In order to carry out the fusion, the bed for the graft must first be prepared. Using either a drill (*1*) or rongeurs (*2*), the bed is formed in the occiput and in the posterior arches of the atlas and the axis. A metal wire is passed through the drill holes in the occiput (*3*) for superior anchorage, while two other wires are passed under the laminae of the axis (*4*)

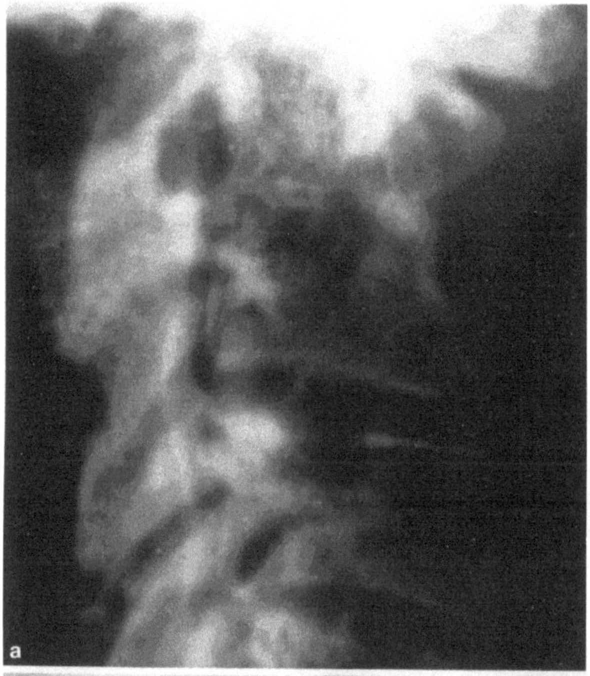

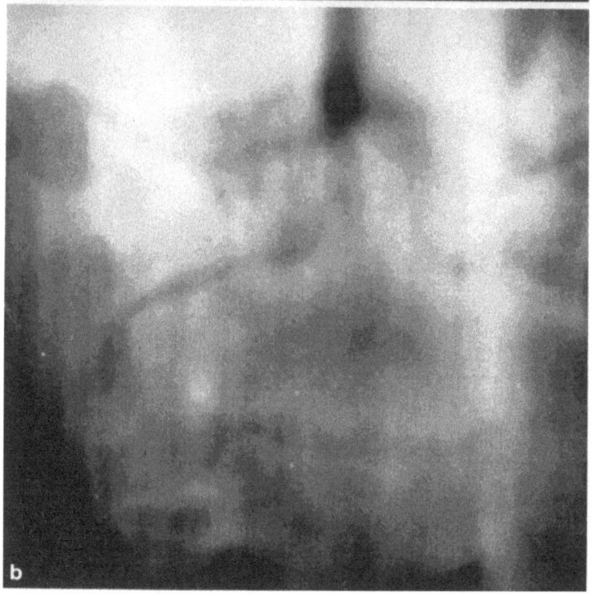

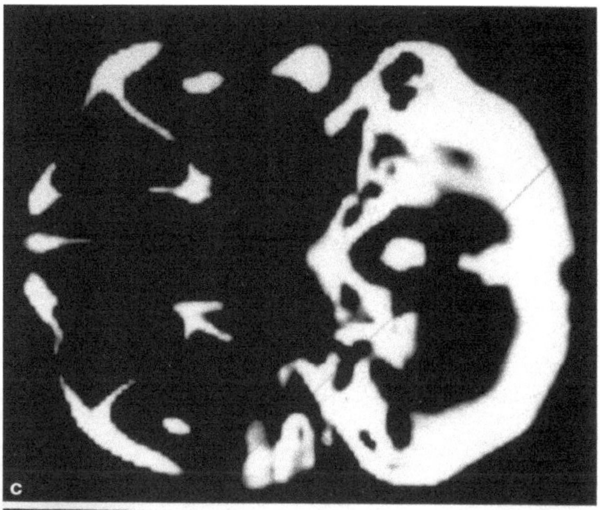

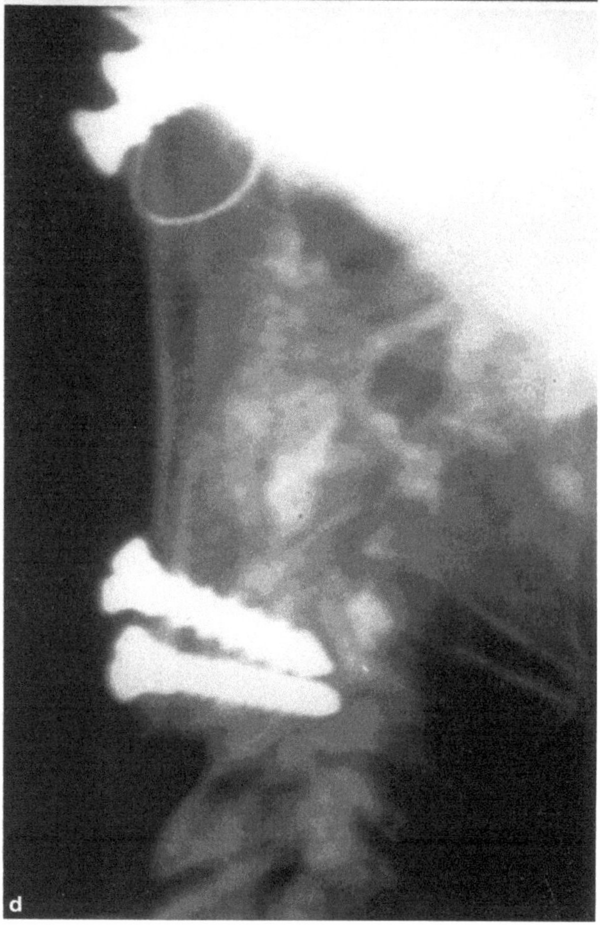

Fig. 9.84 a–d. Radiological imaging in a 54-year-old female patient. **a** Radiograph and **b** laminogram showing that the stenosis is associated with invagination of the odontoid process. **c** Computed tomograph showing the odontoid process within the foramen magnum in association with evidence of instability. **d** Posterior arthrodesis was achieved using two osseous buttresses fixed with screws to the cranial bone and to the lateral masses of C3. This was undertaken after the foramen magnum had been enlarged and the occipitoatlantoaxial membrane had been opened with dural release

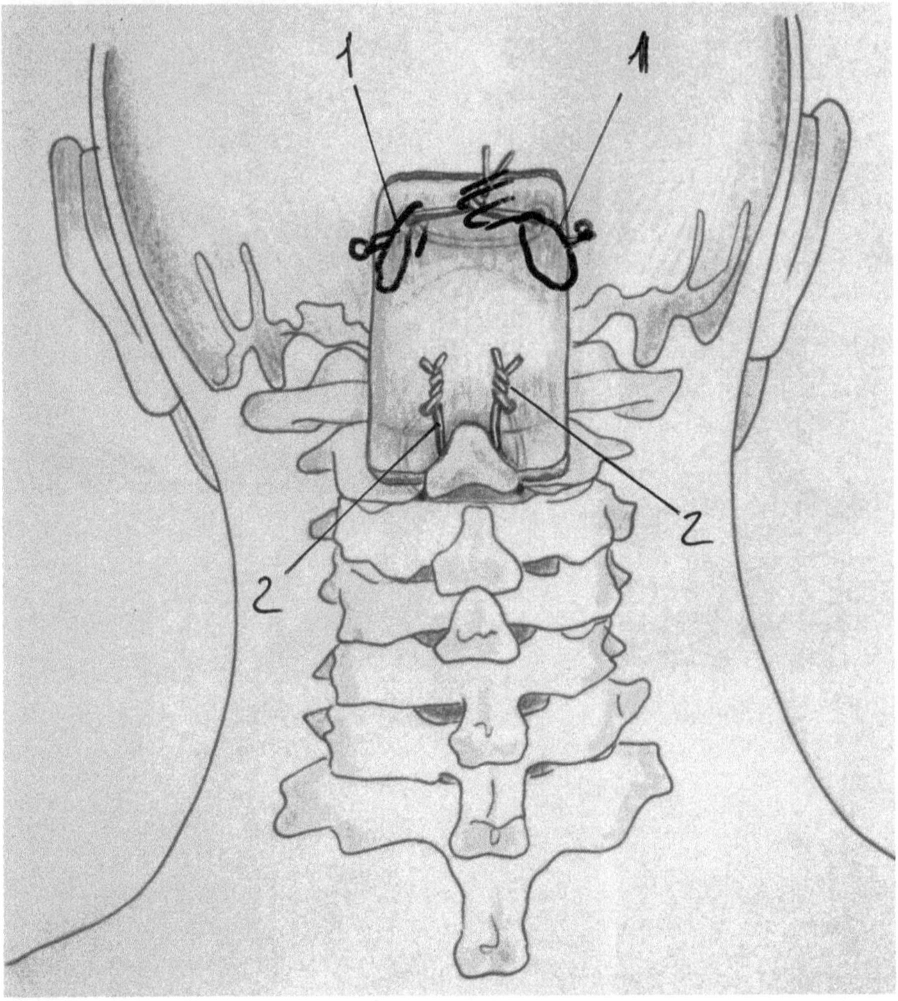

Fig. 9.85. A shaped corticocancellous graft is fixed with metal wires both proximally (*1*) and distally (*2*)

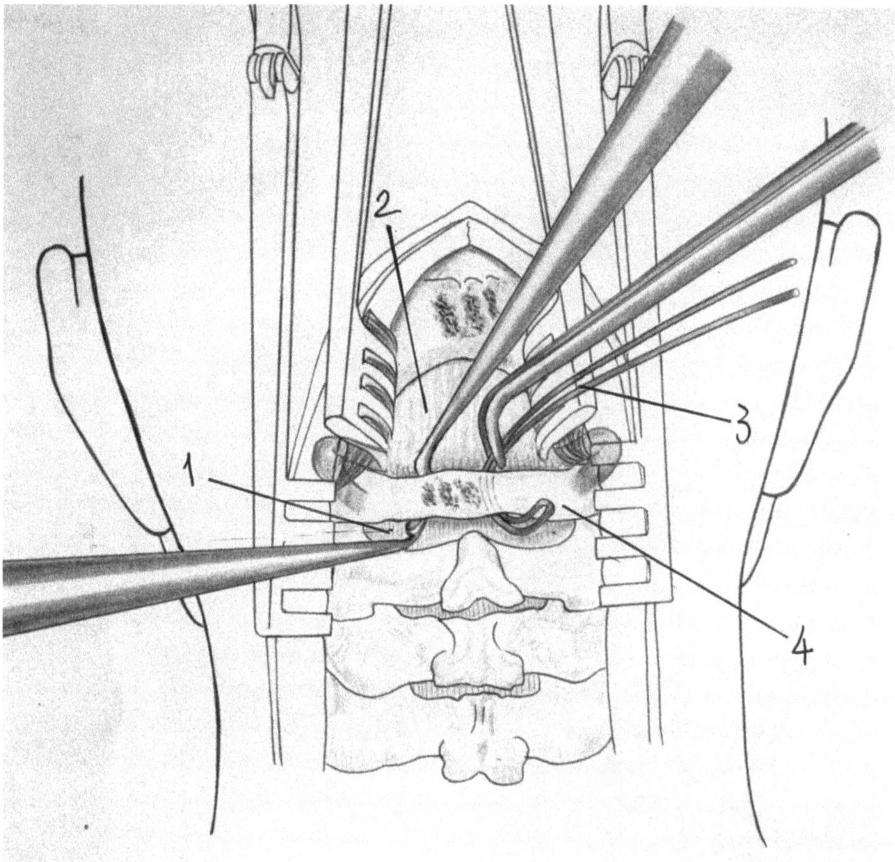

Fig. 9.86. The method of passing the wires under the arch of the atlas. The atlantoaxial membrane (*1*) and the atlanto-occipital membrane (*2*) are detached using blunt curets. The metal wire is doubled (*3*) and slid around the anterior surface of the arch of the atlas (*4*)

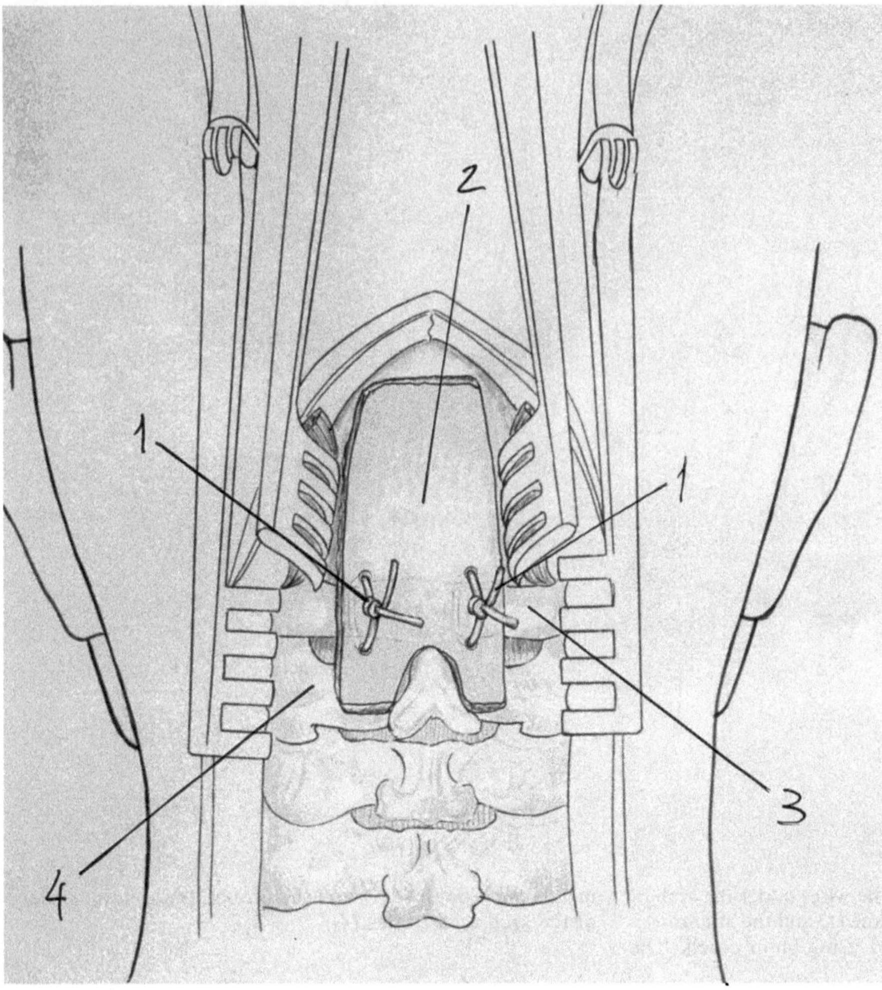

Fig. 9.87. Another method of achieving fusion by fixing the graft with only two metal wires (*1*). The wires passed under the atlas permit approximation of the graft to the occiput (*2*), the atlas (*3*), and the axis (*4*). If this method is used, use of a halo is essential

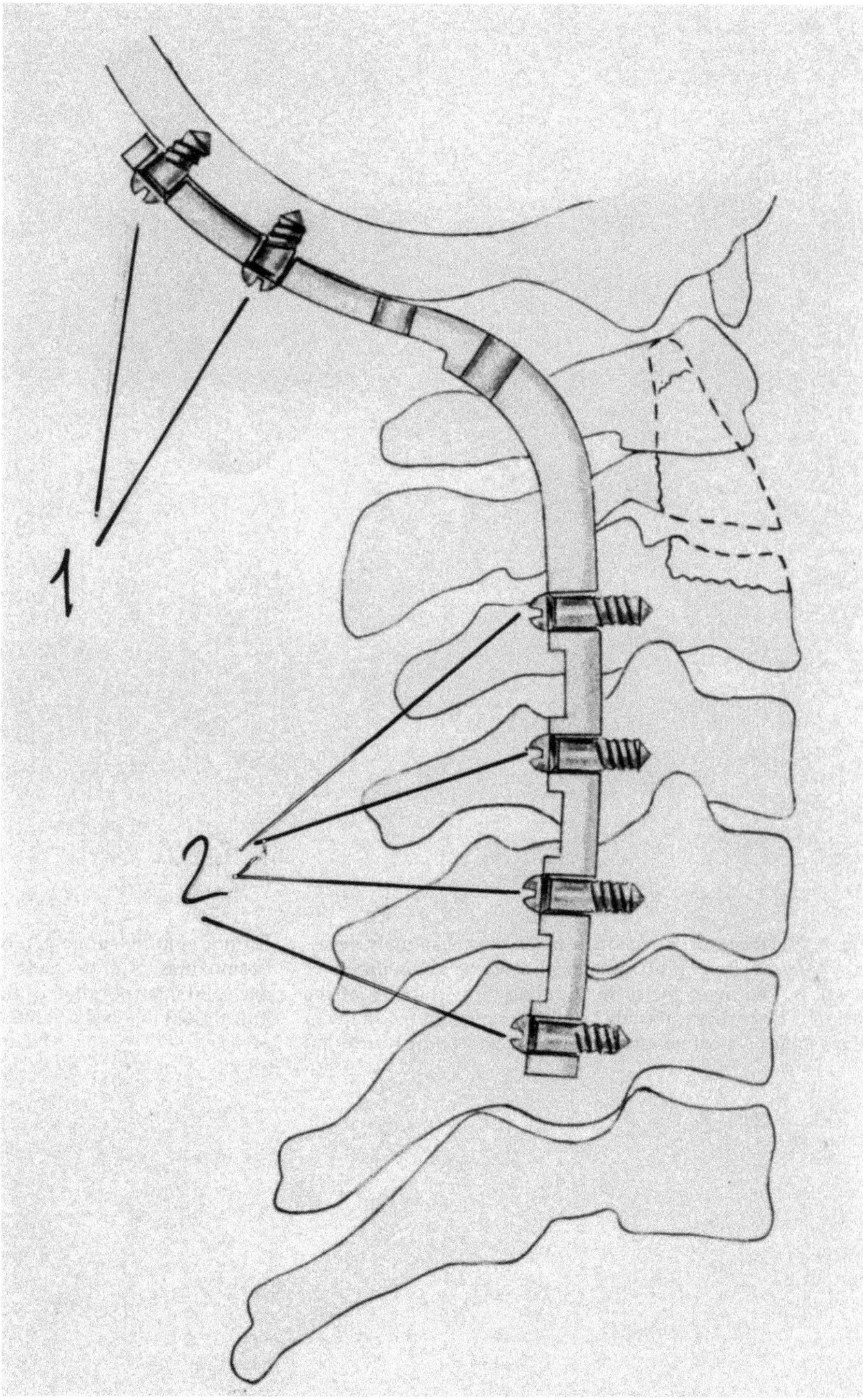

Fig. 9.88. In order to achieve fusion between the occiput and the cervical spine, Roy-Camille plates must be applied in pairs. Fixation is achieved by screws in the occiput (*1*) and in the lateral masses of the vertebral bodies (*2*). The distal extent of the fusion will be decided on the basis of the severity of the instability

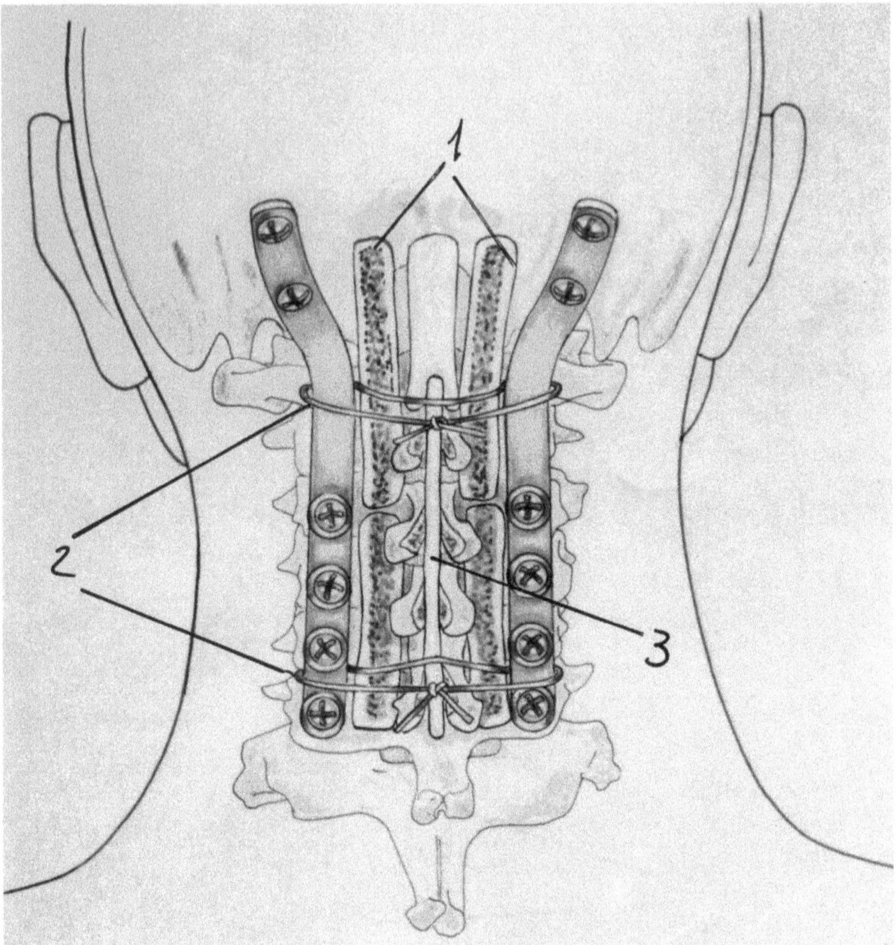

Fig. 9.89. Once the plates are in place, it is absolutely necessary to apply bone graft. The graft must be abundant since it will be the main factor in the long-term stability of the fusion. The corticotrabecular graft is applied in the shape of linear plugs (*1*), which are held in position by ligatures that form a binding suture (*2*), both in the upper regions at the occiput and lower down on the laminae. In order to encourage solid incorporation of the graft and eventual fusion, the graft is laid in a bed created by opening the spinous apophyses (*3*)

Stabilization of the Upper Cervical Spine

A variety of methods have been described by many authors for the fusion and stabilization of the high posterior cervical spine at the levels C1–C3. These basically vary in the type of internal fixation, the type of cerclage, and the length of diffusion. Several methods of internal fixation have been described, including the use of fascia lata, metal wires, and nonresorbable nylon or silk ties. All of these have been used with or without autoallograft bone.

The types of cerclage used also vary:

Simple cerclage is usually a wire or tie passing under the arch of the atlas or of the axis. These however tend not to provide a biomechanically true stability in flexion-extension, or rotation of the head on the neck, as has been well demonstrated by White.

Double cerclage involves cerclage above the posterior arch of the atlas, with the wire or ties anchored lower down in the spinous process or the laminae of the axis. Double cerclage is certainly capable of providing a better biomechanical support than simple cerclage, but does not provide the required and dependable stable immobilization in both the sagittal and horizontal planes.

Single or double cerclage with autograft does provide a more solid anchoring of the graft biomechanically. The grafts are in apposition to or locked into the atlas and the axis in a variety of ways. The top of a single graft (cortico-trabecular) is shaped in such a way as to interlock with the posterior arch of the atlas, while its lower portion sits astride the spinous process of C2. When two cortico-trabecular grafts are used, these are locked on either side of midline onto the atlas and axis, obviously with two wires one for each of the grafts (Figs. 9.90–9.92).

With regard to the length of the fusion, the well-known techniques limit this to the level of C1 and C2 (for lesions involving the atlas and the axis). It is obviously the intention to immobilize the least number of spinal levels. We prefer to use a technique that, in addition to providing fixation and stabilization, permits the reduction of any displacement that might be present in individual cases such as:

- The extension of the fusion from C1 to C3 (not just C1–C2).
- The use of nonresorbable ties. These are softer and may hence be more easily used than the metal wire, which is more rigid and with with there is a greater risk of failure.
- The use of a corticotrabecular autograft from the iliac wing which shaped specifically and accurately to fit exactly from C1–C3 (Figs. 9.50, 9.93, 9.94).

The steps for the basic procedure are as follows: First, the atlanto-occipital membrane and the atlantoaxial membrane must be detached above and below, respectively, to obtain access to the arch of the atlas, around which the tie must be passed to anchor the graft. Then a tress of nonresorbable ties is prepared and slid under the arch of the atlas, using an appropriate curved instrument. After the inspinous ligaments have been released the spinous process of C2 is partially removed. The bed of the graft is given a wedge shape.

The graft is obtained from the iliac wing prior to the procedure. It is then shaped into the appropriate rectangular shape to fit precisely into the upper region of the defect created as its bed and to wedge under the arch of the atlas. A more central groove allows it to interlock with the remaining spinous process of C2 which has been shaped to form the outline of this groove. The lower end of the graft locks astride the spinous process of C3. On the side of the graft, grooves are prepared for the passage of the wire or ties that are used to eventually anchor it in position (Fig. 9.92).

If the graft is accurately placed in this way, the upper end sits astride the posterior arch of the atlas and the lower end is locked astride the posterior arch of C3. On its lower surface the graft adapts to the modeled shape of the spinous process of C2. When it is brought into place by the ties, it is anchored between the atlas and C3 in such a way, that it does not apply any hyperextensive tension between C1 and C2, since its lower end is anchored onto the lower vertebra. In fact, the way in which it sits on the spinous process of C2 supplements the stability produced by the surgery, while maintaining only the desirable degree of diasthesis between the arch of C1 and the lamina of C2. The wire or ties pass over the graft, extend downwards to cross under the spinous process of C2, and, when they are brought up and around the spinous process and out, are tied over the surface of the graft, thereby adding further compression.

The final result is a solid and biomechanically stable fusion in both the sagittal and horizontal planes if the procedure is carried out as described. The atlas is in a good position, with respect to the axis, for fusion without any hyperextension that would result with simple cerclage (with or without bone graft). The latter would not produce an adequate interlock between the laminae of C1 and C2. The only disadvantage of this type of procedure is obviously, that in order to immobilize two levels, three vertebrae are in fact immobilized. Clinically, this may not be biomechanically significant since this procedure is carried out to achieve fusion of C1–C2 in order to prevent the rotatory movement of the neck. The achievement of a biomechanically stable and secure fixation that deals with the clinical situation far overshadows the far less significant loss of mobility between C2 and C3.

The use of nonresorbable ties as opposed to metal wires is also of great advantage. They are easier to work with and can more easily be passed under the arches for anchorage. Once they are fixed, they provide the required tension without the risk of cutting through the arches, particularly of C1 posteriorly, which is a complication with metal wires. Obviously, if this were to happen, it would be impossible to complete this procedure. In order to deal with such a complication, the fusion would have to be extended to the occiput, or alternatively screw fixation of the lateral masses of C1 and C2 would have to be used to obtain posterior fusion. This technique was described by Magerl et al. (1987) and is carried out by first identifying and exposing the posterior facet joints of C1 and C2 completely. The joint is opened and the articular surfaces exposed. Using a Kirschner wire inserted through the joint, all the soft tissues may be upwardly retracted, including the greater occipital nerve and its venous plexus. While keeping the joint under visual control, the screws are introduced from the base of the articular process of C2 in an oblique direction so that they will penetrate the articular masses. The screw will be visible as it crosses the articular space. The use of an image intensifier is essential in following the penetration of the screw and in determining the length of the screw that should be used. Once the screws are in place, the fusion can be completed with the appropriately shaped graft between C1 and C2, which is held in place in the usual fashion by a metal wire.

A further possibility is to fuse the lateral masses of the atlas and the axis using internal fixation as described by Barbour (1971). The approach to the atlantoaxial joint is described in Chap. 8 (pp. 134). Once the atlantoaxial joint has been opened, the articulating cartilage is removed with curved curets until the subarticular bone is exposed. This step is essential to the success of the arthrodesis. In order to fix the atlantoaxial joints, the screw is inserted from the anterolateral surface of the lateral mass of the atlas in an inferoposterior direction. The optimum inclination for tapping the bone is approximately 25° from the horizontal and 10° from the posterior. The use of the probe described by Simmons and du Toit (1978) is very useful in this maneuver. The contralateral side must then be prepared. The head is first placed in a neutral position and then rotated towards the opposite side where the same approach and steps are followed (Fig. 9.95). With this double approach, direct access is obtained simultaneously to the transverse apophysis of the Atlas, the lateral masses, and the atlantoaxial joints bilaterally. Special attention should be paid to the determination of the length of the screw that will be necessary. This may need to be done under fluoroscopy.

Following the fusion, the patient should be immobilized for 90 days. This is a difficult and complex surgical undertaking and the indications must therefore be very specific. Basically, it should be limited to those cases in which it is not possible to obtain posterior fusion and the occipitocervical articulation cannot be sacrificed.

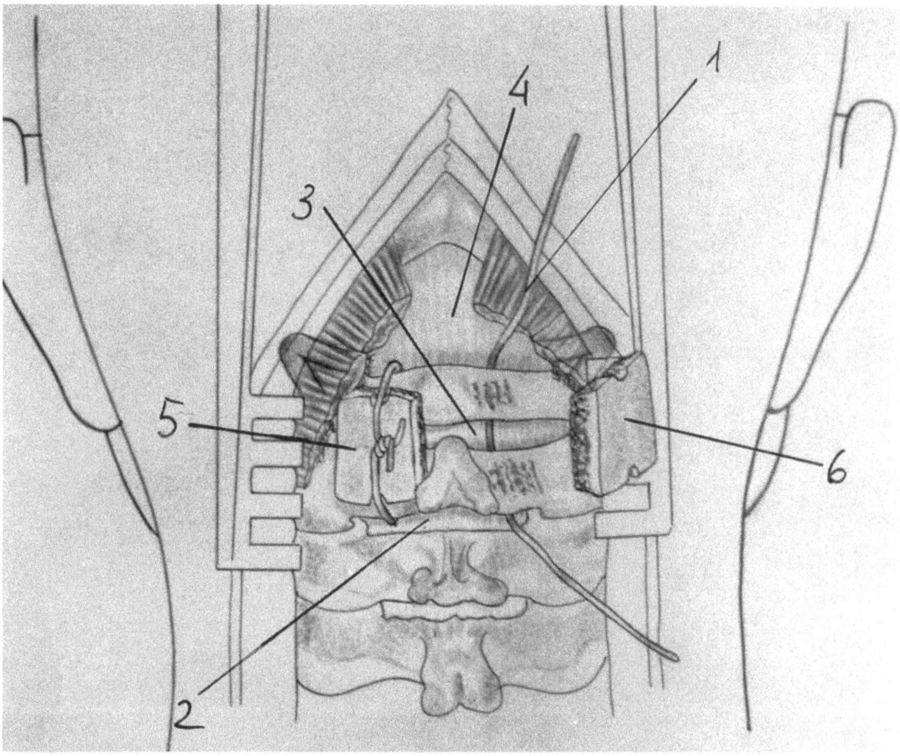

Fig. 9.90. A method of achieving arthrodesis at the C1–C2 level using a metal wire (*1*), which is anchored on the arch of the atlas, passes through the graft (*2*) and then under the spinous process of C2. The prepared graft is shaped to interlock with the posterior arch of C1 in such a way that, with tying of the wire, the distance between the atlas and the axis is maintained (*3*)

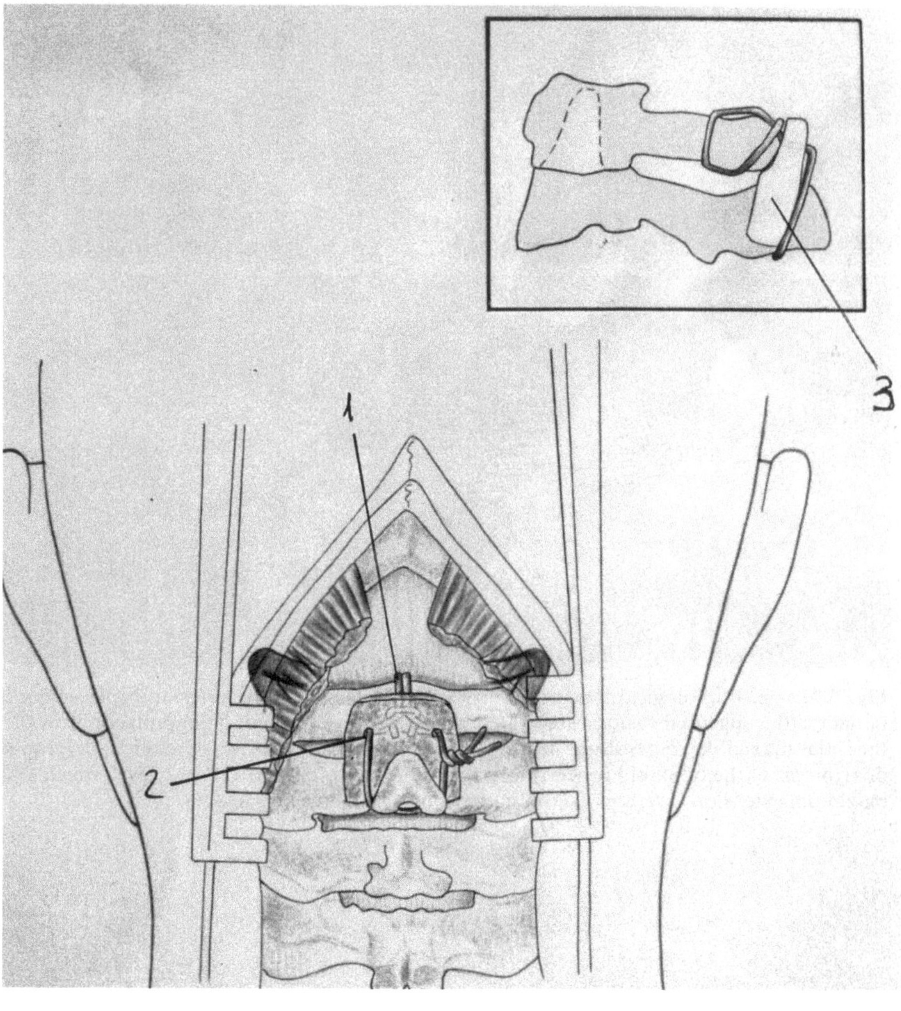

Fig. 9.91. The method by which fusion between C1 and C2 is achieved with grafts that are shaped and fixed between C1 and C2. The metal wire is passed under the lamina of C1 and C2 (*1*) after completion of dissection that includes detachment of the ligamentum flavum from C2 and C3 (*2*) and of the atlantoaxial (*3*) and atlanto-occipital (*4*) membranes. One graft (*5*) is already fixed in place with the wire. A prepared and shaped graft (*6*) is ready to be placed in the host bed once the surfaces have been prepared for fusion

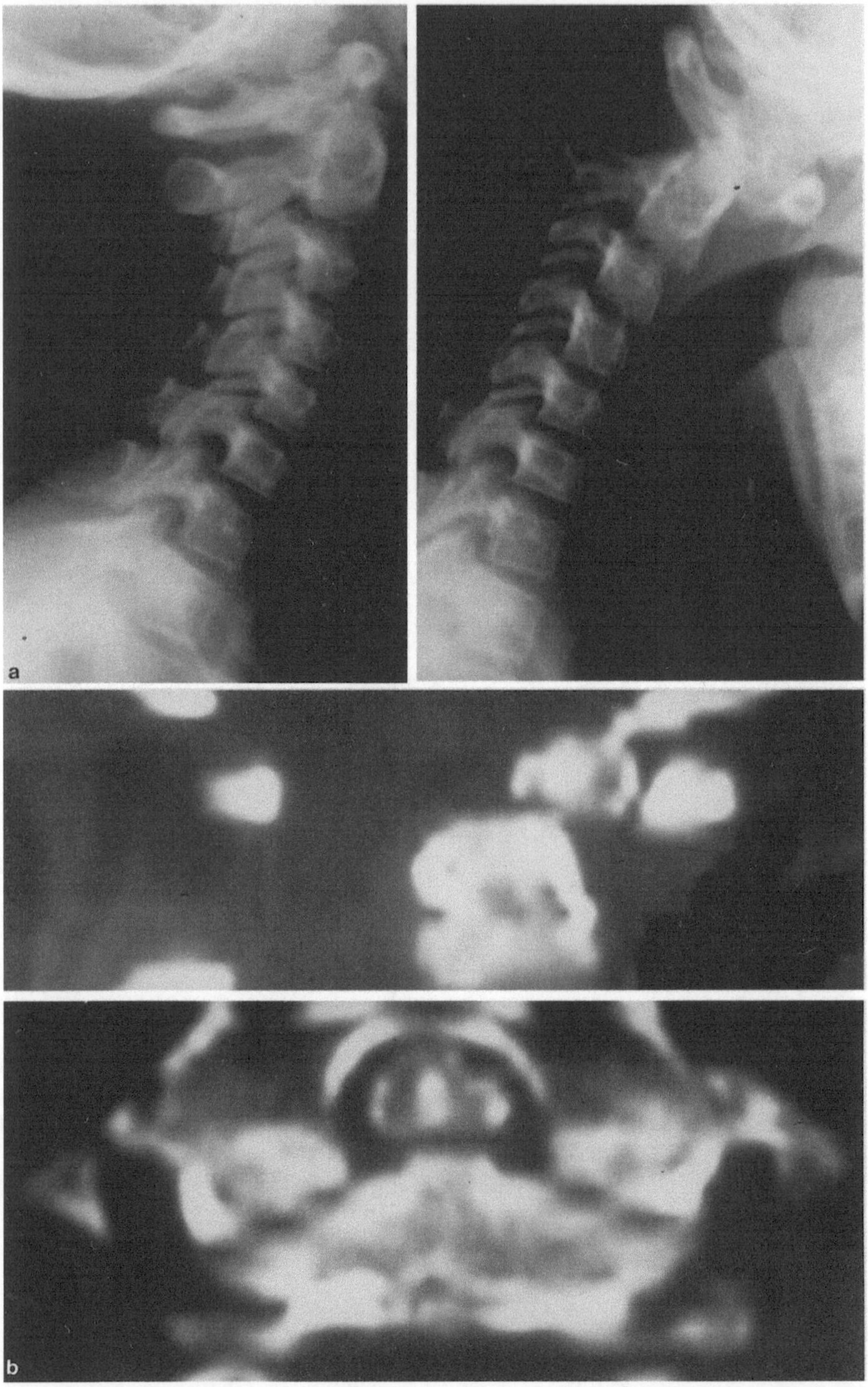

Fig. 9.92a–c. Radiological imaging in a 9-year-old female patient with congenital stenosis associated with instability at the atlantoaxial level resulting from a congenital pseudoarthrosis of the odontoid process. **a** In the radiographs in maximum extension (*left*) and maximum flexion (*right*), note the anterior displacement of the arch of the atlas. **b** Computed tomograph confirms the radiographic images. **c** Postoperative, dynamic radiographic images showing the arthrodesis at C1–C2 level which was achieved using bone graft and wires

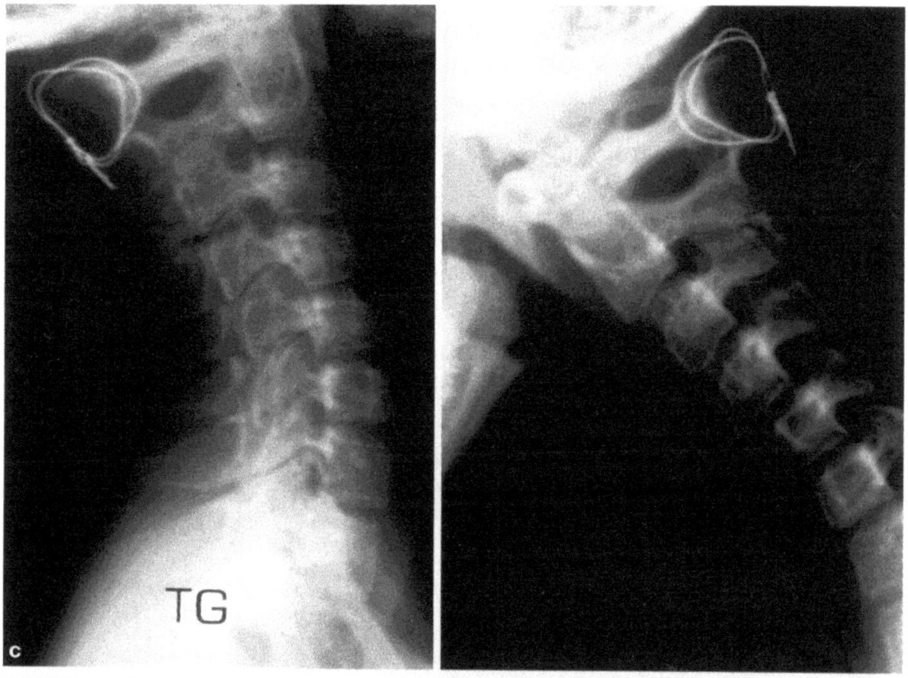

Fig. 9.92c.

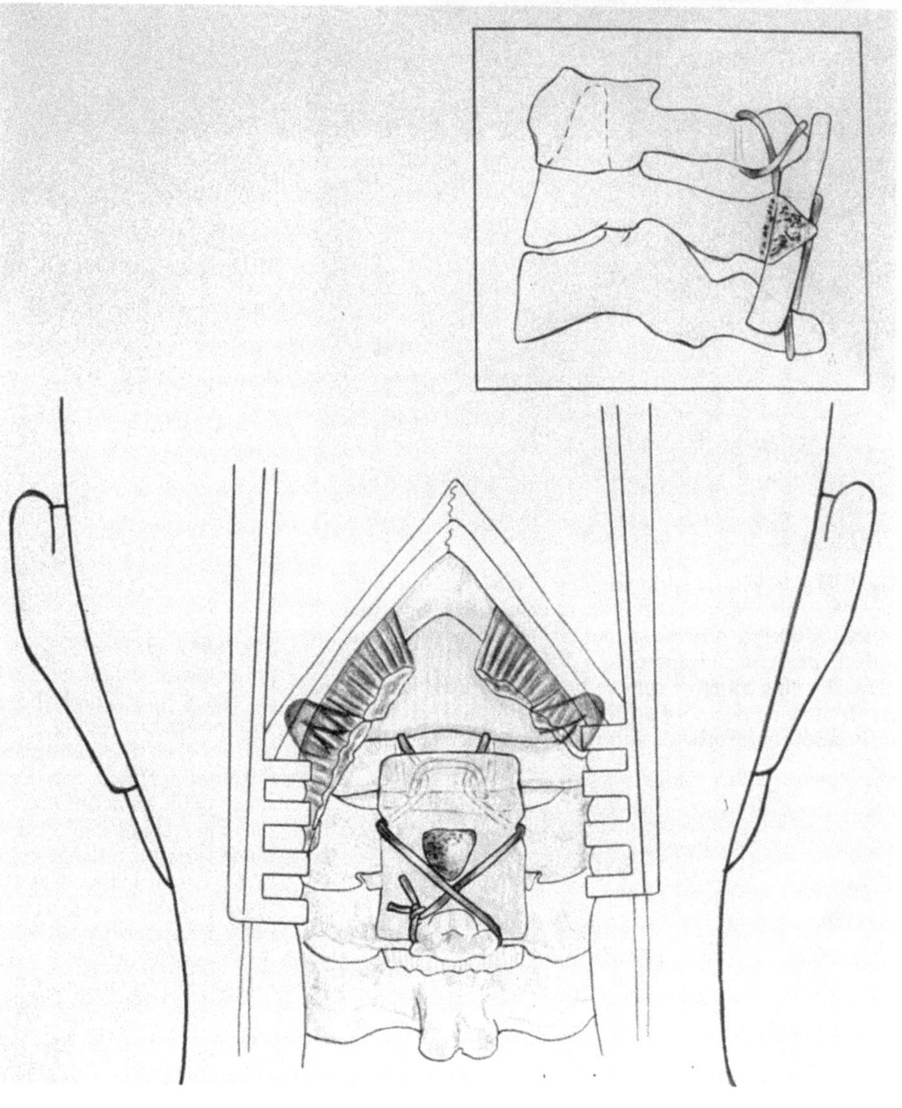

Fig. 9.93. Two views of the positioning and fixation of the graft in fusion of

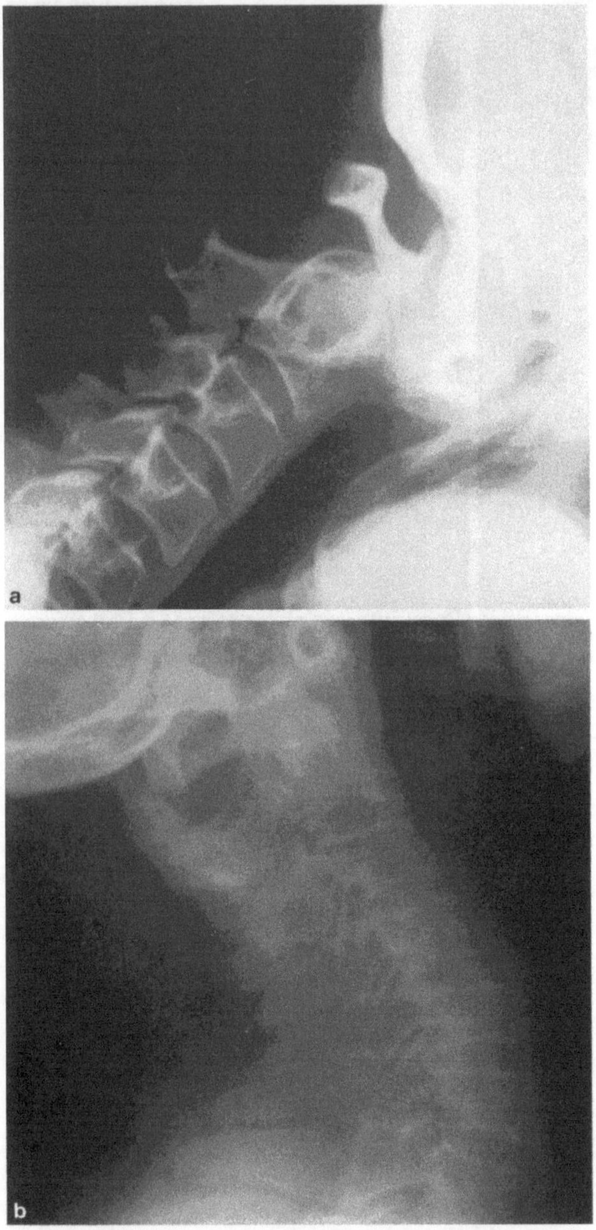

Fig. 9.94 a, b. Radiological imaging in a 61-year-old patient. Post-traumatic stenosis on activity associated with fracture of the odontiod process. Anterior flexion of the head reversed the acute tetraparesis. **a** Preoperative radiographic view, showing anterior subluxation. **b** Postoperative radiograph showing posterior arthrodesis with stabilization, bone graft, and nonresorbable sutures

Fig. 9.95 a–d. Radiological imaging in a 58-year-old male ▶ patient with established pseudoarthrosis of the odontoid process. **a** Radiograph showing stenosis of the cervical canal with posterior slipping of the atlas and the fractured odontoid process. The radiographic views here are in maximum flexion (*right*) and maximum extension (*left*). **b** Myelogram showing the posterior arch of C1 compressing the cord, with the latter being impinged upon anteriorly. **c** Arteriogram taken to confirm the position of the vertebral artery. Fusion of the lateral masses was achieved with screws. **d** Transoral (*left*) and lateral (*right*) views show good position of the posterior arch of the atlas with respect to the occiput and C2. The pseudoarthrosis is reduced with approximation of the dislocated fragment to its base

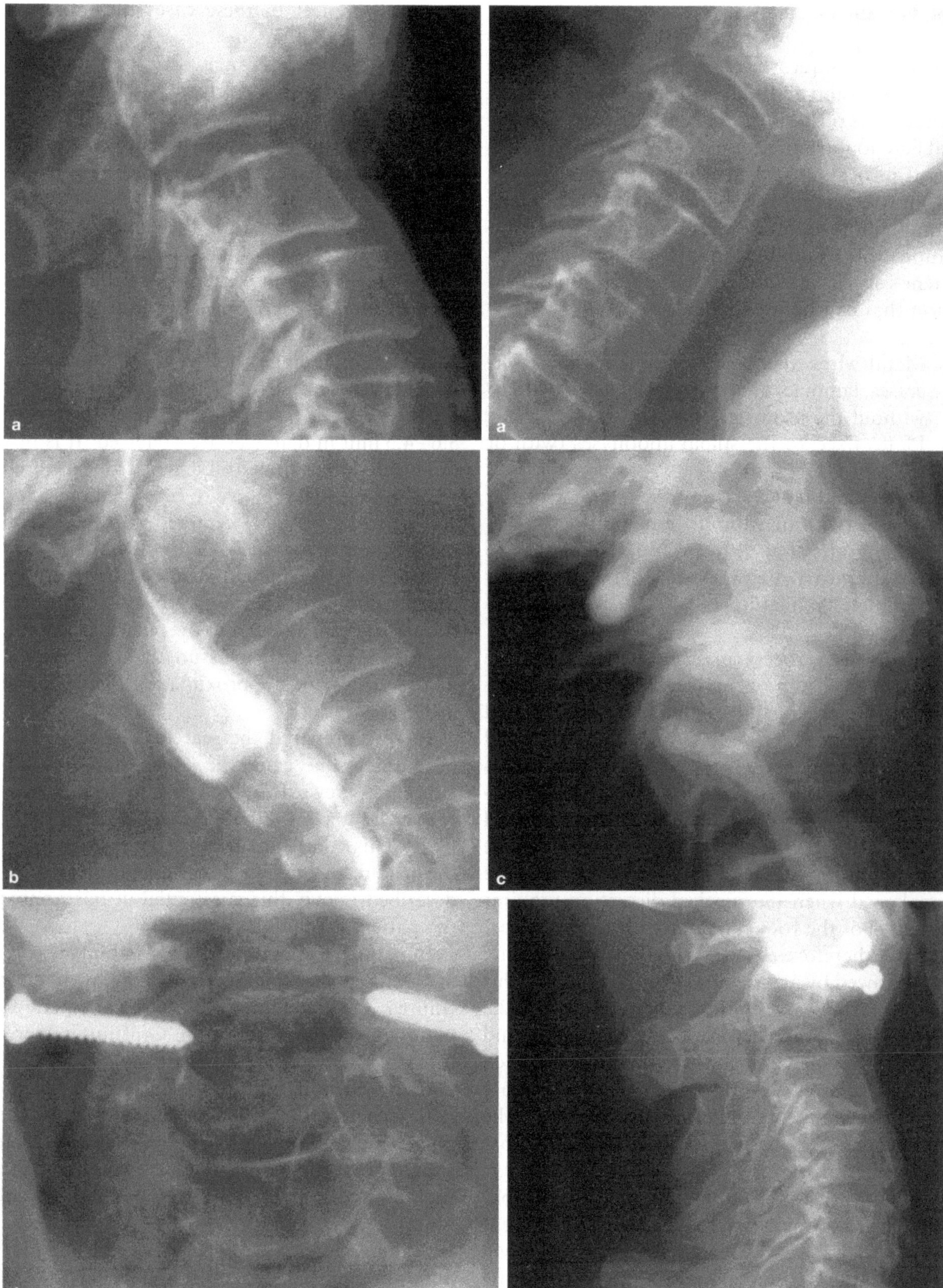
a
a
b
c
d
d

Stabilization of the Lower Cervical Spine

Many techniques have been described for the surgical fusion and stabilization of the lower cervical spine posteriorly. The discussion is restricted here to the more common surgical procedures used in dealing with the instability that results from widening of the spinal canal (postlaminectomy), in posterior decompressions, and in situations of instability that lead to functional stenosis. The methods of internal immobilization that can be used include:

- Metal wires anchored onto the spinous processes, laminae, or apophyseal masses (with or without the use of grafts)
- Plates fixed to the spinal apophyses (with or without bone graft)
- Screws and plates fixed to the lateral articular masses (with or without bone graft)
- Bone grafts shaped to fit and anchored onto the lateral articular masses with metal wires or nonmetallic ligatures

The disease process in each patient and the broader spectrum of cervical stenosis will determine the need and indication for internal stabilization. After wide laminectomy, internal stabilization is needed to achieve extensive decompression of the cord and nerve roots, particularly when the bony dissection has extended widely as far as the lateral articular masses. The lateral apophyseal joints and their supports are weakened when the surgical dissection requires opening of the root canal laterally. In these cases, it is therefore essential that the laminectomy be followed by an attempt at stabilization. If this is not carried out, within a few months of the procedure, severe deformities (swan neck) and instability will be encountered, both of which can be progressive and which will have more severe consequences causing the status of the patient to become worse than it was before surgery.

In these cases, one must rely on the availability of strong and intact structures still present beyond the surgical dissection, which will provide the starting point for any procedure. The lateral apophyseal masses are therefore the preferred choice. In these cases the following procedures can be used.

Plates and screws may be used together with autograft, as described by Roy-Camille (Fig. 9.96). The point of special interest for the purposes of our discussion is the fact that the plates tend to have screw holes placed approximately 13 mm apart, which corresponds to the average distance between the lateral articular masses of the cervical spine. The plates with two, three, four, or five holes are specifically shaped to maintain a predetermined lordosis which can only be modified on the operating table by a few degrees. For tapping the screws, the hole must be drilled much narrower than the diameter of the screws to be inserted there. Again, screws of 3.6–4.5 mm in diameter are preferred. It is recommended that small drill bits (2.8 mm) be used since these allow the hole to be drilled in such a way as to be perfectly centered into the lateral mass. Using a low-speed drill, the holes should be drilled on the characteristic site, i.e. on top of the hill of the articular mass. Obviously, the hole should be perpendicular to the plane of the joint, angled 15° externally to assure that the direction of the drill avoids approximating the vertebral artery.

Having prepared the seat for the screws on both sides, one can proceed gradually to advance the screws. It is important to do this slowly in order to permit the vertebrae to adapt to the plate. This can be assisted by the movement of the head rest from outside the operating area. As described above, this is essential in positioning the patient on the operating table.

In patients being treated for instability associated with stenosis, unlike in patients with acute trauma, the plate alone will not be adequate to maintain the immobilization. Grafting is therefore an essential part of the management. The corticocancellous bone graft is placed on the lateral aspect of the articular masses besides the plate (Figs. 9.51, 9.96). The seat of the graft should obviously be prepared in such a way as to permit good contact of the graft to the subjacent bone.

Stabilization may also be achieved using graft and wires passed through the articular masses (Fig. 9.97; Callahan et al. 1977; Sim et al. 1974;

Stauffer and Kelly 1977; Murphy and Southwick 1989). Since in the primary procedure the lateral articular masses have already been exposed, in spite of the wide laminectomy, immobilization is relatively straight forward and is achieved following the techniques which are amply described in the literature. Basically, immobilization is obtained with using two osseous bars removed from the posterior iliac crest and from the external surface of the iliac wing. Again, as noted, the curvature of the iliac crest and iliac wing are well adapted to preserve the lordosis of the neck. Once the graft has been appropriately shaped, it is anchored onto the lateral masses using wires. A hole is drilled on the inferior apophyseal mass of each vertebra. The anterior articulating facet is protected with a spatula. The holes should be drilled only on the vertebrae that are to be fused. Very fine metal wires or, as is our preference, tresses of nonresorbable ligature are passed through the holes in anticipation of the graft around which they will be tied. Since as a result of the laminectomy that has been previously carried out, the cord and roots are exposed and in full visual control, it is relatively easy and straight forward to undertake the steps that lead to the preparation for the ligature. This would certainly be far more difficult if the laminae were still in place.

The use of an H-shaped graft was described by Murphy and Southwick (1989). Once the laminectomy has been completed, an H-shaped corticotrabecular graft may be placed with the ends astride the spinous processes, just proximal and just distal to the level of the laminectomy. The graft is held in place by wires (Fig. 9.98).

In cases of instability associated with functional stenosis, internal immobilization is also indicated. The circumstances are usually associated with serious and progressive ligamentous disruption or with rheumatoid arthritis. In these cases, one usually expects the osseous components such as the lamina and the spinous processes to be intact. This favors the use of internal fixation through plates or cerclage wires in order to achieve immobilization.

No enyclopedic discussion of all the known or described methods will be described here. Many of these methods such as the use of plates anchored onto the spinous processes have been abandoned because the do not provide sufficient stabilization or provide only temporary stabilization and lead to plate failure. The principal methods which are still in use have already been described. These are the plates and screws method described by Roy-Camille (Figs. 9.99, 9.100) and the articular apophyseal fusion method with autograft. Another method is the use of wires passed through the spinous processes with cerclage and either bone or cement. This technique is obviously best applied in cases of neoplasms (Denaro 1988; Figs. 9.101–9.103).

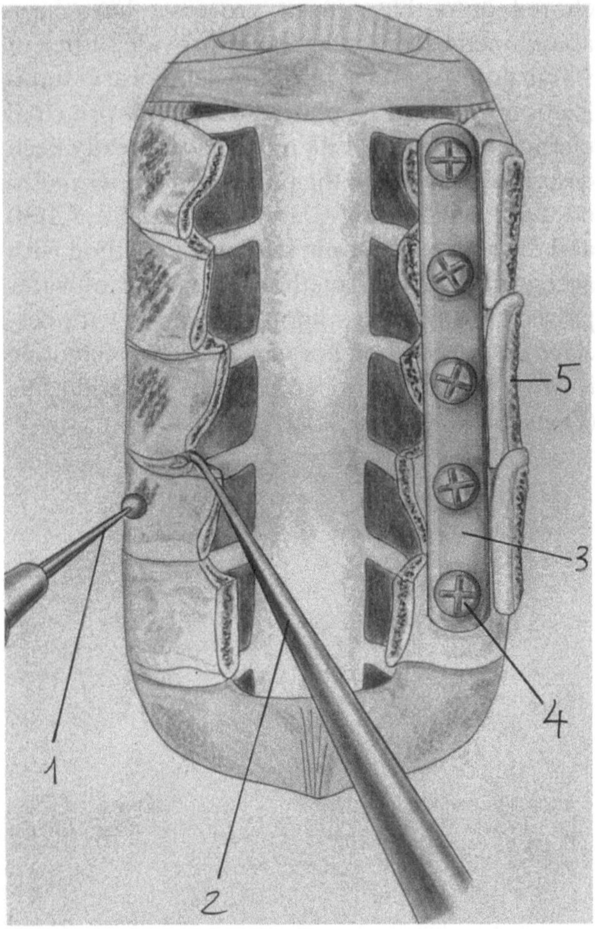

Fig. 9.96. In many cases where extensive lateral decompression is necessary [using drills (*1*) or curets (*2*) to remove a large portion of the lateral masses], stabilization of the vertebral column is essential. A suitable method is the use of malleable Roy-Camille plates (*3*) which are fixed to the articular masses with screws (*4*). In such cases corticotrabecular grafts are placed along the external surface of the articular masses (*5*)

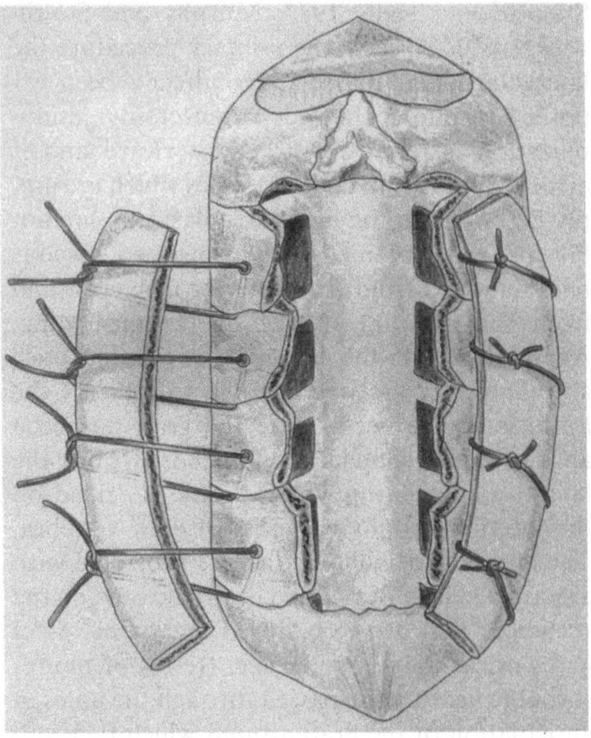

Fig. 9.97. Posterolateral facet fusion after laminectomy according to Murphy and Southwick (1989)

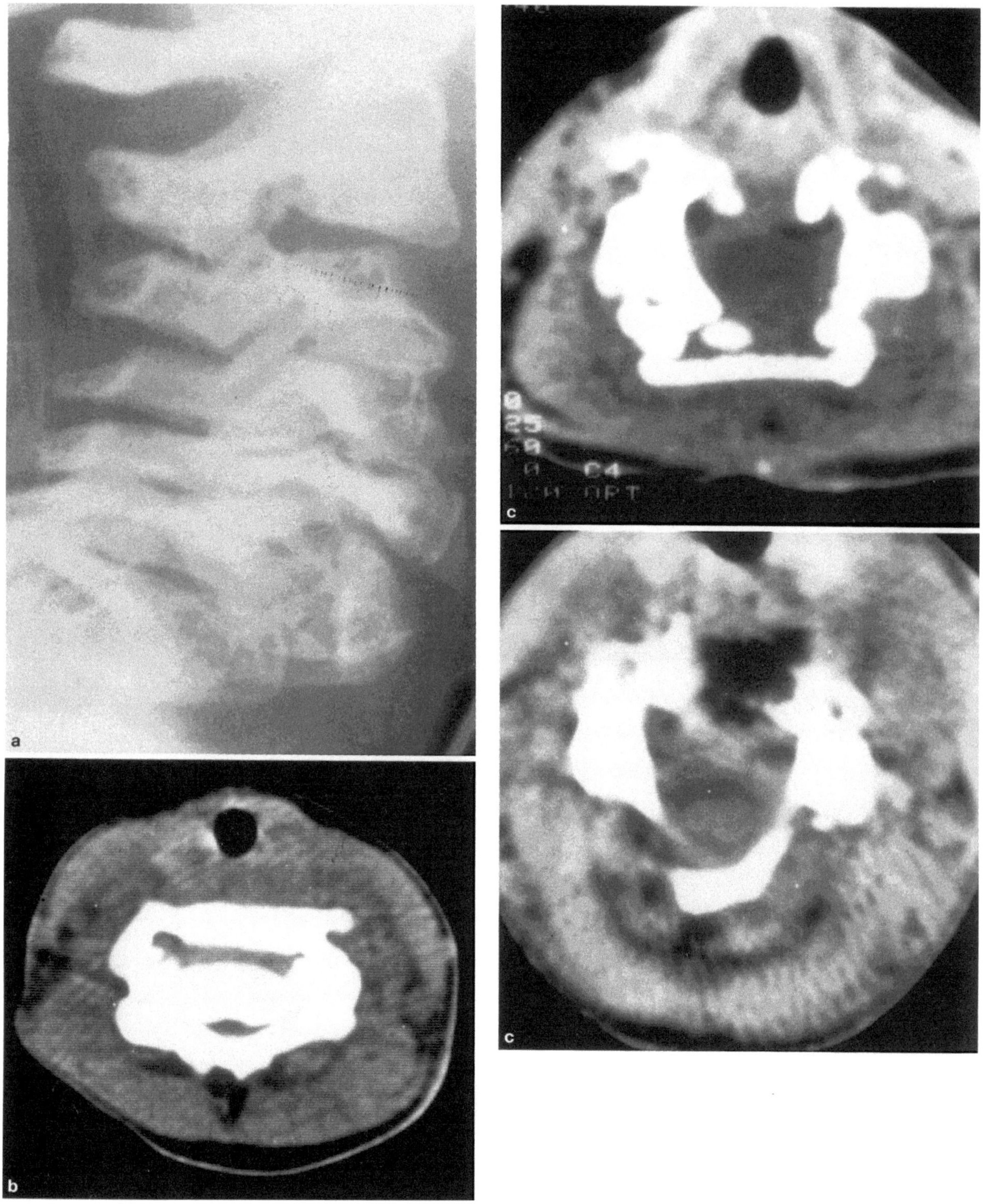

Fig. 9.98. a–d. Radiological imaging in a 4-year-old patient with congenital stenosis. **a** Radiograph showing congenital stenosis and listhesis of the vertebral bodies, with elongated pedicles. **b** Computed tomograph indicating marked stenosis of the canal. **c** Postoperative computed tomographs indicating enlargement of the canal anteriorly and posteriorly. Posterior fusion was obtained using an H-shaped graft. **d** Control radiographs at 3 month follow-up showing maximum extension (*left*) and maximum flexion (*right*). (From Ceciliani and Denaro 1985)

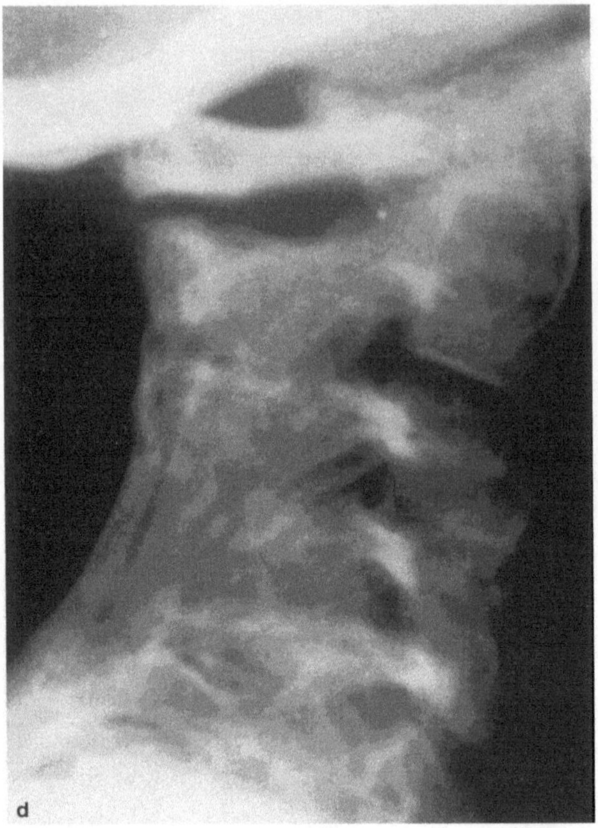

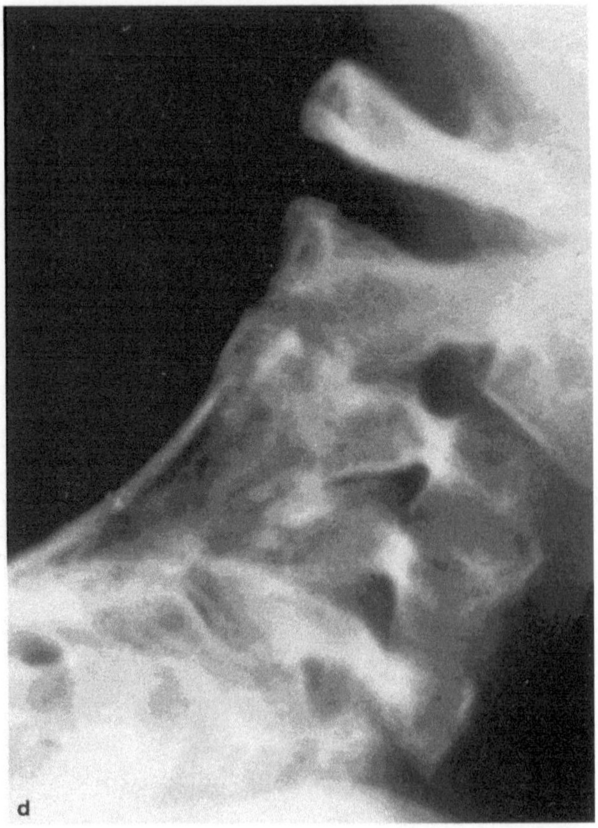

Fig. 9.98 d.

Fig. 9.99 a–d. Radiological investigation in a 26-year-old male patient. Functional stenosis as a consequence of a whiplash injury. **a, b** Dynamic X-rays showing the signs of instability: interspinous widening, facet joint subluxation, posterior disk opening, anterior listhesis of the upper vertebrae. **c** Posterior stabilization using Roy-Camille plates screwed onto articular masses and bone graft. **d** X-rays taken 1 year later, showing fusion by arthrodesis and partial reabsorption of a bracket protruding from C6 ▶

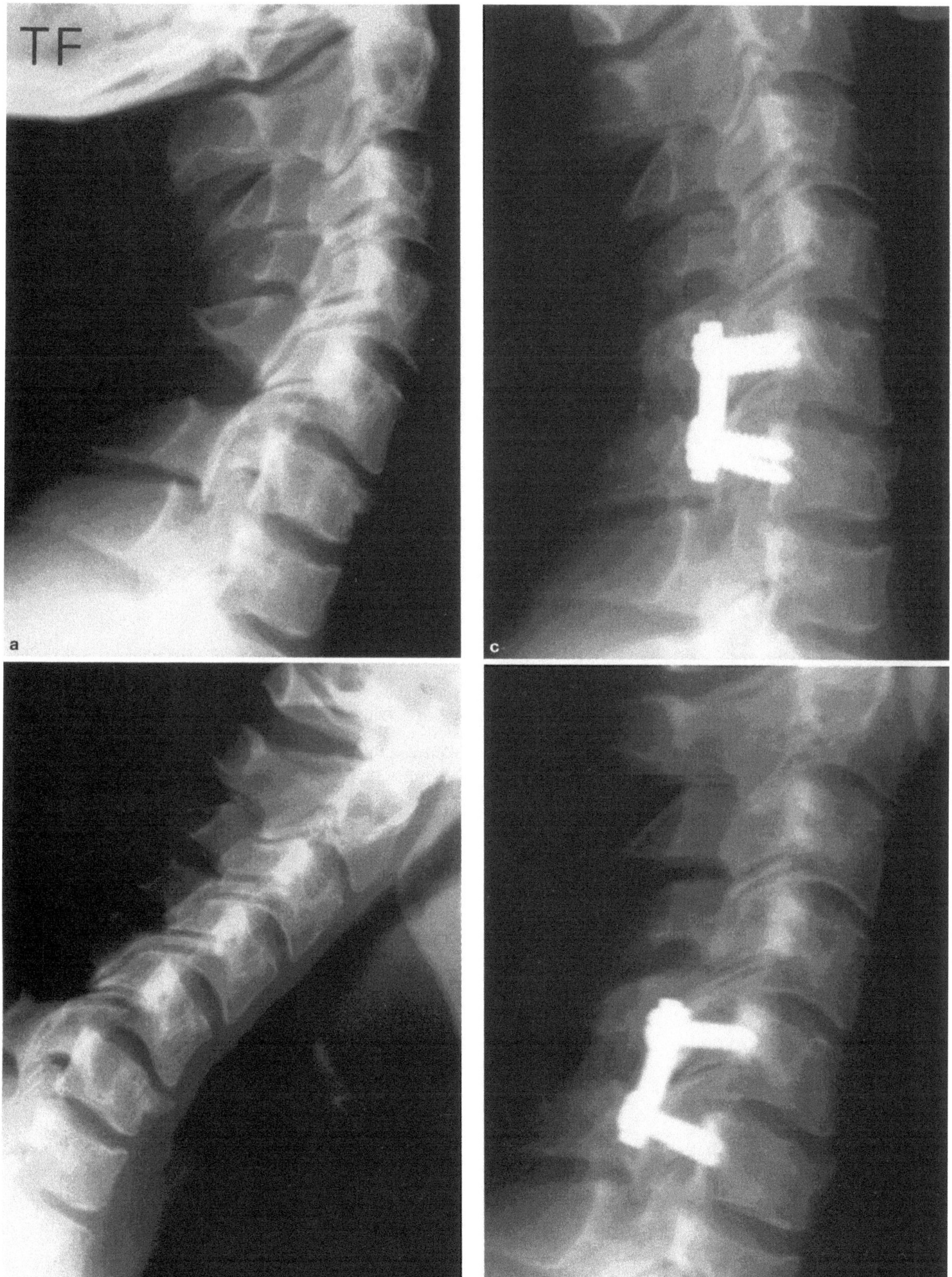
TF
a
b
c
d

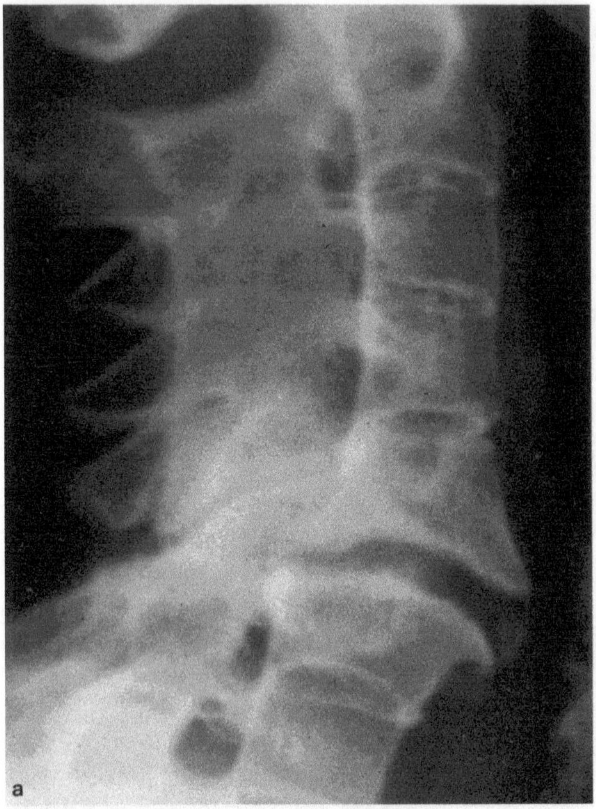

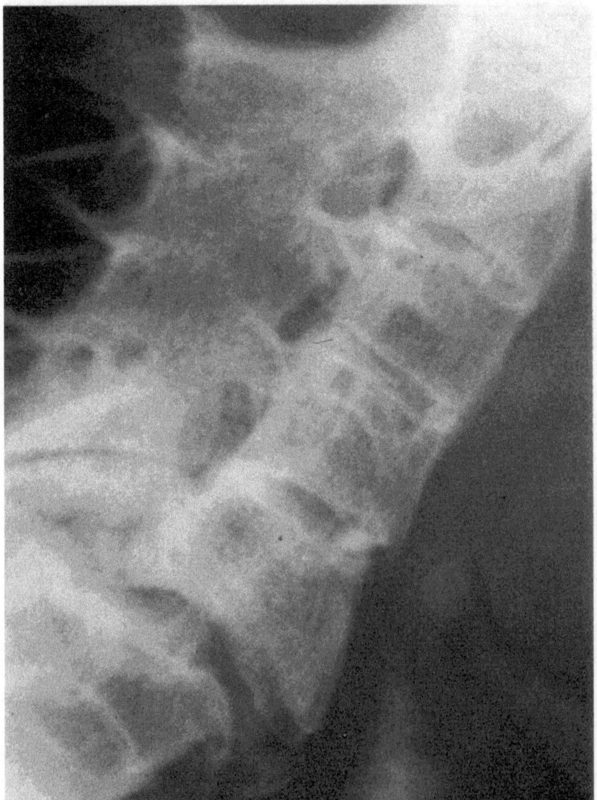

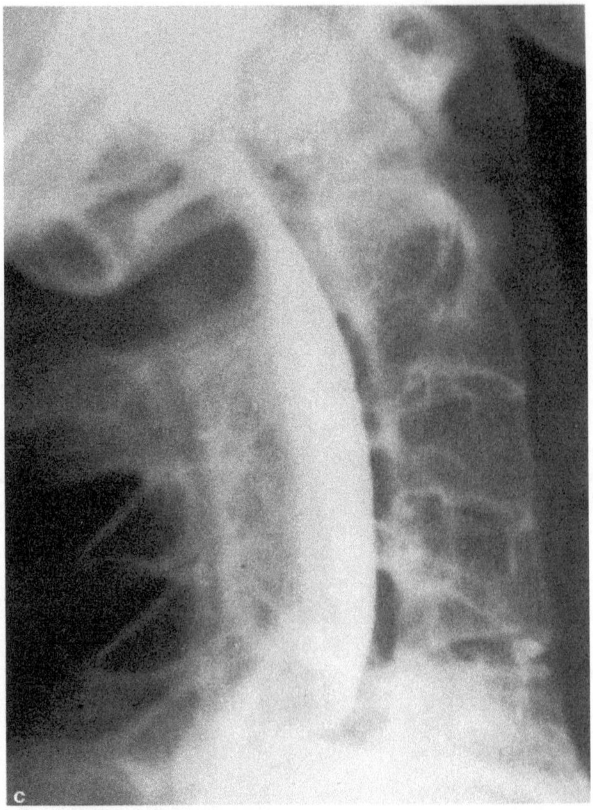

Fig. 9.100 a–d. Radiological investigation of ankylosing spondylitis in a woman aged 41 years who was treated using a combined anterior and posterior approach. **a** The ankylosing spondylitis can be seen on the radiograph. The stenosis is of a combined pathogenesis and involves the C5–C6 level. **b** View in flexion shows worsening of the stenosis. **c** This is confirmed by myelogram in flexion. The surgical procedures were carried out at one sitting. First, the posterior stabilization was carried out with two Roy-Camille plates. **d** After this and using an anterior approach (presternocleidomastoid) decompression with Cloward instrumentation was performed. This involved the removal of the posterior osteophytes and fusion using graft and stabilization with plates and screws. The postoperative myelogram shows that decompression and widening of the canal have been achieved

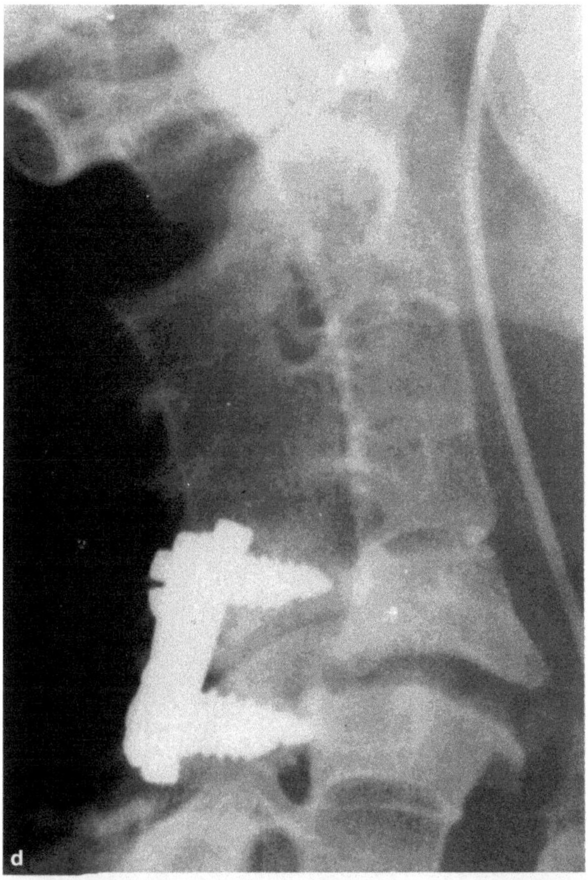
d

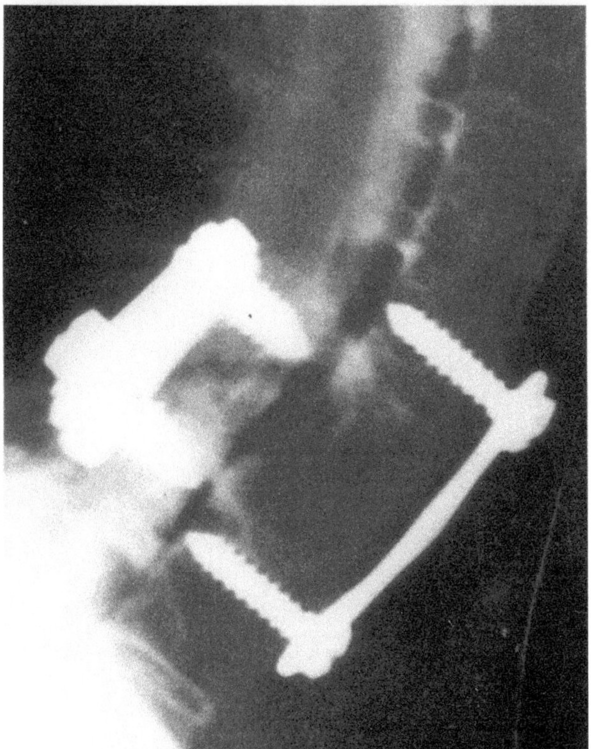
d

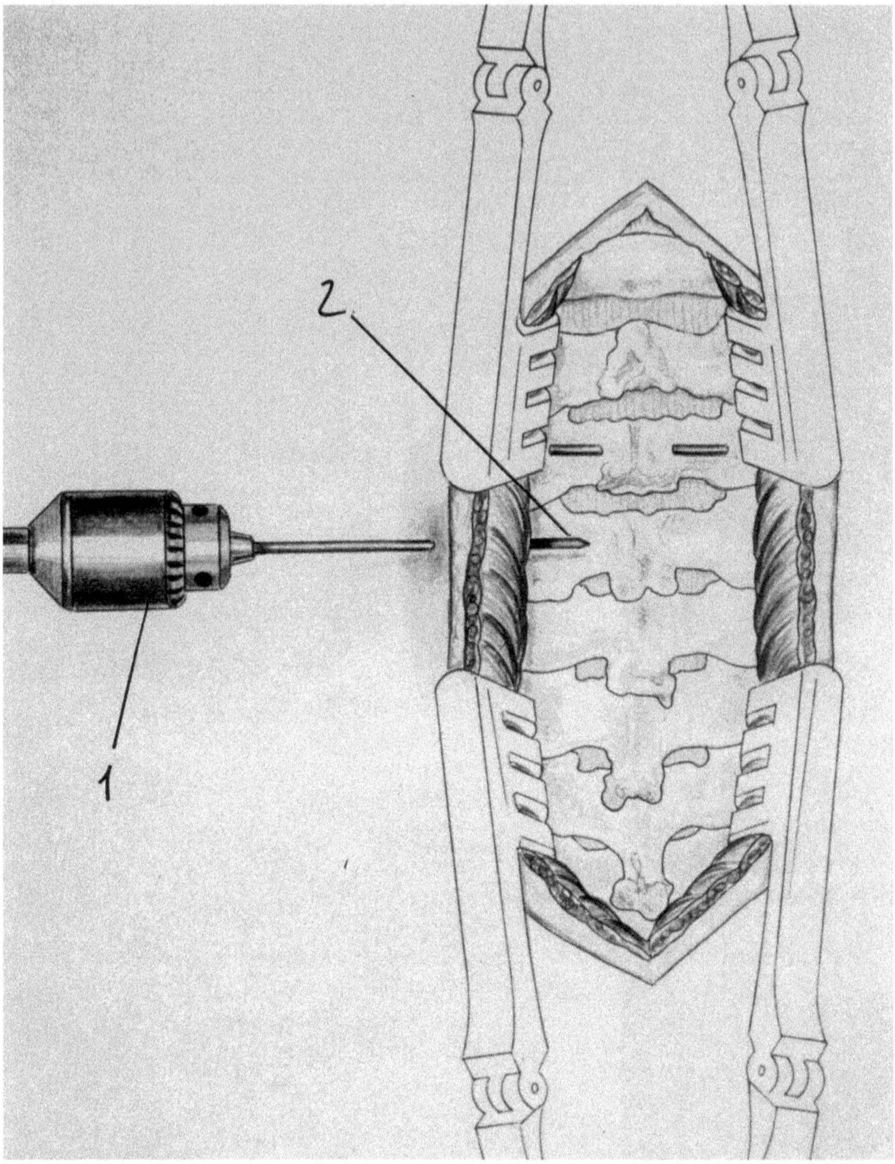

Fig. 9.101. Kirschner wires (*1*) are passed transcutaneously in a transverse direction, through the bases of the spinous process (*2*) of the region to be stabilized

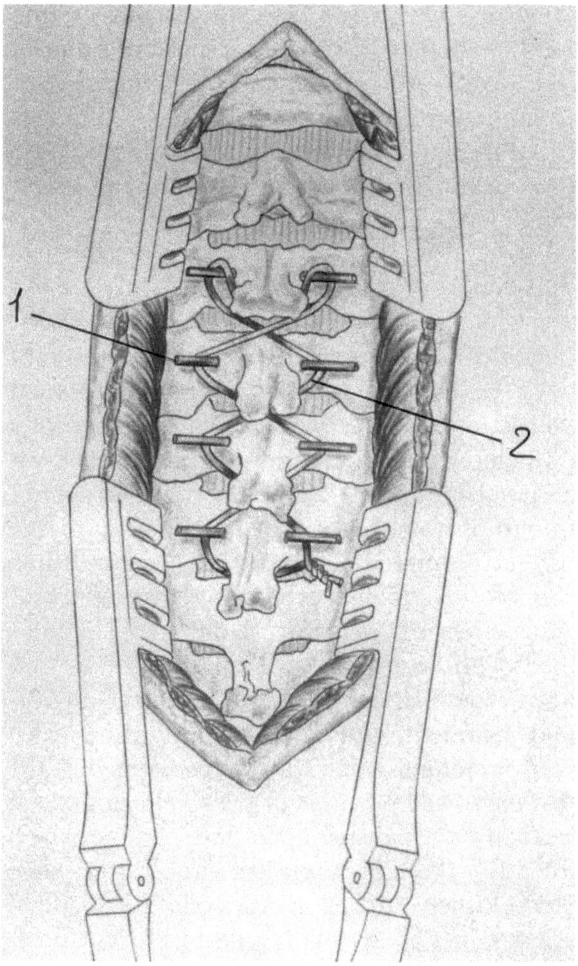

Fig. 9.102. Kirschner wires (*1*) are cut and pulled together by means of figure-of-eight wiring (*2*)

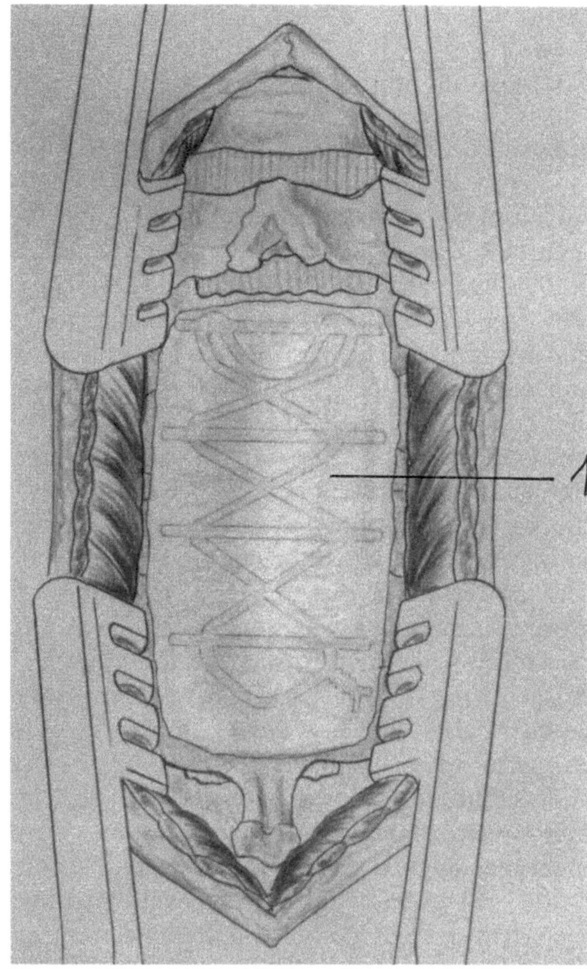

Fig. 9.103. Further stabilization is achieved using acrylic cement (*1*), moulded to the laminae and spinous processes with wires enclosed

Expansive Open-Door Laminoplasty

H. Hirabayshi and K. Satomi

Extensive cervical laminectomy has usually been performed in the treatment of cervical radiculomyelopathy due to cervical canal stenosis, spondylosis, ossification of the posterior longitudinal ligament, and spinal cord tumor. In 1986, a new procedure for cervical laminectomy was introduced by Miyazaki and Kirita as a safer method of posterior decompression of the spinal cord. This procedure consists of simultaneous middorsal division and excision of the laminae, which have previously been thinned with an air drill to prevent the spinal cord from being compressed at the upper laminar edge. In fact, the results of these operations have been improving in Japan ever since the air drill was introduced to be used for laminectomy, replacing the ordinary rongeur. Other authors (Hirabayshi et al. 1972), however, reporting on the long-term (over 10 years) follow-up of 54 laminectomized patients with cervical disk lesions, noted that the patients' symptoms were sometimes aggravated by relatively mild acute trauma to the neck and by the development of osteoarthritic changes in the laminectomized spine. Moreover, postlaminectomy malalignment of the cervical spine was found in 43% of the laminectomized patients in our clinic 20 years ago (Fig. 9.104, Arima 1969).

In order to avoid such postlaminectomy disadvantages as postoperative fragility of the cervical spine owing to acute neck trauma, posterior spur formation on the vertebral body, and malalignment of the cervical lateral curvature, all of which may constitute new pathology supplementing the original disorders, a new surgical technique called expansive open-door laminoplasty was devised by Hirabayashi in 1977 to replace ordinary laminectomy of the cervical spine (Hirabayashi 1978, 1987; Hirabayashi et al. 1981). Hirabayshi observed pulsation of the dura mater at the open-door stage of the laminectomy prior to removing the laminae en bloc. Since then, we have routinely used expansive open-door laminoplasty for posterior decompressive surgery (Fig. 9.105).

In 1973 Oyama and Hattori (see also Oyama et al. 1987) first introduced expansive laminoplasty to prevent postlaminectomy invasion of the laminectomy membrane (Fig. 9.105). This procedure has not been widely accepted because of the technical difficulties of the operation.

Indications

The indications for expansive open-door laminoplasty are the same as those for ordinary cervical laminectomy, i.e., cervical spinal canal stenosis in which the anteroposterior diameter of the spinal canal is under 12 mm, as shown in lateral radiographs, continous type ossification of the posterior longitudinal ligament, and multiple spondylotic lesions over four intervertebral spaces. In cases of spinal canal stenosis combined with localized spondylotic lesions and mixed type ossification of the posterior longitudinal ligament, anterior decompression with anterior spinal fusions may be performed at the most narrowed portions of the spinal canal 3–4 weeks after expansive open-door laminoplasty. Recently, the laminoplastic procedures have been routinely applied in cases of cervical spinal cord tumor and syringomyelia to prevent postoperative malalignment in the cervical spine. For lesions localized lateral to the spinal cord such as hourglass tumors, ordinary open-door laminoplasty is indicated. For lesions localized middorsally, bilateral open-door laminoplasty with mid-dorsal splitting is indicated since it provides the amount of intra- or extradural space necessary to remove the tumor (Fig. 9.106) and set the shunt tube into the syrinx as a drain for the cerebrospinal fluid.

Technique

The patient is placed in a prone position, tilted cranially upwards at an angle of 30° to minimize blood loss from congestion during surgery. The neck is flexed and the nuchal level maintained horizontally. In this position, care must be taken to assure that the patient's eyeballs are not compressed by the face support frame. A median approach between the paraspinal muscles must be performed correctly to minimize local bleeding. The prominent spinous processes of C6 and C7 are the landmarks of the midline and may be identified by palpation. The neck muscles should be separated from the spinous processes and laminae with a raspatory. During this procedure, the surgeon must retract the muscles so that the operative field may be sufficiently developed laterally.

A recent development of this technique is not to cut the spinous processes at all in order to preserve the inter- and supraspinous ligaments (Fig. 9.107a), and to drill bony gutters bilaterally along the medial margin of the facets. Holding the drill firmly with both hands, the surgeon makes a preliminary bony gutter as a guideline on the side to be opened. This bony gutter is then cut down gradually with a cutting bur (Fig. 9.107b). During these procedures, bone wax should be rubbed effectively onto the spongy bone to stop any osseous bleeding. It is safer to deepen the bony gutter with a diamond bur rather than a steel bur to avoid damaging the dural tube. After the medial side of the bony gutter has been thinned enough to be cut with a thin-blade Kerrison rongeur, the exposed portions of the ligamentum flavum between the laminae at both upper and lower ends of the laminoplasty are removed hemilaterally. Then the medial walls of the bony gutter are completely resected with the Kerrison rongeur on the open side. Prior to beginning the procedures on the hinge side, the base of the spinous process below the lower end of laminar door is partially resected using a drill, and the tip of the process is pushed towards the hinge side to preserve the inter- and supraspinous ligaments.

The bony gutter on the hinge side is then drilled slightly more lateral than on the open side to prevent the laminar hinge from being unstable or disjointed (Fig. 9.107c). After a preliminary bony gutter has been made, the spinous processes are pushed tentatively to check the stability of the hinge. If the medial wall is too thick for the laminae to be opened, this cortex should be redrilled thinner with the diamond bur. When the laminar door is ready to be opened, stay sutures which prevent the door from being closed are stitched through the bases of the spinous processes, the deep muscles, the capsules around the facets, and through a small intraosseous hole at the facet of the hinge side (Fig. 9.107d). It is very difficult to do this after opening the laminar door.

The laminar door is then opened. The resected border of the laminae is elevated, like opening a door, using a large Kerrison rongeur as if the corner of the retractor were the fulcrum of a lever (Fig. 9.107e). When each lamina has been elevated, the remaining ligamentum flavum and any adhesive fibrous band between the dura mater and the inner surface of the laminae are divided with scissors from the open side. At the final stage, the stay sutures are tied around the bases of the spinous processes through the ligamentum flavum to keep the laminar door open (Fig. 9.107f). Until now there have been no known cases in which these procedures could not be completed because of severe adhesion between the dura mater and the inner surface of the laminae. However, venous bleeding from the epidural space has been experienced in some cases with severe stenosis of the spinal canal.

The dural pulsation can now be seen. This indicates that the enlargement of the spinal canal is sufficient for posterior decompression of the compressed spinal cord without removing the laminae (Fig. 9.108). Postoperatively, the patient should be kept in bed for 2–5 days and then should ambulate with a cervical brace for 3–6 months.

Patients

We have so far operated on a total of over 150 patients with this method; the follow-up period was a maximum of 11 years and on average 4 years. Of a total of 90 patients, 55 had ossification of the posterior longitudinal ligament, 22 had spinal canal stenosis, and 13 had multiple level spondylosis. The range of laminoplasty extended from C2 to T1, the levels between C3 and C7 being the most frequent in this series. The average operation time was approximately 1.5 h (20 min per lamina). The average blood loss was 450 ml in each operation, and 90 ml per lamina.

Operative results were estimated by the recovery rate of activity according to daily living criteria (Japanese Orthopedic Association, JOA, score) which have been established for the evaluation of operative results in patients with cervical myelopathy. A recovery rate of over 75% is described as excellent, over 50% is good, over 25% is fair, and less than 25% is unchanged. Of our 90 patients, most gained good results, with an average recovery rate of 58% for ossification of the posterior longitudinal ligament and 54% for spondylosis.

Complications

As far as complications of expansive open door laminoplasty are concerned (Fig. 9.109), the clinical symptoms did not worsen severely except in one patient who developed a transient Brown-Séquard syndrome. However, weakness of the muscles innervated by the C5 and C6 segments has occurred on the open side, possibly as a result of traumatic use of the Kerrison rongeur. Four cases of this were recognized, but the patients recovered well and had no disturbance in their daily life. On the hinge side, three patients developed similar transient paresis caused by detachment of the hinge due to overdrilling of the bony gutter (Fig. 9.110). One patient still has segmental paresis of C5 and C6, possibly as a result of reclosure of the opened laminae, and two patients have paresis of unknown etiology.

On the other hand, three patients with ossification of the posterior longitudinal ligament complained of severe persistent scapular pain. This was caused by the extreme dorsal stretching of the C5 and/or C6 nerve roots resulting from the tethering effect of the thick posterior longitudinal ligament (Fig. 9.111). The width of the spinal canal increased by 3–5 mm on average compared with the preoperative anteroposterior diameter seen on lateral view radiographs; this was considered sufficient to be defined as a good operative result (Table 9.1).

The laminar doors failed to remain open in several of the initial 15 cases because the aforementioned stay sutures between and around the spinous processes and the facets had not been applied. Conventional laminectomies were required as a second operation in two patients whose clinical symptoms had been temporarily alleviated by the initial expansive laminoplasty, but worsened again when the laminar door reclosed.

Discussion

Variations of Expansive Laminoplasty

Expansive laminoplasty is here defined as a technique for expanding the cross-sectional area of the stenotic spinal canal and reconstructing the spinal canal osteoplastically. Accordingly, floating laminotomy and suspension laminotomy are outside the scope of this discussion. Expansive laminoplasty is divisible in three types: open-door laminoplasty (Hirabayashi and Satomi 1987; Kimura et al. 1982; Nakano and Tamita 1980), mid-dorsal laminoplasty (Iwasaki 1987; Iwasaki et al. 1982), and Z-plasty (Fig. 9.105; Miyasatza et al. 1981a; Oyama and Hattori 1973; Oyama et al. 1987; Watanabe et al. 1987). There are two modifications of open-door laminoplasty with bone grafting in the opened space, namely, Itoh's modification with wiring (Itoh et al. 1982, 1985; Hoh and Tsuji 1987; Tomita et al. 1988) and Matsuzaki's modification with screws and wiring (Matsuzaki et al. 1982, 1987). Mid-dorsal laminoplasty had Kurokawa's modification with midlongitudinal or midsegmental bone graft and wiring (Hoshino et al. 1987; Kurokawa et al. 1984, 1986). Three types of Z-plasty may be performed: on the lamina using Hattori's method (Hirabayashi et al. 1981; Oyama and Hattori 1973; Oyama et al. 1987), between each lamina using Sakou's reciprocal method, and between two segmental laminae using the Chiba University technique (Miyasaka et al. 1981a; Watanabe et al. 1987).

Comparison of Expansive Laminoplasty and Laminectomy

Effectiveness of Decompression. CT shows that the metrizamide ring which was compressed flat before surgery has recovered its round shape after expansive laminoplasty (Fig. 9.108). Considering that the dorsal portion of the dural tube is already swollen and pulsating during surgery, it is hardly necessary to say that expansive laminoplasty is no less effective in decompressing the spinal cord than laminectomy. In fact, many investigators (Hoh et al. 1985; Kimura et al. 1982) agree that expansive laminoplasty is no less effective than laminectomy treating cervical stenotic myelopathy.

The decompression of nerve roots achieved during these surgical techniques may now be compared. Whereas facetectomy and foraminotomy are possible with laminectomy, they are not desirable with expansive laminoplasty because they may weaken the hinge: they are not impossible, however, even on the hinge side. Accordingly, the nerve roots may only be easily decompressed on the open side using open-door expansive laminoplasty. Therefore, expansive laminoplasty does not compare favorably with laminectomy for bilateral radiculopathy. However, we have never encountered any case where open-door expansive laminoplasty was precluded in treating cervical myelopathy because of combination with bilateral radiculopathy. We think in fact that anterior decompressive surgery is indicated in such cases.

Postoperative Support of the Neck. Since both laminectomy and expansive laminoplasty are invasive, they both cause a certain amount of damage to the posterior structures. In the literature (Cattell and Clark 1967; Jenkins 1973; Sim et al. 1974), postoperative malalignment of the spine has been reported as a complication of laminectomy in infants. We have had patients with a poor long-term postlaminectomy result because of spinal fragility resulting from the lack of posterior osseous protection against cervical trauma and progressive spondylotic changes at the intervertebral disk level (Hirabayashi et al. 1972).

Malalignment of the sagittal plane, notably kyphosis, can arise from various conditions, such as the loss of spinous processes and laminae and myoligamentous dynamic changes caused by decreased cervical muscle and ligament force due to loss of their anchoring (Fig. 9.104). The preservation of the C2 spinous process, which exerts the greatest dynamic effect on the anchoring muscles, and the reconstruction of the anchoring muscles by proper suturing are indispensable maneuvers in both techniques (Arima 1969). In this respect, expansive laminoplasty has an advantage over laminectomy since osseous and ligamentous loss is smaller with the former technique. In point of fact, we have not encountered any cases where marked kyphosis or swan-neck deformity is newly formed after open door expansive laminoplasty; we only noticed mild kyphosis in 5% of patients.

In patients with hourglass tumor or syringomyelia, laminectomy sometimes resulted in postoperative malalignment of the cervical spine; cervical lordosis was, however, well maintained postoperatively after laminoplastic treatment (Fig. 9.106). It is desirable for the kyphotic curvature of the cervical spine to be changed into lordotic curvature with expansive laminoplasty, because the effects of decompression on an anteriorly compressed spinal cord are usually considerable. In fact, it has been clearly shown in ossification of the posterior longitudinal ligament that preoperative kyphosis is one of the factors that may lead to a poor operative outcome.

We have always kept strictly to a mid-dorsal approach between the bilateral paravertebral muscles and two-layer muscle suturing in our operative procedures in order to restore the function of the nuchal ligament and paravertebral muscles in the cervical spine. Furthermore, recent attempts have been made to preserve both supra- and interspinous ligaments and hemilateral ligamentum flavum on the hinge side above the upper and below the lower edges of the opened laminae (Fig. 9.112). There is, so far, no evidence to corroborate the superiority of expansive laminoplasty over laminectomy with regard to the vulnerability of the spinal cord to cervical trauma, but, at least theoretically, it may be easily imagined that expansive laminoplasty, with which it is possible to reconstruct the spinal canal, is more advantageous than laminectomy in protecting the spinal cord from cervical trauma.

As for progressive spondylotic changes at the intervertebral disk level, expansive laminoplasty may be considered to be more advantageous from the standpoint of postoperative supportability and restriction of motion in the cervical spinal column. It should not be overlooked that expansive laminoplasty exerts a braking effect that reduces the incidence of dynamic factors leading to disorders of the posterior spur of the vertebral body. This braking effect may also be seen faintly in laminectomy patients as a reduction in the range of motion resulting from postoperative contracture and ossification around the level of the spine operated on. After expansive laminoplasty, however, the intervertebral joints are liable to become more rigid when the lateral gutter of the laminae on the hinge side undergoes osseous fusion. As a matter of fact, after expansive laminoplasty patients demonstrate one-third of their preoperative range of motion in our clinic (Table 9.2).

These dynamic advantages of expansive laminoplasty are also considered to be beneficial, since they inhibit the postoperative progression of ossification in the patient with ossification of the posterior longitudinal ligament. We have indicated elsewhere three factors that favor the postoperative progression of ossification of the posterior longitudinal ligament (Hirabayashi et al. 1981), namely, biological stimulation, dynamical compensation, and mobility. As far as surgical intervention is concerned, the biologically stimulative factor is unavoidable in both procedures. Expansive laminoplasty does, however, have a definite advantage over laminectomy in the sense that the former inhibits the dynamically compensatory and mobile factors. In our series, the frequency of nongrowth cases of ossification of the posterior longitudinal ligament after operation was three times higher in the expansive laminoplasty than laminectomy. Postoperative ossification was far less frequent after expansive laminoplasty (Figs. 9.113, 9.114).

Safety of Surgery. It is hardly necessary to say that the safety of surgery has a critical bearing on the postoperative prognosis of patients. Knowing that prognosis depends on the skill of the surgeon in most cases, the safety of surgery and danger of complications in each of the techniques under discussion will be compared.

The main complications observed after open-door laminoplasty were motor weakness in muscles innervated by the C5 and C6 segments and scapulalgia, presumably of radicular origin. A study of these symptoms suggested that traumatic maneuvering of the Kerrison rongeur, detachment of the hinge, and reclosure of the enlarged laminae were the probable causes (Fig. 9.109). With both operative techniques, the Kerrison rongeur or drilling should be maneuvered with meticulous care when decompressing the spinal cord. It is controversial as to which side laminotomy is safer: mid-dorsal or lateral.

There is no danger of disjointing the hinge at all with laminectomy, but expansive laminoplasty may permit the hinges to be detached unilaterally after the open-door procedure and bilaterally after the mid-dorsal procedure. Be that as it may, strict observance of the surgical procedures and thorough familiarity with the technique are the keys to prevention of hinge detachment. With laminectomy there is no danger either that the opened laminae reclose after surgery. Even with expansive laminoplasty, such a danger may be completely avoided by grafting bone into the opened laminae or employing Z-plasty as well. At any rate, it can now be safely said that there is no danger of reclosure in open-door expansive laminoplasty, because the position of enlarged spinal canal is held by silk thread through the base of spinous processes from the facets or capsules of the intervertebral joint to prevent the door from being closed.

Difficulty of Surgery. The proverb says "practice makes perfect" and surgery is a case in point. Apart from the familiarity factor, the two surgical techniques can be compared to some extent with respect to the number and nature of maneuvers required.

Generally speaking, laminectomy can be said to be simpler than expansive laminoplasty, but as is obvious from its historical development, our own open-door expansive laminoplasty, which ends in the stage preceding en bloc laminectomy, compares favorably with laminectomy as far as operating time and blood loss are concerned, even allowing for the time required for ligation to prevent reclosure.

All other expansive laminoplasty procedures are, by contrast, not only difficult to perform, but are also more time consuming than laminectomy (Fig. 9.105). Kurokawa's mid-dorsal bone graft (Hoshino et al. 1987; Kurokawa et al. 1984, 1986), Ito's procedure with wiring (Itoh et al. 1982, 1985; Itoh and Tsuji 1987), and Matsuzaki's procedure with iliac bone graft (Matsuzaki et al. 1982, 1987) seem to demand far greater skill and longer operating time. Hattori's technique (Kawai and Hattori 1980; Oyama and Hattori 1973; Oyama et al. 1987), among others, is extremely difficult since it involves thinning the entire laminae for Z-plasty.

Conclusion

1. Cervical expansive laminoplasty has the same decompressive effect as laminectomy.
2. Expansive laminoplasty provides better postoperative support than laminectomy.
3. It is hard to say which is superior, laminoplasty or laminectomy, in technical safety and simplicity, but our own open-door expansive laminoplasty can be said to be the simplest of all laminoplasties.
4. Our own open-door expansive laminoplasty seems to be a rational modality for common cases of cervical spinal stenotic myelopathy. Other expansive laminoplasties with bone grafting seem to be indicated in special cases with a high degree of instability such as cerebral palsy.

Table 9.1. Optimal widening of anteroposterior diameter

Width (mm)	Cases (n)	Recovery rate
< 2	12	41%
3–5	23	70
> 6	9	63

Table 9.2. Range of motion at involved disk levels

Surgical procedure	Disks decompressed (n)	Preoperative	Postoperative	Decreasing rate[a]
Laminectomy	61	7.0°	3.3°	52.8
Expansive laminoplasty	117	6.1°	2.4°	61.2

[a] $p < 0.01$

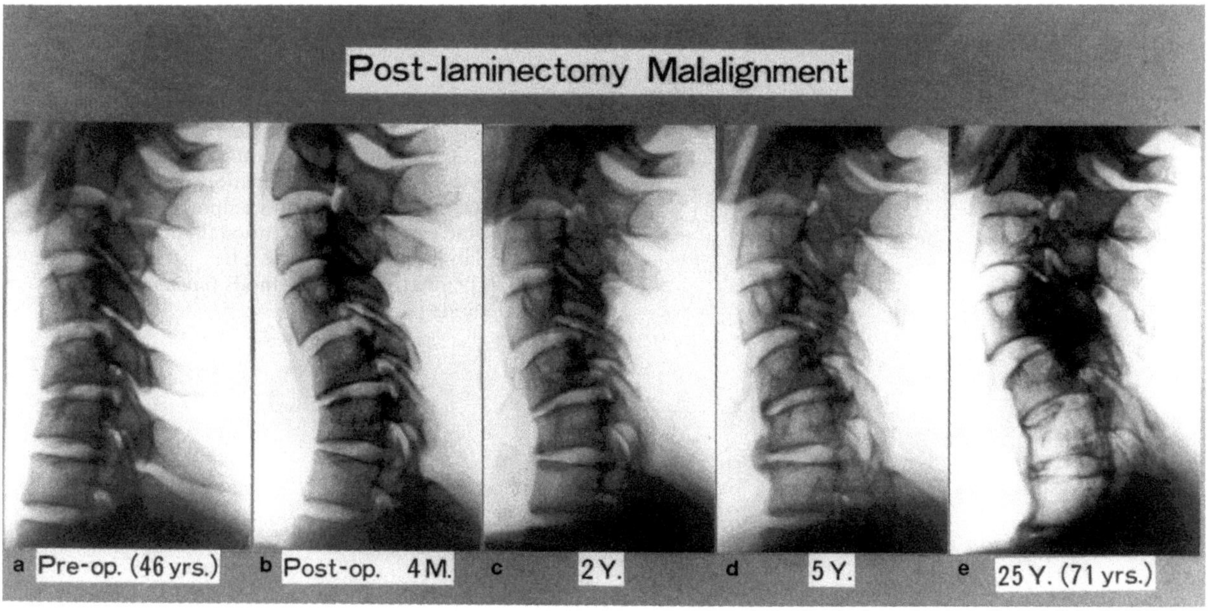

Fig. 9.104 a–e. Postlaminectomy malalignment. **a** Laminectomy from C4 to C6 was performed to remove a spinal cord tumor in a 46-year-old patient. **b** Kyphotic deformity from C5 to C7 appeared 4 months after surgery. **c, d** This deformity progressed, as shown at 2 years and 5 years follow-up, and **e** was completely ankylosed 25 years after operation

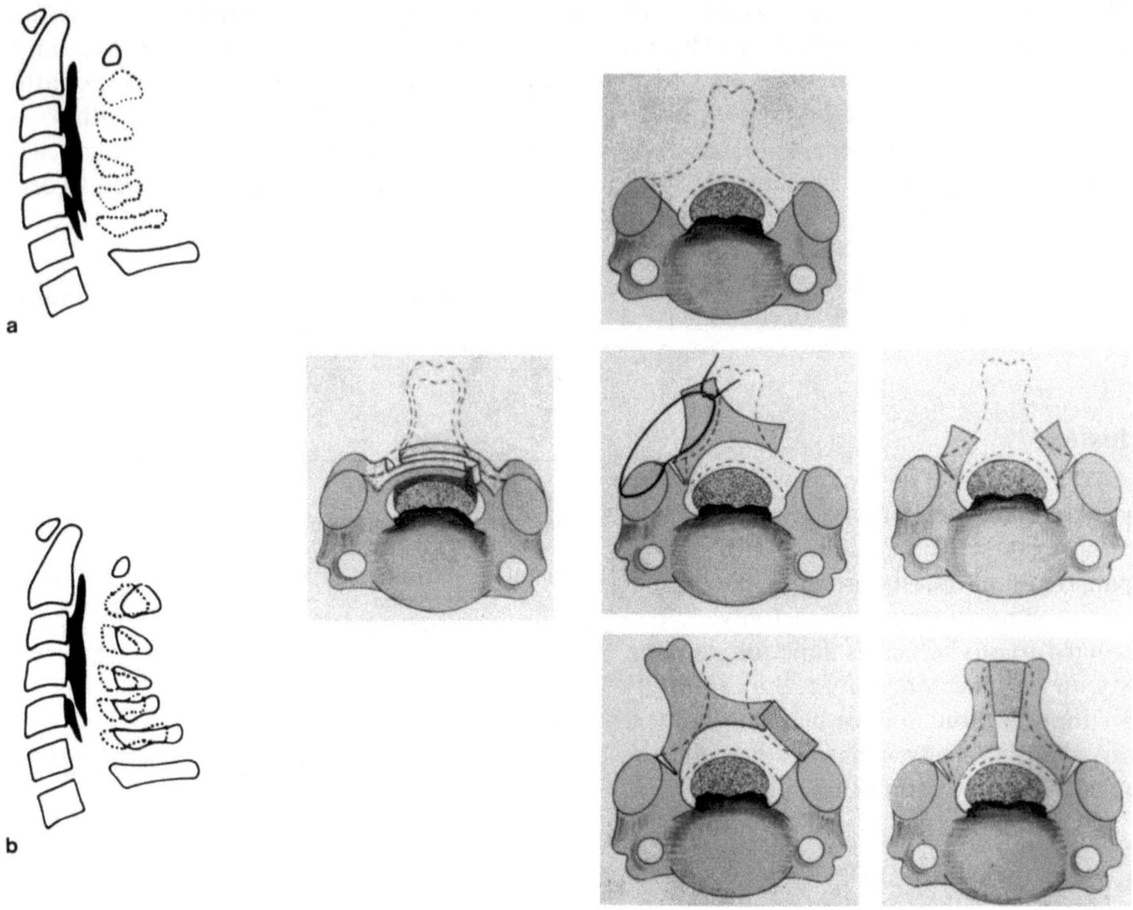

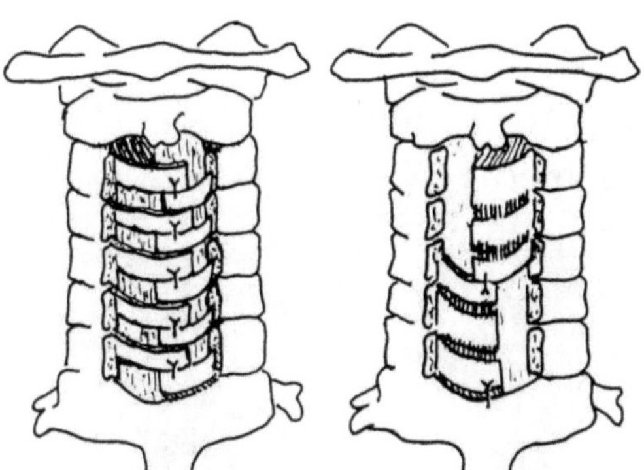

Fig. 9.105 a, b. Schematic presentation of posterior decompressive surgeries for cervical ossification of the posterior longitudinal ligament. Posterior decompressive surgery in the cervical spine consists of conventional laminectomy (**a**) or expansive laminoplasty (**b**). The latter is classified into Z-plasty (*left*) hemilateral open methods (*middle*), and bilateral open methods (*right*)

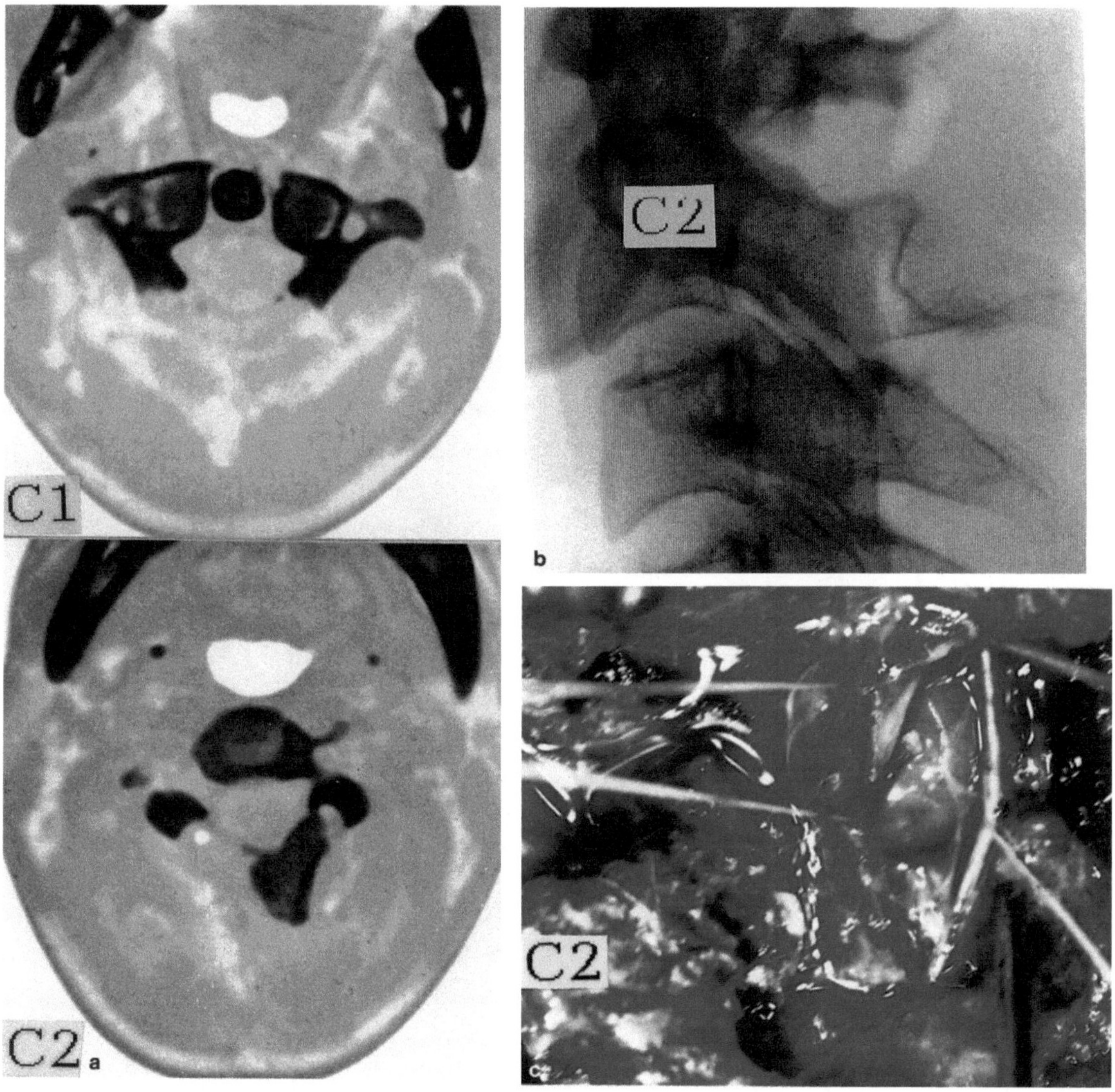

Fig. 9.106 a–c. Removal of spinal cord tumor using expansive laminoplasty. **a** Postoperative CT shows total laminectomy of C1 (*top*) and right hemilaminectomy and hemilateral expansive laminectomy (opened to the left) of C2 (*bottom*). **b** Postoperative lateral view shows normal alignment in the upper cervical spine. **c** Intraoperative view shows intradural and extramedullary tumor located at right side of the dorsum of the spinal cord

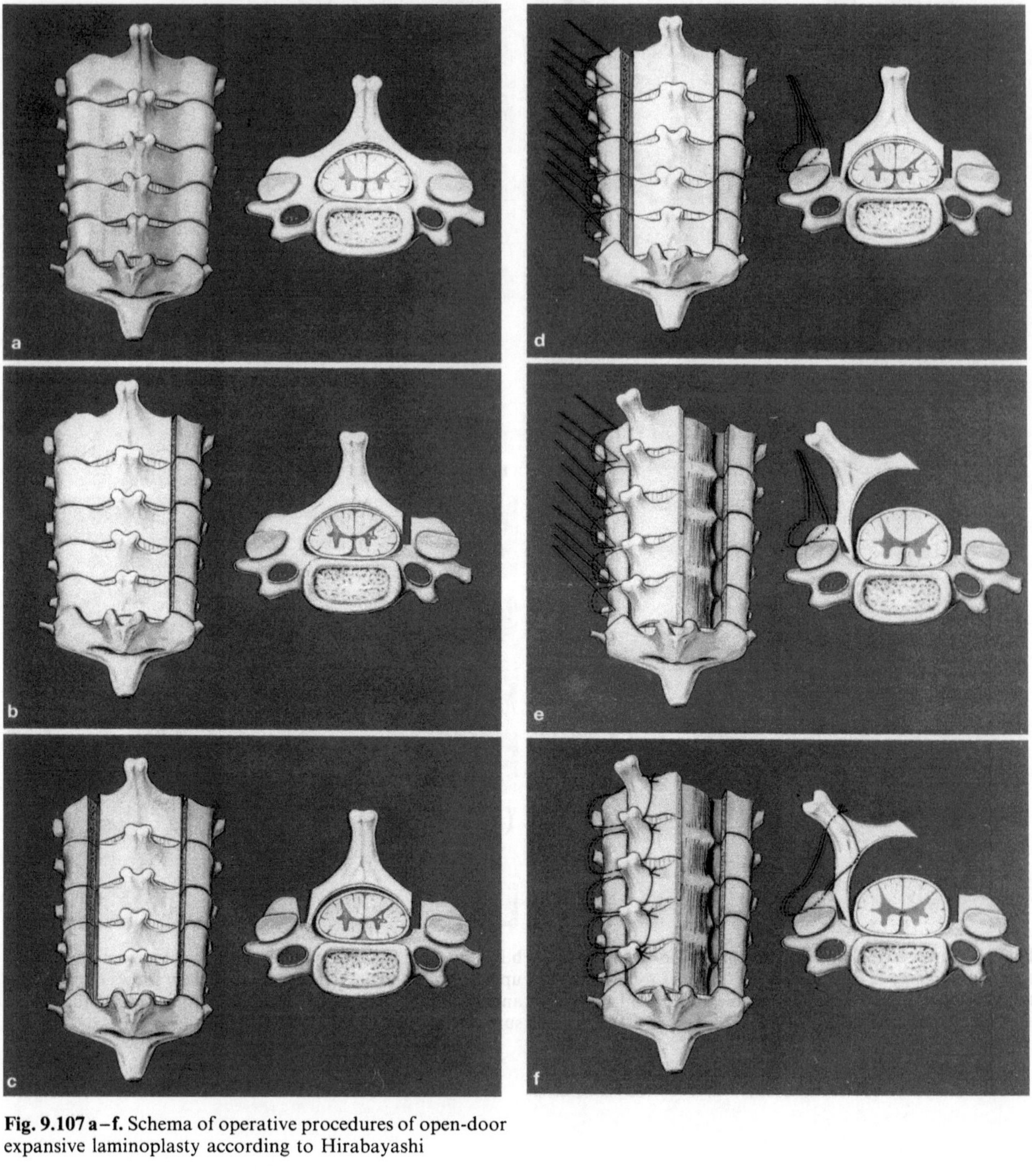

Fig. 9.107 a–f. Schema of operative procedures of open-door expansive laminoplasty according to Hirabayashi

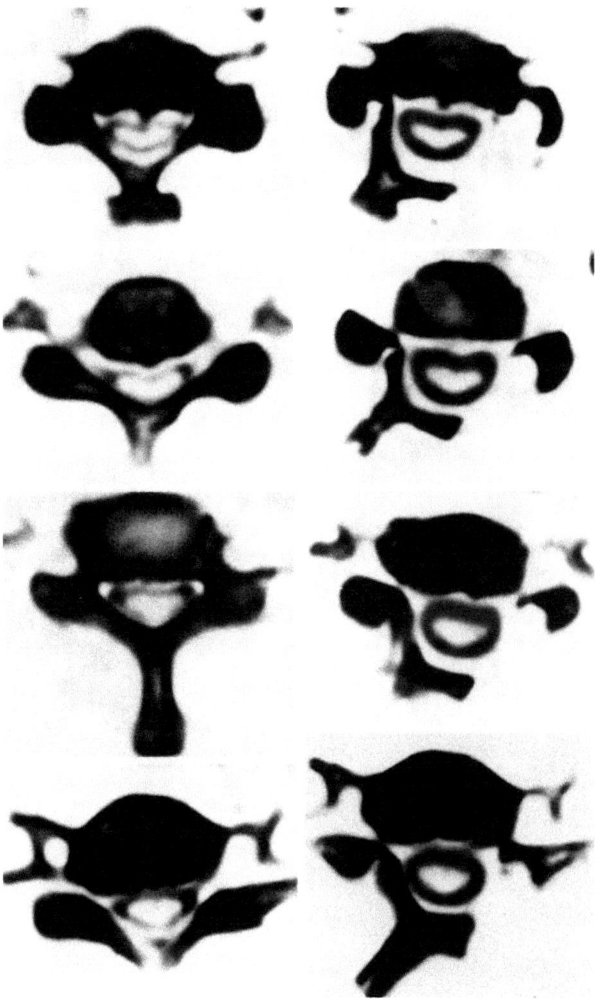

Fig. 9.108. Pre- and postoperative CT myelograms. The decompressive effect of expansive laminoplasty is clearly shown in pre- and postoperative CT myelograms in a 59-year-old male patient with cervical myelopathy due to spinal canal stenosis

SYMPTOMS		CAUSES		PREVENTIVE CHECK POINTS
Radicular back pain	↖	Disjoint of hinge	↗	Strict observance of operative procedures
	↙			
Segmental paresis	←	Traumatic handling	→	Atraumatic skill
	↖	Reclosure of opened laminae	↘	Supporting sutures around spinous processes or Bone grafting at open side
Tractal paresis	↙			

Fig. 9.109. Complications of open-door expansive laminoplasty and preventive check points

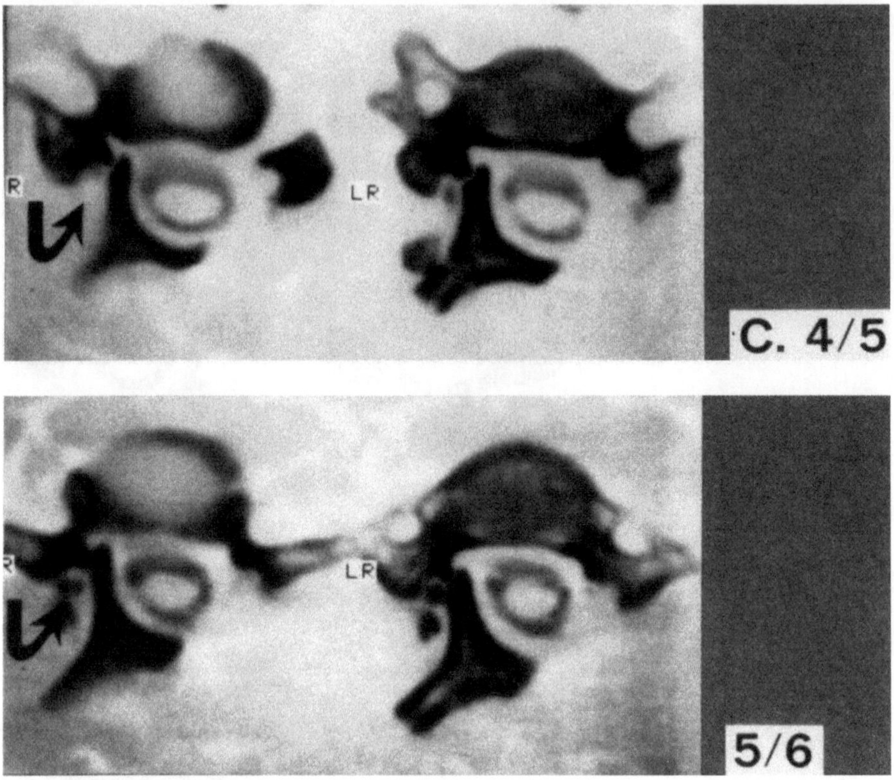

Fig. 9.110. Disjoint of hinge causing transient paresis of the roots of C5 and C6 in a 35-year-old male patient

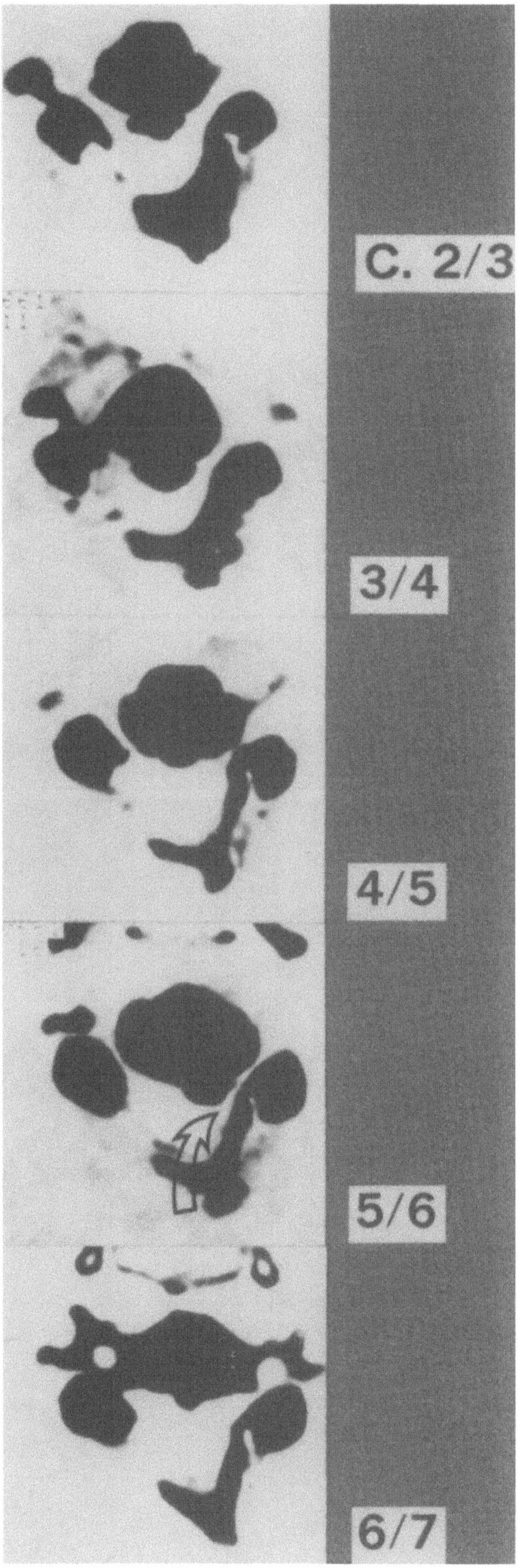

Fig. 9.111. Tethering and compressive effect causing neck pain in a 60-year-old male patient

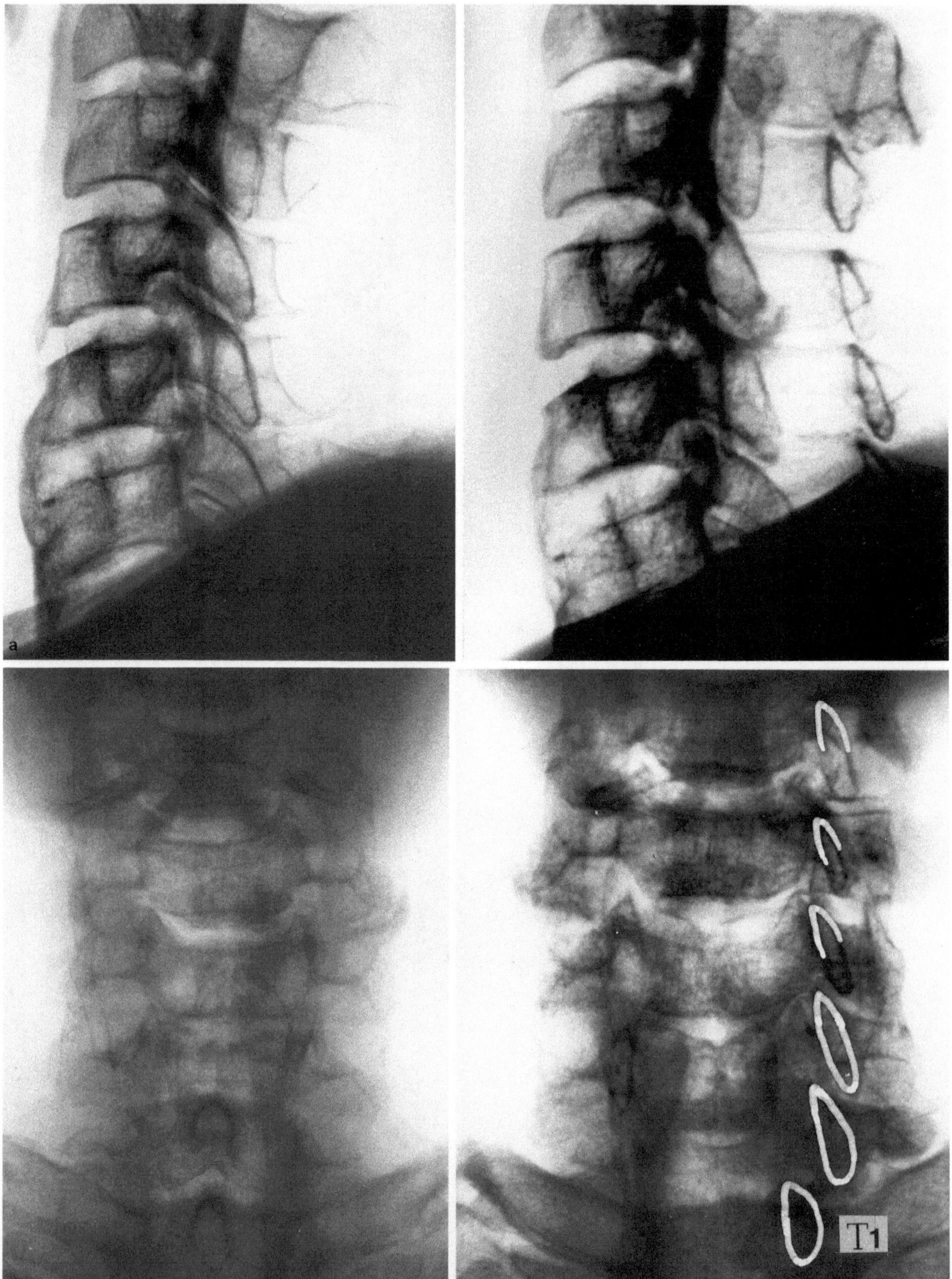
T1

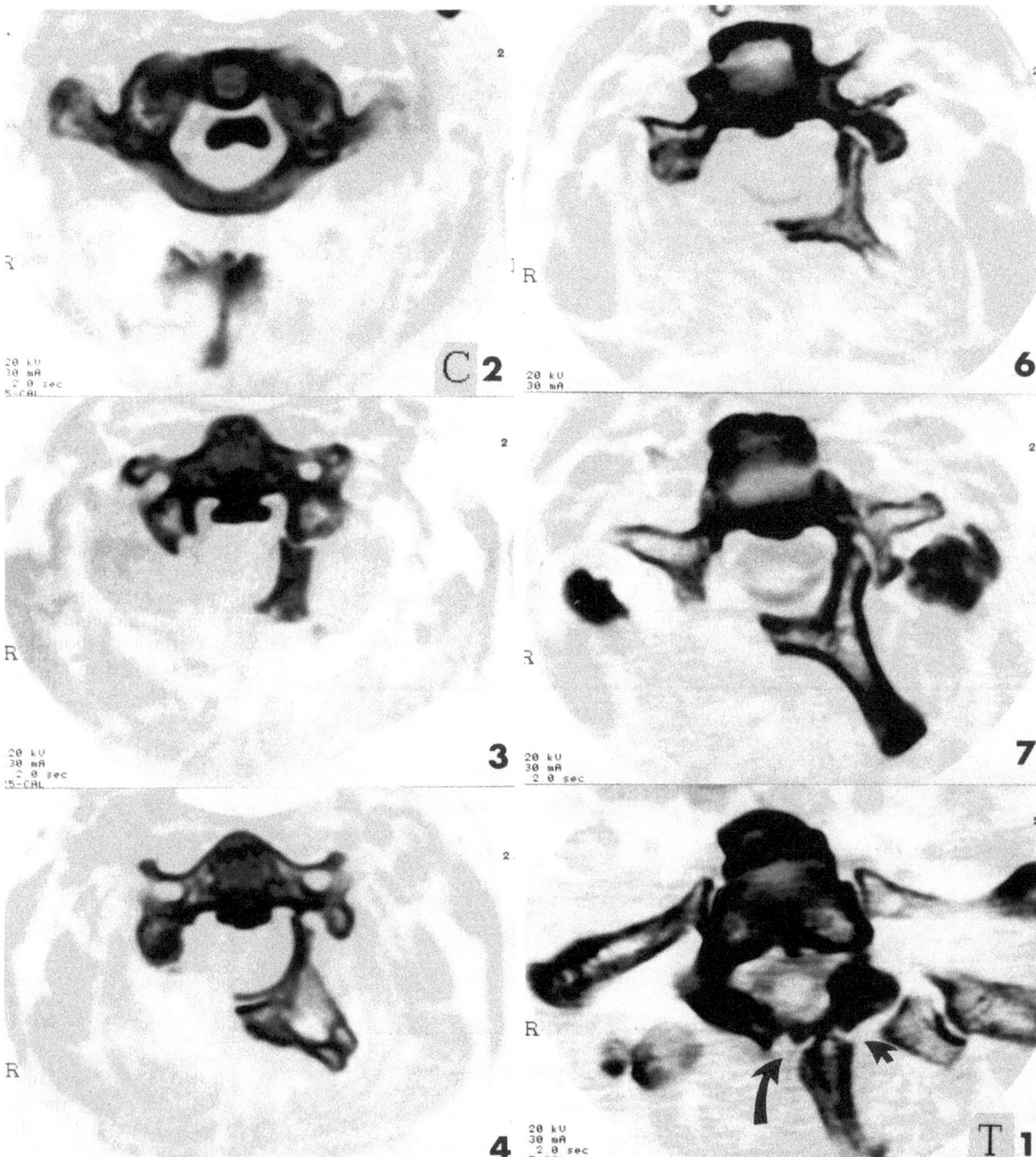

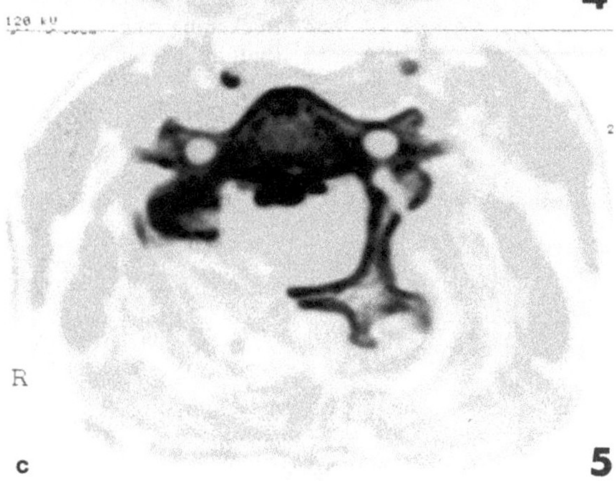

Fig. 9.112 a–c. Pre- and postoperative plain X-ray and CT in a patient with ossification of the posterior longitudinal ligament (C1–C6, mixed type). **a** Lateral views show that the spinal canal is enlarged after expansive laminoplasty (C2–C7, right side opened). **b** Anteroposterior views show that the spinous processes of the enlarged levels are shifted to the left with T1, which is fractured artificially. **c** Postoperative CT shows that the laminar doors with the spinous processes from C3 to C7 are sufficiently opened to the left, and that T7 spinous process has been bent to the left by drilling and pushing to preserve the inter-and supraspinous ligament through all the levels

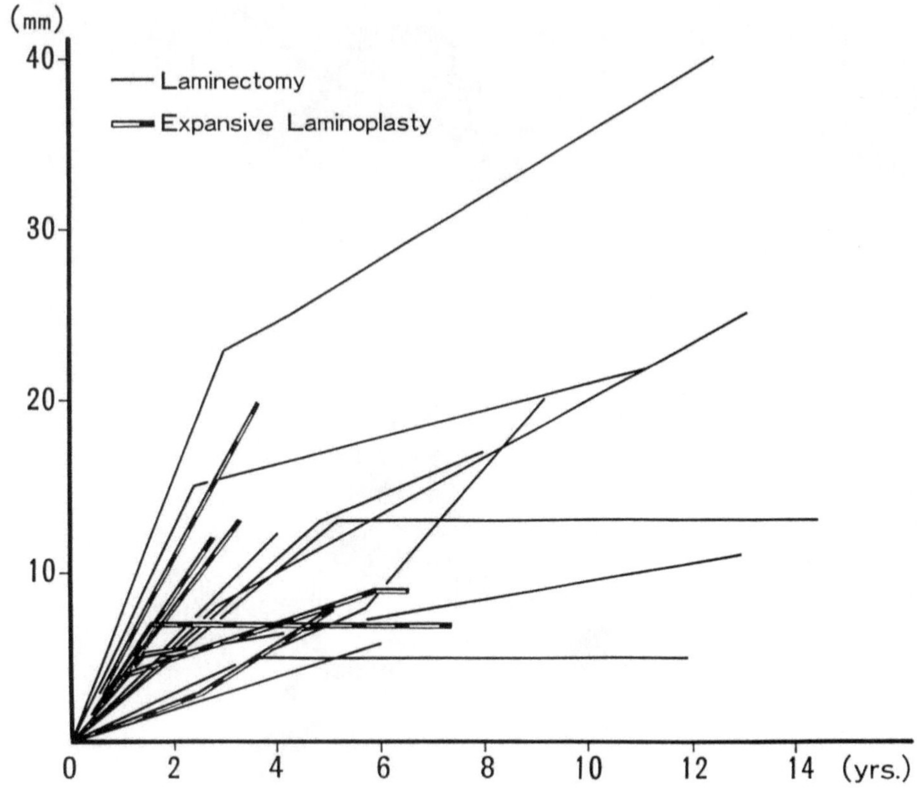

Fig. 9.113. Postoperative increase in ossification of the posterior longitudinal ligament. After expansive laminoplasty the extent of longitudinal thickening of the posterior longitudinal ligament is less than after laminectomy

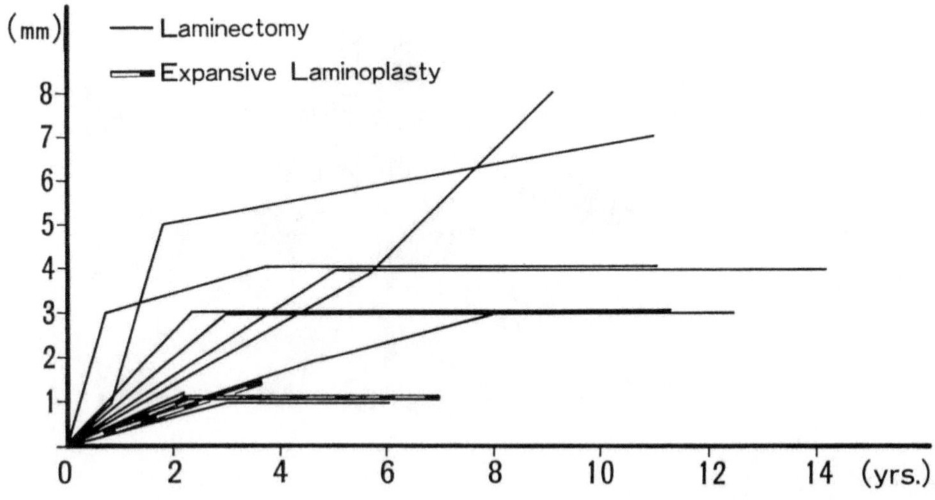

Fig. 9.114. After expansive laminoplasty, the posterior longitudinal ligament is subject to less thickening tranversely than after laminectomy

Bone Grafts

In surgery of the cervical spine it often becomes necessary to use bone graft. Under normal circumstances, it is used for the following reasons:

- As tissue that permits the restoration of the height and structure of a destroyed vertebral body.
- As a simple buttress or support for internal fixation with plates and screws to assure the stability of the fusion. This implies that the bone graft will eventually achieve osseous fusion, while the immediate stability is achieved through internal fixation with plates and screws.
- To fill in a large gap in the bone and act as a support across this gap.

It becomes apparent, therefore, that grafts are used for two fundamental purposes: mechanical (cortical bone), and biological by filling and rebuilding a segment of the bone (spongy and corticotrabecular). For these reasons, autograft bone is unique and nonreplaceable. Cement and allografts are less ideal and therefore the second choice whenever possible.

Banked allografts tend to delay fusion and, because of the greater degree of resorption to which they are subject, they may actually weaken the restoration, resulting in collapse and deformity, and often produce kyphoses and pseudoarthroses (nonunion) with an eventual risk of neurological consequences. These same consequences pertain to an even greater degree to heterografts which should therefore never be used in stabilizing and repairing the cervical spine.

The use of acrylic cement seems to be totally unjustified in degenerative diseases. It may well have the potential for causing injury to the cord, the nerves, and other parameningeal structures because of the heat generated during polymerization. There are very few good data on the eventual outcome of implanted cement on a long-term basis. Cement should be restricted to cases of tumors, in particular in patients with a poor or very limited prognosis in whom the purpose of surgery is to obtain an immediate restoration of the stability and continuity of the spine. It can also be very useful if a considerable volume of tissue has been removed to eradicate a large lesion. We have no experience with the use of cement where the follow-up period is longer than 3 years after implantation. Since autograft is easily available, the use of cement in cases of degenerative arthropathy of the spine is definitely to be discouraged.

Choice of Donor Site

The iliac crest, the tibia, and the fibula are the common donor sites for grafts in spinal surgery.

Iliac Crest Grafts

The most common source of graft is the iliac crest. This site that has the potential to provide mainly cortical, mainly cancellous, or both cortical and cancellous graft. The ideal site for harvesting is the anterior portion of the crest and the posterior iliac wing, the latter being the part that can provide the greater amount of bone. It is important to begin harvesting of the graft from the front and work towards the back. The incision must start at least 5 cm from the anterior superior iliac spine. If the graft is taken too far anteriorly, the muscles that insert into the bone may disrupt the bone at the anterior superior iliac spine. The major muscular pull will be from the tensors of the fascia lata and the sartorius muscle. The choice of site will also depend on the patient's position on the operating table (whether supine or prone) and on the type of graft required by the operative procedure.

The most commonly used corticocancellous grafts are discussed below.

Bicortical Cylindrical Graft As Required By the Cloward Instrumentation (Fig. 9.115). In operations using Cloward instrumentation, the aim is to achieve full arthrodesis at the operative level following anterior decompression. The graft must therefore have good mechanical characteristics; the size of the graft and the thickness of its cortical components are very important features. The graft should be taken from the medial portion of the iliac wing, which at this point has a slight posterior curvature. This is the site at which the bone is thickest. The graft should be removed carefully from under the iliac crest with the appropriate instrumentation. Bone taken more distally will be of lesser thickness and will not be suitable for use as a dowel graft that will achieve arthrodesis in distraction.

Another feature which is of practical importance is the angle at which the graft is separated from the ilium. The drill should always be applied at right angles to the external cortical surface of the iliac wing. In order to achieve this, it must be tilted downwards by 30–40° to meet this requirement in each case. This orientation of the drill is necessary in order to avoid an oblique surface along one edge of the graft, a feature which would make the graft unsuitable as a dowel to slot into the host site.

Once it has been released from its bony attachment, the graft must be cleared of all soft tissues and shaped and filed along its sides into an elliptical shape. The hole drilled between the two adjacent vertebral bodies is spherical, but when distraction is applied, it also assumes an oblique elliptical shape. The graft must therefore be shaped to fit the elliptical shape of the drill hole which can be achieved in distraction. In addition, the graft should be approximately 5 mm larger in diameter than the drill bit used to produce the drill hole in the vertebrae so that distraction is maintained after the distractor has been released and the graft is in place. A practical point that is also of at least theoretical clinical value is to drill a hole through the full thickness of the center of the graft. This is done to ensure that any bleeding that occurs posteriorly (behind the graft) may be drained through this hole, avoiding the development of a fully contained hematoma.

Once the graft has been obtained, it should be mounted on the carrier (see Fig. 9.14) which is used to insert the graft at the host site. This graft carrier has two lateral wings that come to rest on the lateral arms of the distractor, thus limiting the advance of the graft and avoiding its being inserted too deeply.

Errors. The graft removed may be too small if it is taken from the more distal portion of the iliac wing where the bone is thinner. Because of the mechanical and biological inappropriateness of such a graft, an additional graft must be obtained from a more suitable and better selected area.

If the graft is the same size as the drill holes in the vertebral bodies, it will provide very little stability and will lead to failure of the arthrodesis because it may be easily mobilized postoperatively and lead to collapse of the two adjacent vertebral bodies.

The graft may be placed too deeply in the drill hole if it is too small, either because the depth was inappropriately assessed or because the instrumentation used was inadequate. This may have serious consequences, particularly if the graft protrudes posteriorly into the canal. If this happens, the graft should be immediately removed. In the majority of cases, this can be achieved with relatively simple technical steps. Without distraction, a self-tapping screw is threaded into the center of the graft. This is relatively easy because this is an area with spongy bone. With a pair of sturdy pliers, the screw is firmly gripped. Distraction is applied and the graft can then be removed.

Tricortical Rectangular Graft For Smith-Robinson Type Vertebral Fusion

In order to obtain a tricortical bone graft (Fig. 9.116), a full thickness resection of a portion of the iliac crest must be undertaken. It must be remembered that the purpose of this exercise is to obtain a graft that is uniform in thickness. Since saws generate heat that may produce necrosis and tissue denaturing, it is better to use chisels, which must be sharp. The iliac crest is stripped of all soft tissues. The technique involves driving the first chisel into the bone approximately 2 cm from the crest. This first chisel is left in place and a second chisel is inserted into the bone more distally. This is followed by a third chisel yet more distally to complete the separation at the base. A modification that is sometimes practical is the use of drill holes along the resection margin on both cortices so that the chisel can more easily and less traumatically transect the bone. This may well avoid disruption of the graft and result in a straight linear margin of resection. Once the graft has been obtained, it is shaped and filed. Here again it must be emphasized that the diameter of the graft must be larger than that of the drilled hole, and the graft must be shaped in order to maintain the distraction between the two opposing vertebral bodies after its insertion.

Errors. The major error is harvesting a graft from the more anterior part of the iliac wing where the bone is too thin. Other errors involve inaccuracies in the size of the graft and the insertion of the graft too deeply in the drill holes with a risk of posterior protrusion into the canal.

Tricortical Graft For Multiple Vertebral Resections

The length of a tricortical graft for multiple vertebral resections must be 4–8 cm. In order to obtain a graft of such size, the skin incision must be proportionally longer (Fig. 9.117). This can only be achieved with an incision parallel to the iliac crest and placed approximately 1 cm below the superior surface of the crest. Muscles must be detached from the abdominal surface and from the external surface of the iliac wing to expose the entire iliac crest. The central iliac crest is the preferred zone for harvest. The graft is obtained using chisels as described above. The chisels, one at each end of the graft being harvested, must reach a depth of approximately 2 cm into the bone. The graft length must exceed the length of the host trench in the vertebrae by at least 2 cm in order to meet the requirements of the final preparation and shaping prior to insertion. Saws should be avoided in order to preclude unnecessary tissue damage, as noted above. The outline of the graft can be marked in the iliac crest using a series of drill holes to specifically define the margins, which can then be cut with the chisel. Again emphasis must be placed on obtaining well-defined linear and intact resection margins.

Once the graft has been harvested, its bed must be subjected to careful and complete hemostasis. This will require packing with ample bone wax. Closure must be undertaken scrupulously in well-approximated layers in order to avoid the formation of potential cavities in the abdominal wall, which all too frequently result in hematomas and fluid cysts in the wound if the deep muscular layers have been closed too loosely. Suction drainage is essential postoperatively. Very often patients continue to complain of pain and discomfort in the donor area in the iliac region long after the surgery.

The final preparation of the graft is quite important. It must be assured that all soft tissues have been stripped from the bone and that the periosteum has been totally removed. The bone will be curved and asymmetrical and will vary in thickness depending on the exact source on the iliac crest. The steps for shaping the graft must be carried out by hand. The use of a vice made out of sterilizable steel and either placed on or anchored to the instrument table will be of particular use during these steps (Figs. 9.118, 9.119). Once the graft is well anchored, files of different sizes and coarseness may be used to shape the walls in such a way as to straighten the graft. In addition, the shape and configuration that is achieved should assure that the length exceeds the undistracted bony groove in the vertebral bodies by 10–15 mm.

Particular care must be used in the shaping the interlocking ends (Fig. 9.119). The ends must obviously be shaped in such a way as to interlock with the appropriate portions of the prepared vertebral bodies. During distraction, the dowel graft is slotted to interlock perfectly with the vertebral bodies. This assures that the graft is well seated and fully stable. If this technique is carried out accurately, the use of internal fixation may be avoided, as recommended in the literature.

Errors. Should the graft be obtained from the anterior portion of the iliac wing, then it will be excessively curved, too thin, and impossible to accurately shape to fit the requirements of the host site. In cases of posterior extensive multilevel fusion (Fig. 9.96) the posterior iliac crest is a good donor site. Strips of tricortical grafts may be obtained through tangential resection of the iliac crest (Fig. 9.120).

Fibular Grafts

The fibula is composed of solid, primarily cortical bone and as such is quite advantageous when mechanical strength and support are required from a graft. However, it is straight and very difficult to model and, as such, is not fully adaptable to maintaining the existing cervical lordosis.

Nevertheless, it is the preferred type of graft in cases in which immediate mechanical support is required. As such, it is primarily used in the management of vertebral destruction by tumor. Even though the fusion achieved produces a straight cervical spine, fibular grafts have been successfully used as described in the literature (Whitecloud and La Rocca 1978). In harvesting the graft, great care must be taken to avoid the all too frequent injuries to the external popliteal branch of the sciatic nerve. This complication can be avoided as follows:

1. Obtain the graft from the metaphysis and away from the head and neck of the fibula where the nerve crosses.
2. Avoid penetrating into the muscular structures of the anterior compartment of the leg during the stripping of the bone.
3. It is preferable at this site to use a Gigli saw and avoid the use of chisels which may produce contusions of the nerve with the final "give" as the bone is divided.

Tibial Grafts

The proximal metaphysis of the tibia is a well-known source of bone graft (Fig. 9.122). This site provides primarily cortical bone, although corticotrabecular bone can also be obtained. The antermedial surface is a good donor site. The surgical steps are well established. The perimeter of the graft is first outlined with drill holes after the bone has been stripped. Chisels are used to elevate the bone. This type of graft is such as to be well suited in the management of vertebral destruction by tumor and in cases requiring solid support and immediate stability.

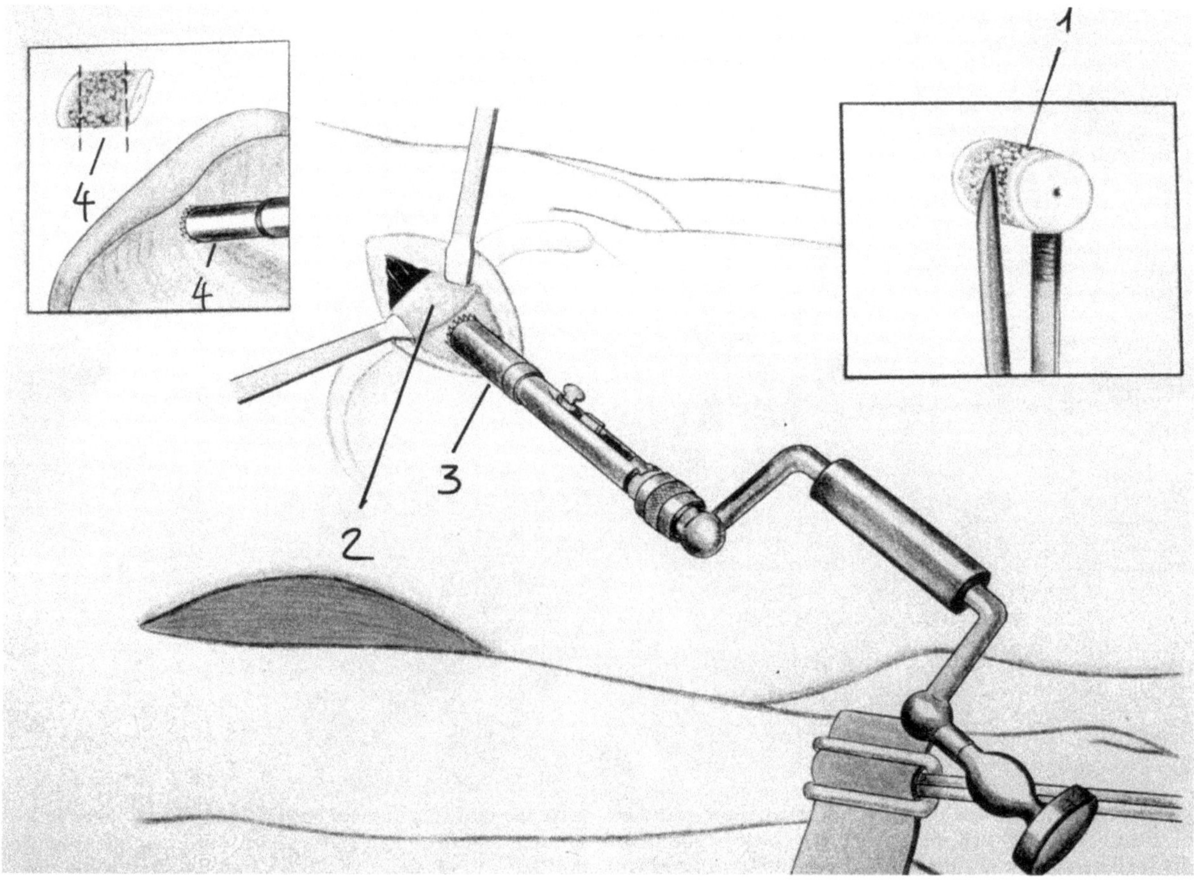

Fig. 9.115. Method for obtaining the cylindrical graft from the iliac crest (*1*). The graft obtained with the appropriate Cloward drill is taken from immediately under the cortex of the iliac crest approximately in the midzone of the crest (*2*). This provides a graft with a good amount of centrally placed spongiosa wedged between the inner and outer cortical plates (*1*). The angle of the drill is important; it must be placed perpendicular to the cortical plane (an inclination of 45°; *3*). If an angled graft is obtained, it may not be geometrically or mechanically acceptable (*4*)

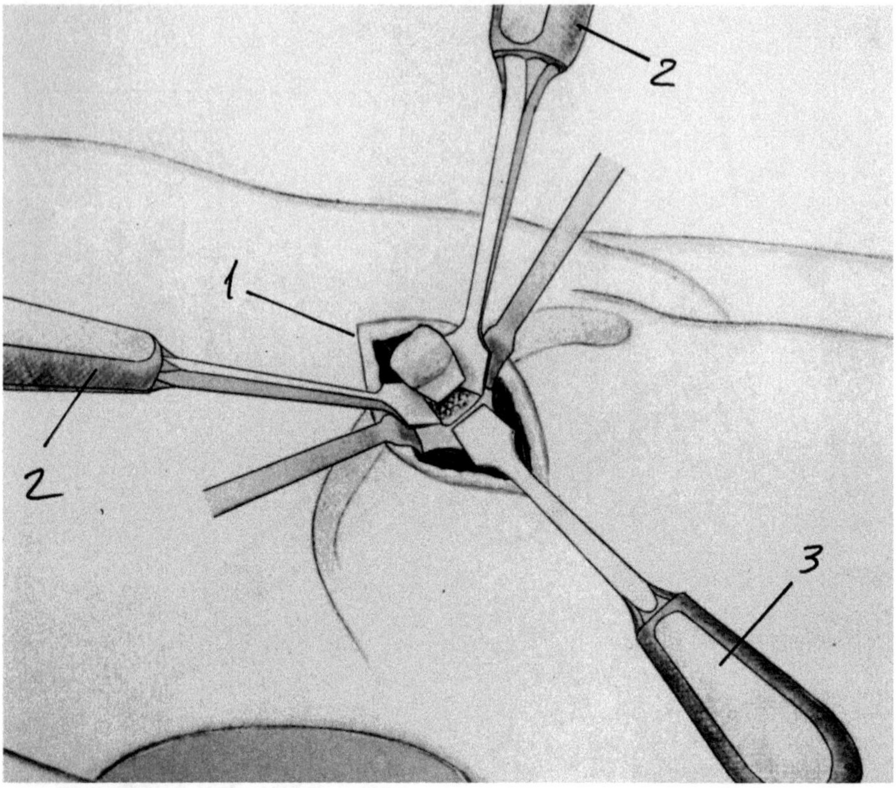

Fig. 9.116. The position of the longitudinal incision over the iliac crest (*1*) that is used in harvesting a corticotrabecular graft for intervertebral arthrodesis. Two chisels are used to raise the graft (*2*), measuring the depth of the bone with a third chisel (*3*), which is then used to lift the graft from the bottom

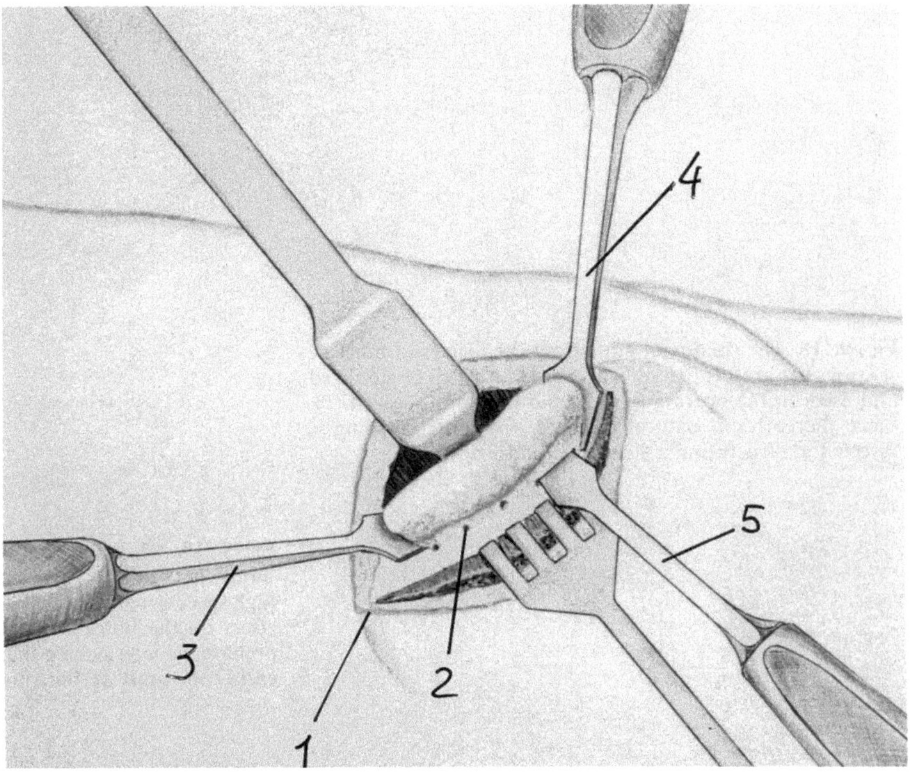

Fig. 9.117. When it is necessary to obtain a tricortical graft from the iliac crest following a corpectomy, the incision (*1*) should be parallel to the iliac crest. The abdominal muscles and the gluteal muscles are detached on their respective sides. The iliac crest is exposed and full depth drill holes (*2*) are used to delineate the margin of the resection. Chisels are placed proximally (*3*) and distally (*4*), and are then used as levers to hold and raise the graft, while a third scalpel (*5*) is used to cut the graft in between the drill holes

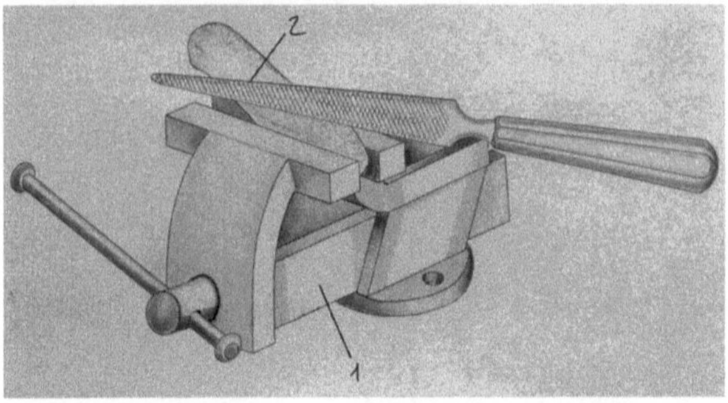

Fig. 9.118. The tricortical graft from the iliac crest must be shaped. The graft is placed in a vice (*1*), that can be sterilized and used on the operating table, and filed on the sized (*2*). Since the cortex is naturally curved, the initial shaping is directed at structuring a straight cylindrical draft

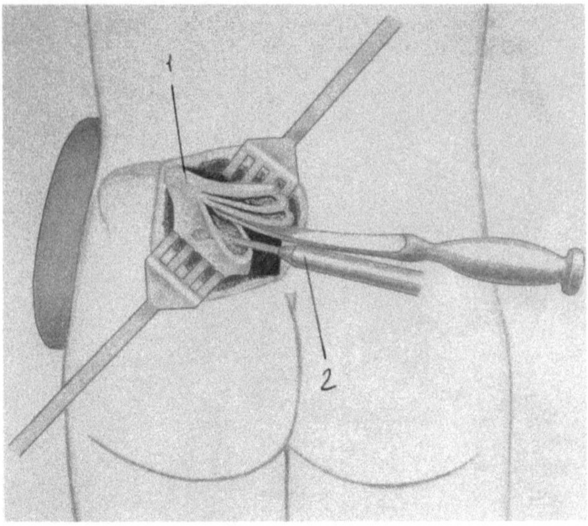

Fig. 9.119. Additional shaping of the graft with the hand file. Drills, particularly air drills, should be avoided since their high speed generates heat which has a necrotizing or burning effect on the bony tissue. Hand-held files (*1*) are used to prepare the interlocking shape at the proximal and distal (*2*) end of the graft as illustrated

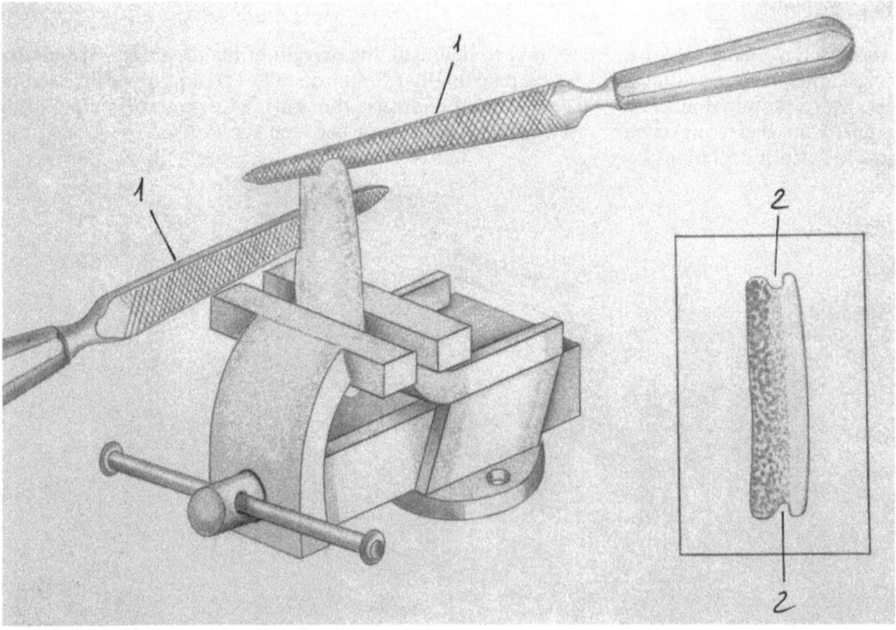

Fig. 9.120. In the case of posterior fusions, long slices of corticocancellous bone (*1*) are required as well as abundant trabecular bone, which can then be obtained with a curved curet (*2*)

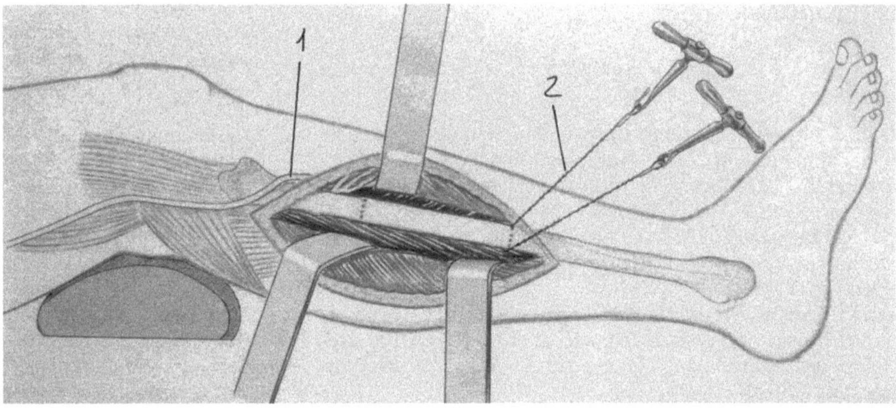

Fig. 9.121. Fibular grafts are relatively easy to obtain. After cutting through the soft tissues, one strips the periosteum, taking care not to injure the external popliteal nerve (*1*) that crosses the neck of the fibula from back to front. The diaphysis makes the best graft. The bone is severed use Gigli's saw (*2*) or, if this is not available, using a chisel to join the drill holes in the cortex. A fibular graft which is composed primarily of cortical bone is recommended when immediate stabilization is required

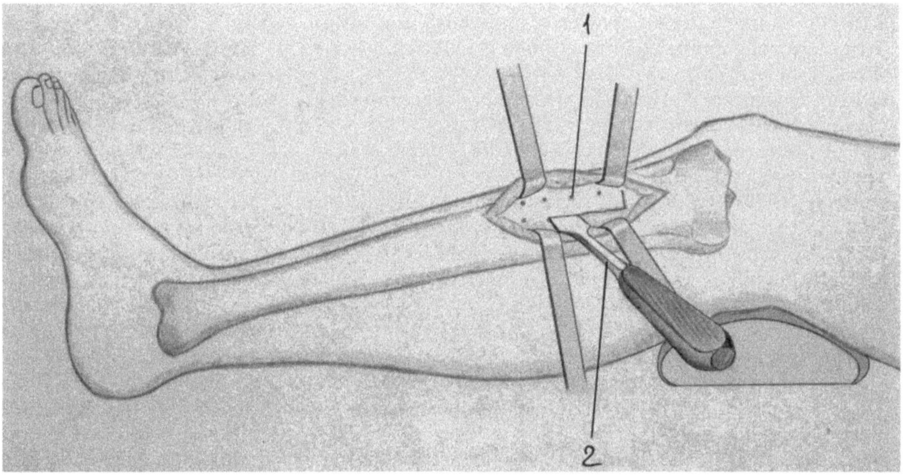

Fig. 9.122. To obtain a corticotrabecular graft from the tibia, the area of choice is the medial aspect of the proximal metaphysis. The cortex is quite thick and it is advisable to outline the bone to be taken as graft with drill holes (*1*). The chisel (*2*) is then used to remove the graft as this method is less likely to disrupt the cortex margins

References

Arima T (1969) Postlaminectomy malalignments of the cervical spine (in Japanese) NoShinkei Gaisho 1:71–78

Barbour JR (1971) Screw fixation and fractures of the odontoid process. S Aust Clin 5:20–24

Boni M, Denaro V (1982a) The cervical stenosis syndrome with a review of 87 patients treated by operation. Int Orthop 185:195

Boni M, Denaro V (1982b) Traitement chirurgical des cervico-arthroses. Révision à distance (2–13 ans) des 100 premiers cas opérés par voie antérieure. Rev Chir Orthop 68:269–280

Boni M, Cherubino P, Denaro V, Benazzo F (1984) Multiple subtotal somatectomy. Technique and evaluation of a series of 39 cases. Spine 9:358

Bailey RW, Badaley CE (1960) Stabilization of the cervical spine by anterior fusion. J Bone Joint Surg 42(A):565

Callahan RA, Johnson RM, Margolis RN et al. (1977) Cervical facet fusion for control of instability following laminectomy. J Bone Joint Surg [Am] 59:991

Cattel HS, Clark GL (1967) A Cervical kyphosis and instability following multiple laminectomies in children. J Bone Joint Surg [Am] 49:713–721

Ceciliani L, Denaro V (1985) Cervical spine surgery in children. Med Biol Environ 13 (1):429–442

Cervical Spine Research Society (ed) (1983) The cervical spine. Lippincott, Philadelphia

Denaro V (1988) Treatment of metastases and systemic tumors of the cervical spine. Neuroorthopedics 6:101–110

Denaro V, Kehr P (1990) In: Louis R, Weidner A (eds) Cervical spine II. Marseille 1988. Springer, Berlin Heidelberg New York Tokyo, pp. 131–138

Dereymaeker A, Ghosez JP, Henkser R (1963) Le traitement chirurgique de la discopathie cervical. Résultats comparés de l'abord postérieur (laminectomie) et de l'abord ventral (fusion corporéal) dans une cinquantaine de cas personnels. Neurochirurgie 9:13

Epstein JA et al. (1963) Cercical spondylotic myelopathy: the syndrome of the narrowed canal treated by laminectomy, foraminotomy, and the removal of osteophytes. Arch Neurol 8:307

Fineschi G (1962) Verhandlungsrichtlinien bei den zervikalen Diskushernien. Verh Dtsch Orthop Ges

Frykholm R (1951) Lower cervical vertebrae and intervertebral discs. Surgical anatomy and pathology. Acta Chir Scand 101:345–359

Harada Y, et al. (1974) Instability after extensive laminectomy in the cervical spine (in Japanese) Rinsho Seikeigeka 9:909–911

Hirabayashi K (1978) Expansive open-door laminoplasty for cervical spondylotic myelopathy (in Japanese). Shujutsu 32:1159–1163

Hirabayashi K (1987) Expansive open-door laminoplasty (in Japanese) Shujutsu 41:499-508

Hirabayashi K, Satomi K (1987) Expansive open-door laminoplasty for cervical spinal stenotic myelopathy. State Art Rev 1:517–532

Hirabayashi K et al. (1972) The posterior and anterior operation in treatment of cervical disk lesions including cervical spondylosis: a long term follow-up study (in Japanese). Chubu Seisaishi 15:786–788

Hirabayashi K et al. (1981) Operative results and postoperative progression of ossification among patients with ossification of cervical posterior longitudinal ligament. Spine 6:354–364

Hoshino Y et al. (1987) Enlargement of spinal canal by the sagittal splitting of spinal processes (in Japanese). Shujutsu 41:489–497

Itoh T, Tsuji H (1987) En-bloc laminoplasty (in Japanese). Shujutsu 41:509–518

Itoh T et al. (1982) Expansive laminoplasty in the cervical spine (in Japanese). Chubu Seisaishi 25:112–114

Itoh T et al. (1985) Technical improvements and results of laminoplasty for compressive myelopathy in the cervical spine. Spine 10:729–736

Iwasaki Y (1987) Expansive laminoplasty in the cervical spine (Nara method) (in Japanese). Shujutsu 41:471–478

Iwasaki Y et al. (1982) Expansive laminoplasty in the cervical spine (in Japanese). Bessatsu Seikeigeka 2:228–233

Jenkins DHR (1973) Extensive cervical laminectomy, long-term results. Br J Surg 60:852–854

Jung A (1963) Résection de l'articulation unco-vertébrale et ouverture du trou de conjugaison par voie antérieure dans le traiement de la névralgie cervico-brachiale. Technique opératoire. Mem Acad Chir 89:11–13, 361–367

Jung A, Kehr P, Magerl F, Weber BG (1974) The cervical spine. Primary and posttraumatic disorders. Advances in surgical management. Huber, Bern

Kawai N, Hattori S (1980) Enlargement of the cervical canal indication and the technique (in Japanese). Sekei Saigai Geka 23:39–44

Kehr P (1984) Anterolateral approaches to the cervical spine for management of cervical vascular and radicular syndromes. In: Contemporary neurosurgery, vol 6. Williams and Wilkins, Baltimore, pp 1–6

Kehr P (1987) Combined anterolateral and anteromedial approaches of the lower cervical spine. In: Kehr P, Weidner A (eds) Cervical spine I. Springer, Berlin Heidelberg New York

Kehr P, Jung A (1985) Chirurgie der Arteria vertebralis an den Bewegungssegmenten der Halswirbelsäule. In: Die Halswirbelsäule (Funktionelle Pathologie und Klinik der Wirbelsäule) Fischer, Stuttgart

Kimura I et al. (1982) Expansive open-door laminoplasty on CT (in Japanese) Rinsho Seikeigeka 17:32–42

Kurokawa T et al. (1984) Enlargement of spinal canal by the sagittal splitting of spinal processes for cervical spondylotic myelopathy (in Japanese). Rinsho Seikeigeka 19:483–490

Kurokawa T et al. (1986) Enlargement of spinal canal by the sagittal splitting of spinal processes – new modification and results (in Japanese) Besattsu Seikeigeka 9:30–32

Magerl F et al. (1987) Stable dorsal fusion of the cervical spine using hook plates. In: Kehr P, Weidner A (eds) Cervical spine I. Springer, Berlin Heidelberg New York

Miayazaki K, Kirita Y (1986) Extensive simultaneous multisegment laminectomy for myelopathy due to the ossification of the posterior longitudinal ligament in the cervical region. Spine 11:531–542

Miyasaka H et al. (1981a) Operative results for the cervical spondylotic myelopathy – anterior surgery and expansive laminoplasty (in Japanese). Besattsu Seikeigeka 2:43–50

Miyasaka H et al. (1981b) Long-term follow-up after laminectomy for ossification of the posterior longitudinal ligament in the cervical spine (in Japanese). Niseikaishi 55:985–986

Matsuzaki H et al. (1982) Cervical canal-expansive laminoplasty with unilateral fusion (in Japanese). Besattsu Seikeigeka 2: 249–254

Matsuzaki H et al. (1987) Cervical canal-expansive laminoplasty with unilateral fusion (in Japanese). Shujutsu 41: 529–536

Murphy MJ, Southwick WO (1989) Posterior approaches and fusion. In: Cervical Spine Research Society (ed) The cervical spine. Lippincott, Philadelphia, pp 775–791

Nakano N, Tomita T (1980) Enlargement of cervical spinal canal for cervical spondylotic myelopathy (in Japanese). Seikeigeka 31: 453–461

Oyama M, Hattori S (1973) A new method of cervical laminectomy (in Japanese). Chubu Seisaishi 16: 792–794

Oyama M et al. (1987) Operative procedures of osteoplastic spinal canal enlargement (Yamaguchi method) (in Japanese). Shujutsu 41: 479–487

Roy-Camille R, Mazel CH, Saillant G (1987) Treatment of cervical spine injuries by a posterior osteosynthesis with plates and screws. In: Kehr P, Weidner A (eds) Cervical spine I. Springer, Berlin Heidelberg New York, p 163

Saito T, Yamamuro T et al. (1989) Simulation study by finite element of posterior decompressive surgeries to prevent postoperative malalignment in the cervical spine (in Japanese). Rinsho Seikeigeka 24: 461–469

Senegas J et al. (1975) Technique de décompression médullaire antérieure dans les stenoses canalaires étendues. Rev Clin Orthop 61: 219–223

Sim FH et al. (1974) Swan neck deformity following extensive cervical laminectomy. J Bone Joint Surg [Am] 56: 564–580

Simmons EH, Du Toit G (1978) Lateral atlo-axial arthrodesis. Orth Clin N. Am 9: 1101

Smith GW, Robinson RA (1958) The treatment of certain cervical spine disorders by the anterior removal of the intervertebral disc and interbody fusion. J Bone Joint Surg 40(A): 607

Stauffer ES, Kelly EG (1977) Fracture dislocation of the cervical spine: instability and recurrent deformity following treatment by anterior interbody fusion. J Bone Joint Surg [Am] 59(1): 45

Tomita K, Nomura S et al. (1988) Cervical laminoplasty to enlarge the spinal canal in multilevel ossification of the posterior longitudinal ligament with myelopathy. Arch Orthop Trauma Surg 107: 148–153

Tsuzuki N, Tanaba H et al. (1989) Cervical expansive laminoplasty preserving spinous processes and ligaments complex (in Japanese) Rinsho Seikeigeka 24: 387–396

Watanabe T et al. (1987) Expansive laminoplasty (Chiba) for the cervical spondylotic myelopathy (in Japanese). Shujutsu 41: 519–527

White AA, Panjabi MM (1978) The clinical biomechanics of the spine. Lippincott, Philadelphia

Whitecloud TS III, La Rocca SH (1976) Fibular struct graft in reconstructive surgery of the cervical spine. Spine 1: 33

CHAPTER 10

Causes of Poor Results

The approaches and surgical methods that are used to deal with cervical stenosis have been discussed. In each chapter, the risks of complications that result from incorrect surgical technique have been indicated, but, unfortunately, poor results may also be the result of incomplete preoperative assessment of the patient, an inappropriate approach, a poor choice of technique or type of decompression, of immobilization, or of vertebral body reconstruction, and operations carried out at the incorrect spinal level. It must be emphasized that surgery should only be carried out when the indications are unequivocally present. Obviously, this represents a broad and variable set of circumstances that are difficult to classify and describe. Only those known to be the more common errors and those that have a real probability of significant iatrogenic consequences will be covered here.

Errors in Diagnosis

If cases of trauma, tumor, and rheumatic diseases are excluded, then the problems that fall in the category of errors in diagnosis arise from the cases of degenerative arthrosis of the cervical spine, associated with myelopathy because of organic stenosis. The need for careful clinical assessment of the patient cannot be overemphasized. The neurological examination, the duration and pattern of development of the symptoms and signs, and a full knowledge of the patient's clinical history must be ascertained before any investigation can be undertaken.

On the basis of the clinical findings, the need for specific radiological investigations such as CT and MRI is determined. EMG and SEP studies will help to orient and localize the level and type of disease process. If this stepwise progression is followed methodically, one of the major causes of misdiagnoses will be avoided. A complete assessment is needed in order to specifically identify the presence of syringomyelia, amyotrophic lateral sclerosis, sclerosis, calcification, and plaque formation, etc. in a differential diagnosis. A correct diagnosis does not just happen, it is the result of a methodical search for clinical symptoms and the institution of correct clinical and investigative studies. These must be correlated with the symptoms and physical findings of the patient. This combined effort will minimize the risk of errors in diagnosis.

Incorrect Level of Surgery

Obviously, the confirmation of the level at which a surgical decompression is to be carried out is important, yet failure to do so is one of the more frequent errors. There is no problem when the neurological investigations and findings confirm the level at which there is cord impingement. There are however many cases in which multilevel abnormalities are present and in these cases the clinical symptoms may not necessarily correspond to the area identified by the investigation. It may be that the pathogenetic mechanisms are vascular in origin and the symptoms and signs may therefore occur outside the area of the lesion; a higher or lower spinal level may then be involved. In addition, there may be coexisting pathogenetic features that must be carefully assesed. This multifocal involvement gives rise to clinical situations that are difficult to specifically localize and which require meticulous investigation and correlation. All imaging techniques including CT and MRI assess the static features of the spine and cord. The clinical situation however arises because of function that requires movement. For this reason myelograms and computed tomographic myelograms in various anatomical positions must always be included in the assessment of these patients. This is probably the most useful way of confirming and identifying the anatomical levels requiring surgery and will help to determine the type of surgery and the extent of decompression needed.

Indications

In spite of correct diagnosis and careful peoperative assessment of the patient, in selected cases one may have to undertake a surgical procedure in the absence of specific indications. The indications for surgery are always specifically related to the cause of the stenosis but may not always be clearly delineated and classified, particularly in cases of trauma, tumors, or rheumatic diseases where the surgeon is forced to undertake stabilization after decompression because of the resection of a large tumor and hence segmental reconstruction. One can certainly be much more specific in defining the indications in cases of spondyloarthrosis.

The first step is to recognize the cause of the stenosis: cord compression by posterior osteophytes, posterolateral (uncal) osteophytes, calcification of the posterior longitudinal ligament, hypertrophy and thickening of the ligamentum flavum, malformation of the pedicles or laminae, or by uniform and circumferential narrowing of the canal such as may occur in congenital stenosis. Once the specific cause has been defined, the surgeon is in a position to plan its correction. If there is anterior stenosis produced by osteophytes (and when the symptoms are those of anterior compression) posterior decompression will obviously be inappropriate and produce a poor result. This approach would presuppose that a simple laminectomy (either classical laminectomy or open-door laminoplasty) will provide adequate release of the cord impingement from the ridges of osteophytes that are present anteriorly. This leaves the cause of the cord impingement (stenosis) in place, and, even though the anteroposterior diameter of the canal is increased, the surgical procedure fails to address the specific cause of the stenosis; the results will therefore not be acceptable. Furthermore, even though it is possible (as described by Epstein) to remove posterolateral osteophytes after posterior decompression through a laminectomy, it may be particularly difficult and even dangerous to attempt to remove more centrally placed osteophytes. In these circumstances, the correct approach is the anterior one that would lead to a safe and complete removal of the cause of the stenosis and cord impingement (i.e., the osteophytes which were obviously demonstrable preoperatively with MRI and CT).

The same applies to the obstinate pursual of an anterior surgical approach in order to decompress lesions that are strictly posterior, such as laminar deformity or enlargement of the ligamentum flavum. There is no doubt that the canal is enlarged through a wide corpectomy anteriorly, but, nevertheless, if the specific cause of the symptoms is not addressed then even after surgery has been completed, the specific cause remains exactly where it was preoperatively.

The disputes that are frequently expressed in comparing anterior or posterior decompressions are futile. The discussion should not be as to whether one approach is better than another, but should in fact address whether or not the definitive surgical procedure removes the cause of the patient's problem. If the myelopathy is the result of osteophytes protruding into the anterior surface of the cord, it is appropriate to use either the anterior approach (Cloward instrumentation with or without multiple corpectomies) or a posterior approach following laminectomy (as described by Epstein) to remove the osteophytes. It is however inappropriate to limit oneself to a laminectomy without attempting to remove the anterior osteophytes which are the real cause of the compression, simply on the basis that, having removed the posterior wall of the canal, the canal is now larger and the problem is therefore corrected.

When this precept has been fully understood only features of personal preference remain, which, along with a fully logical approach, will determine the selection of the procedure. Failures therefore will result both from incorrect choice of approach and from incorrect choice of the definitive surgical technique. The argument is somewhat different when dealing with anterior compression because of calcification in the posterior longitudinal ligament. The basic principles, however, remain the same. When there is massive continuous calcification, the ligament is in fact uniformly thickened producing narrowing of the canal over a long distance. In such cases the patient would obviously benefit from an extended widening of the canal which can be achieved through open-door laminoplasty. However, if the calcification of the posterior longitudinal ligament is focal, segmental, mushroom, or hill shaped, then obviously the offending alteration is placed anteriorly and must be completely removed through the appropriate approach. One cannot categorically state what the management should be in all cases of calcification of the posterior longitudinal ligament. The surgical management must be predicated by the pattern and degree of involvement in each individual case.

Incomplete or Inadequate Surgery

In previous chapters complications and technical errors resulting from the various surgical procedures and techniques have been discussed. Here, however, only those techniques are covered, which are directed at the definitive removal of the cause of the stenosis and which do not provide acceptable results if they are not fully carried out. For example, anterior decompression using the Cloward instrumentation (or any other technique) cannot be considered to have been carried out if the posterior and posterolateral osteophytes (uncus) have not been completely removed. The same applies even more to the procedures that do not even reach the posterior cortical wall of the vertebrae, let alone undertake to remove the posterior osteophytes, as can be confirmed by postoperative imaging. The same is also true of a posterior approach where decompression of the canal by laminectomy is not followed by the removal of either posterior or posterolateral osteophytes and where the root canal is not explored (foraminectomy). Therefore, one must regard these as completed approaches, but incomplete and inadequate surgical correction of the disease process. Often the clinical symptoms do not improve after such incomplete procedures.

One of the major factors in the failure of even accurately carried out and complete decompression with removal of all the causes is the failure to provide full stabilization of the involved segments at the end of the surgical procedure. The need for internal stabilization should always be anticipated and planned preoperatively. The following are features that should warn the surgeon that stabilization may be necessary:

- Whenever any degree of instability (trauma, rheumatoid arthritis, degenerative spondylolisthesis) can be anticipated in the preoperative clinical assessment of patients. The same will apply in young patients, particularly those with hypermobile vertebrae.
- Whenever the need for a particularly wide decompression from a posterior approach with the resection carried out to the level of the lateral apophyseal masses is anticipated.

Whenever these lateral masses are weakened by the dissection or disease, they have the propensity to produce deformity after laminectomy (swan neck) and are subject to progressive kyphosis. These circumstances are known to lead to cord injury and the consequences may be even more serious than the symptoms that led to the original surgical intervention. The indication for internal stabilization very seldom occurs introperatively, and if it does it is usually associated with destructive processes such as neoplasms. If in doubt, stabilize!

Inadequate Postoperative Immobilization

Adequate immobilization of the cervical spine is an essential part of the postoperative care of the patient. In order to assure good postoperative results, a technically correct procedure must first of all be carried out. When this involves multilevel corpectomies with massive grafts from the iliac crest, the surgeon is very much dependent on complete postoperative immobilization (halo cast or halo jacket) for immobilization of the graft during incorporation and fusion.

In the literature, many methods of immobilization of the cervical spine are described. My personal experience has convinced me that the only orthotic applications that provide true immobilization of the cervical spine are the halo cast, the halo jacket, or the individually designed Minerva jacket. The specific choice of orthotic immobilization is crucial to the immobilization of the spine in order to permit fusion and avoid undue stress on and mobilization of bone grafts. Partial or complete failure, both in the static state and if there is unacceptable and excessive movement may obviously occur under these circumstances. Cases of excessive movement often result in severe cord injuries. One must also warn against using correct orthotic appliances, but not leaving them in place for a sufficient length of time to assure fusion. Premature removal of the orthotic brace will have serious consequences not the least of which are nonunion, instability, and mobilization of the graft, and may lead to total disruption at the operative site.

Chapter 11

Conclusion

The discussions in this book are intended to provide the reader with the following food for thought: The term "cervical stenosis" is taken here to be a primarily clinical term and the justification for defining it to include all the myelopathic and myeloradiculopathic consequences of a discrepancy between the contents of the vertebral canal and the vertebral canal itself as a container of the cord lies in the fact that such a definition makes it possible to classify the multiple etiological causes of the pathology in one chapter, regardless of whether they are functional or organic (congenital or acquired).

Once the many causes of the stenosis had been described, the discussion continued with the more common approaches and the definitive surgical techniques. From their own personal experience, the authors undertook to describe these techniques and provide practical suggestions. Known complications were detailed along with possible methods of prevention and management. The discussion always attempted to retain an organized, possibly didactic approach in many areas. This was intentional in order to provide well-organized information for the beginner in his or her first steps along the path leading to this subspecialty area.

It must be emphasized that this is a very complex and demanding area of orthopedic surgery that requires the full and dedicated effort of experienced surgeons. This is reflected here in the authors'insistance on specific indications for each and every surgical procedure. It must be realized that any discussion of this subject predicates good knowledge of the clinical signs, the most common etiology, the value and limitation of the clinical, laboratory, and imaging investigations, the surgical approaches, and the specific surgical techniques. The surgeon who lifts a scalpel to enter this area must be a highly dedicated, wise physician enriched by a high level of common sense. It is not sufficient for him to have the mere technical skills. He must also have the capacity to assess the individual circumstances causing the stenosis in each patient and to religiously identify the indications that lead to the choice of definitive management. The choice of the correct surgical technique is often more important than the correct completion of the surgical technique itself: a surgical procedure correctly carried out for the wrong indication can only lead to failure.

There is no way of standardizing the indications for operations. The surgical management of cervical stenosis must address many variable factors, each of which must be fully evaluated, and the overall impact of all parameters must be accounted for in the choice of surgical procedure. Our discussion must therefore be limited to general principles which the surgeon should use in determining the significance of the multiple characteristics presented by an individual patient. No doubt a review of the literature will indicate that there are different schools of thought, not all of which agree on the choice of management for all cases of cervical stenosis. In the past, there were proponents of the posterior approach and proponents of the anterior approach. Each of the two contrasting groups provided a priori indications for the selection of the approach. It is a relief to say that this no longer exists and that the choice of approach depends on the indications for surgery as determined by the cause of the stenosis.

The definitive purpose of surgical intervention must remain the complete removal of the stenosis and all its causes in each patient. Compression from the front predicates an anterior approach, while impingement from the back requires a posterior approach. If the compression is due to a combination of factors from the front and the back, then a combined anterior and posterior approach must be used. The challenge that the surgeon faces is not determined by his choice of approach, but in fact by his ability to use an approach that will give him access in the most direct fashion and permit the complete and safe removal of the cause or causes of the stenosis. The guiding principle must always be to choose the best way to reach the spine that will permit the most direct, full and safest removal of the cause of the stenosis. This is a very important concept that must be fully accepted by the surgeon, for the determination of the surgical procedure to be carried out and the best approach available in order to achieve his purpose will depend on this. There is no doubt that any choice that the surgeon makes will be colored by his experience, skill, and manual dexterity in carrying out the surgical procedure that he has determined to be necessary for each patient. Individual skills and experience in surgery of the cervical spine are essential and their importance cannot be overemphacized.

Subject Index

MIX
Papier aus verantwortungsvollen Quellen
Paper from responsible sources
FSC® C105338

If you have any concerns about our products,
you can contact us on
ProductSafety@springernature.com

In case Publisher is established outside the EU,
the EU authorized representative is:
Springer Nature Customer Service Center GmbH
Europaplatz 3, 69115 Heidelberg, Germany

Printed by Libri Plureos GmbH
in Hamburg, Germany